With my
HIGHEST REGARD
AND ADMIRATION

GARY

MANAGERIAL ETHICS
in HEALTHCARE

MANAGERIAL
ETHICS
in HEALTHCARE
A NEW PERSPECTIVE

EDITORS

GARY L. FILERMAN · ANN E. MILLS · PAUL M. SCHYVE

Foreword by Stephen Shortell

AUPHA

Health Administration Press, Chicago, Illinois

Association of University Programs in Health Administration, Arlington, Virginia

18   17   16   15   14   5   4   3   2   1

Library of Congress Cataloging-in-Publication Data

Managerial ethics in healthcare : a new perspective / edited by Gary L. Filerman, Ann E. Mills, and Paul M. Schyve.
    pages cm
  ISBN 1-56793-603-2

1. Health services administration--Moral and ethical aspects. 2. Public health--Moral and ethical aspects. 3. Medical ethics. I. Filerman, Gary L. (Gary Lewis), editor of compilation. II. Mills, Ann E., editor of compilation. III. Schyve, Paul M., editor of compilation.

RA427.25.M36 2013
  174.2--dc23
                       2013019375

The paper used in this publication meets the minimum requirements of American National Standard for Information Sciences—Permanence of Paper for Printed Library Materials, ANSI Z39.48-1984. ♾ ™

Acquisitions editor: Carrie McDonald; Project manager: Amy Carlton; Cover designer: Marisa Jackson; Layout: Cepheus Edmondson

Found an error or a typo? We want to know! Please e-mail it to hapbooks@ache.org, and put "Book Error" in the subject line.

For photocopying and copyright information, please contact Copyright Clearance Center at www.copyright.com or at (978) 750–8400.

Health Administration Press
A division of the Foundation of the American
    College of Healthcare Executives
One North Franklin Street, Suite 1700
Chicago, IL 60606–3529
(312) 424–2800

Association of University Programs
    in Health Administration
2000 North 14th Street
Suite 780
Arlington, VA 22201
(703) 894–0940

We dedicate this book to the future healthcare administrators who will sustain and enhance the moral core of their organizations.

BRIEF CONTENTS

Foreword xv
      Stephen Shortell
Introduction: Toward a New Perspective xix

1: Introduction to Ethics 1
      Mary V. Rorty

2: Ethics and the Healthcare Organization 19
      Ann E. Mills

3: Ethics and Governance 51
      John F. Wallenhorst

4: The Healthcare Organization, Business Ethics, and
    Stakeholder Theory 79
      Patricia H. Werhane

5: Professional Ethics 95
      Edward M. Spencer

6: Organizational Administration and the Clinical
    Ethics Mechanism: A Question of Respect 121
      Mark H. Waymack

7: Moral Distress and the Healthcare Organization 137
      Ann B. Hamric, Elizabeth G. Epstein, and Kenneth R. White

8: Ethics in Healthcare Quality Improvement 159
      Paul M. Schyve

9: The Healthcare Organization as Employer:
    The Demands of Fairness and the Healthcare Organization 177
      Leonard J. Weber

10: An Introduction to Environmental and Sustainability Issues in Healthcare Management 195
Carrie R. Rich, J. Knox Singleton, and Seema S. Wadhwa

11: External Requirements for Ethics in Healthcare Organizations 205
Ann E. Mills

12: Healthcare Ethics, Public Policy, and the Healthcare Organization 223
Katherine L. Acuff

13: Healthcare Ethics and a Changing Healthcare System 243
Carolyn Long Engelhard

14: Leadership and the Healthcare Organization 265
Gary L. Filerman, Ann E. Mills, and Paul M. Schyve

15: Toward a New Perspective 287
Gary L. Filerman, Ann E. Mills, and Paul M. Schyve

Appendix 293
Glossary 297
Index 305
About the Editors 325
About the Contributors 329

DETAILED CONTENTS

Foreword xv
   Stephen Shortell
Introduction: Toward a New Perspective xix

1: Introduction to Ethics 1
   Mary V. Rorty
   Learning Objectives 2
   Introduction 2
   The Language of Ethics 3
   Moving Beyond the Individual: Ethics and Organizations 8
   The Role of Ethics in Organizational Leadership 10
   Organizations as Ethical Agents: Values and Virtues 10
   Conclusion 14
   Points to Remember 15

2: Ethics and the Healthcare Organization 19
   Ann E. Mills
   Learning Objectives 20
   Introduction 20
   Organizational Statements 22
   Patient Rights and Responsibilities 25
   Genesis of Ethical Tension 33
   Organizational Culture 34
   A Culture of Safety 36
   Barriers to Building Organizational
      Culture and Ethical Climate 38
   A Process for Resolving Ethical Conflict 39
   Controversial Issues and the Healthcare Organization 41
   Conclusion 46
   Points to Remember 47

3: **Ethics and Governance**..51

John F. Wallenhorst

Learning Objectives 51

Introduction 52

Healthcare as a Service 52

Governance Leadership and Duties 54

Board Makeup 58

Areas of Focus 62

Board Effectiveness and Evaluation 71

Conclusion 74

Points to Remember 74

4: **The Healthcare Organization, Business Ethics, and Stakeholder Theory**..79

Patricia H. Werhane

Learning Objectives 80

Introduction 80

Stakeholder Theory 82

Business Ethics and Healthcare Ethics.....................................86

Conclusion 91

Points to Remember 93

5: **Professional Ethics** 95

Edward M. Spencer

Learning Objectives 95

Introduction 96

Defining the Terms..97

Development of Ethical Codes and Guidelines..........................98

Societal Influences on Codes of Ethics and
      Professional Principles 110

Professional Ethics in Today's Healthcare System.....................113

Practical Advice...115

Conclusion 116

Points to Remember 118

6: **Organizational Administration and the Clinical Ethics Mechanism: A Question of Respect** 121

Mark H. Waymack

Learning Objectives 121

Introduction 122

What Is Clinical Ethics? 124

The Emergence of the Clinical Ethics Mechanism.....................125

Administrative Engagement 128

Conclusion 135

Points to Remember 136

7: Moral Distress and the Healthcare Organization 137

Ann B. Hamric, Elizabeth G. Epstein, and Kenneth R. White

Learning Objectives 137

Introduction 138

Understanding Moral Distress..139

Levels at Which Moral Distress Is Experienced 141

Strategies to Address Moral Distress 146

Conclusion 151

Points to Remember 152

Cases and Questions 152

8: Ethics in Healthcare Quality Improvement...........................159

Paul M. Schyve

Learning Objectives 159

Introduction 160

Role of QI in Healthcare 161

A Moral Obligation to Engage in QI 163

Role of the Healthcare Executive in QI 166

Ethical Challenges That Arise in Healthcare QI 168

Addressing Ethical Challenges with QI 170

Conclusion 172

Points to Remember 174

9: The Healthcare Organization as Employer:

The Demands of Fairness and the Healthcare Organization...........177

Leonard J. Weber

Learning Objectives 178

Introduction 178

Mandatory Influenza Vaccinations 179

Nonsmoking as a Condition of Employment 182

Just Compensation 186

Union Organizing 189

Conclusion 191

Points to Remember 192

10: An Introduction to Environmental and Sustainability Issues in Healthcare Management 195

Carrie R. Rich, J. Knox Singleton, and Seema S. Wadhwa

Learning Objectives 195
What Is Sustainability? 196
Linking Environmental Ethics to Healthcare Ethics 196
Wealth Versus Health 197
How to Present Sustainability Without Degrading It 198
Defining Roles in Healthcare Sustainability.........................199
Individual Versus Public Health 201
Impact of Ethics Across the Supply Chain..............................201
Conclusion 202
Points to Remember 202

11: External Requirements for Ethics in Healthcare Organizations.....................205

Ann E. Mills

Learning Objectives 205
Introduction 206
Law and Ethics 207
Compliance Program Guidance.....................208
Incentives to Develop Effective Compliance Programs.............211
Barriers to Creating an Appropriate Culture
    Through Compliance Programs..............................212
Accreditation Standards and The Joint Commission 212
The Evidence.....................214
Moral Behavior and Organizations..............................216
Conclusion 218
Points to Remember 218

12: Healthcare Ethics, Public Policy, and the Healthcare Organization.....................223

Katherine L. Acuff

Learning Objectives 223
Introduction 224
Health and Healthcare Policies 225
Health Policy and the Ethical Context of Leadership 226
Examples of Health and Healthcare Policies
    Affecting Healthcare Organizations 228
Crisis Standards of Care and Medical Liability..........................234

Conclusion 238

Points to Remember 239

13: Healthcare Ethics and a Changing Healthcare System 243

Carolyn Long Engelhard

Learning Objectives 243

Introduction 244

Margin Versus Mission: Historical Overview 244

The Costs of Caring 246

Health Reform and Healthcare Organizations...........................249

Healthcare Organizations:

   Ethical Challenges and Opportunities...............................254

Conclusion 258

Points to Remember 259

14: Leadership and the Healthcare Organization 265

Gary L. Filerman, Ann E. Mills, and Paul M. Schyve

Learning Objectives 266

Introduction 266

Leadership Blindness...268

Moral Imagination...274

Moral Reasoning...276

Conclusion 283

Points to Remember 284

15: Toward a New Perspective..287

Gary L. Filerman, Ann E. Mills, and Paul M. Schyve

Introduction 287

Your Moral Core 288

About Integrity..288

Integrity and Your Organization 291

Conclusion 292

Appendix...293

Glossary..297

Index 305

About the Editors..325

About the Contributors 329

FOREWORD

Managerial Ethics in Healthcare: A New Perspective addresses the core question of professional training for healthcare administrators; namely, what are we about? Why have faculty and the students put in our charge chosen a field intended to manage resources and lead people to restore, maintain, and improve the health of individuals and populations? This book makes a major contribution by asking readers to question their motives for entering the field. Questioning one's motives is a key pathway to the examination of one's values. What do we value as "good" for ourselves, our neighbors, our organization, our community? What do we believe are accepted rules and standards of human behavior; that is, what is morally "right"? This is the domain of ethics—the study of morals as reflected in human behavior.

The book's 15 chapters cover a broad range of issues from multiple perspectives, but a central idea is the importance of maintaining one's personal integrity as a prerequisite to building organizational integrity. Integrity means staying true to one's values, to one's moral core, and using that core as a guide in making difficult decisions that will inevitably involve compromise. Where do you draw the line? For yourself? For your organization? Sometimes you may not know what you really value until you are tested with making a difficult choice. Our espoused values may not be our enacted values.

Current changes in the healthcare environment will increase the importance of personal and organizational integrity in addressing morally complex and ambiguous issues. For example, the Patient Protection and Affordable Care Act is encouraging new payment and delivery models for hospitals, moving away from fee-for-service toward bundled payments, capitated payments, and global budgets. This shift will require significant changes in the business models of how hospitals derive their revenue. In turn, this will give rise to a number of complex decisions involving hospital admission and readmission policies, bed capacity, staffing, and negotiations with physician organizations. How do you reconcile the need to operate a financially viable hospital with meeting community-wide needs that may dictate less use of the hospital as a resource? How do you think about community and population health? For example, do you and the organization have an obligation to enhance the health of the entire community and population above and beyond your current catchment area? Why should you spend resources that may help competing organizations more than yourself even if it might benefit the community at large? What about your strategy to merge with a competing hospital to gain greater economies of scale, efficiency, and improve the quality of care? Do you also have a hidden reason or motive to increase your negotiating power with insurers to raise payment rates? In the era of rapid-cycle gene sequencing and personalized medicine, do you encourage investments that will target new therapies to benefit a few people versus investments in technologies to reduce preterm births and narrow the gap in infant mortality rates among different socioeconomic and racial or ethnic groups?

An important implication of these examples is the increased need for leaders who can manage across boundaries of their own individual organizations. Healthcare is now delivered more by networks of organizations and cross-sector teams involving not only healthcare delivery organizations but also public health and the social service sector. This structure will require leaders who can reconcile the values of different organizations and develop a shared moral core to guide the network enterprise. It will place a premium on what the book calls "moral imagination"—the ability to think of creative alternatives to a morally complex issue that goes beyond the immediate demands of the situation and current ways of thinking about the issue.

A particular strength of the book is its emphasis on the importance of organizational culture for establishing the moral climate of the organization. Culture is reflected in the shared beliefs, norms, values, and behaviors of those in the organization. What behaviors are rewarded? What behaviors are punished? A National Business Ethics Survey (Ethics Resource Center 2011) that included healthcare organizations found that 45 percent of employees surveyed had observed at least one instance of ethical misconduct at work in the past year, 35 percent of those did not report the violation to management, and of those who did, 22 percent experienced some form of retaliation.

The coming decades will strongly test the ethical behavior of our healthcare organizations as they adapt to the increased demand for care and incorporate new biomedical advances while constraining the rate of growth in cost. Meeting this challenge will require an increased awareness of the values guiding one's own moral core and of the organization that one serves. This book provides an important and strong foundation for the preparation of leaders who can meet the challenge.

Stephen Shortell, PhD
Dean, School of Public Health, University of California–Berkeley
Blue Cross of California Distinguished Professor
of Health Policy and Management
Berkeley, California

Reference

Ethics Resource Center. 2011. "National Business Ethics Survey: Workplace Ethics in
    Transition." Accessed May 13, 2013. www.ethics.org/nbes/.

INTRODUCTION: TOWARD A NEW PERSPECTIVE

This book is based on the assumption that students, including you, want to make a positive contribution to the field of healthcare administration, to the healthcare organizations you will serve, and to the diverse stakeholders interacting with healthcare organizations. (The term *stakeholder* means any individual or group, including the community, that is affected by the activities of a healthcare organization.)

The single most important responsibility of a healthcare administrator is to ensure that the moral core of his healthcare organization remains intact as the organization faces increasing challenges to its operations and even its viability. If you, as a healthcare administrator or manager, succeed in preserving and enhancing the moral core of your organization, you will have made a significant and positive contribution.

To achieve this contribution, healthcare administrators and managers need a new perspective that recognizes that every decision they make and every activity they undertake has the potential to compromise or to enhance the moral core of their healthcare organization.

Some debate exists concerning exactly what constitutes the moral core of a specific healthcare organization. But there is no debate about the service mission of all healthcare organizations: to alleviate pain and suffering and help restore the health of their patients. This is, or should be, the foundation of any healthcare organization's mission. This mission is, or should be, the foundation of any healthcare organization's moral core.

The mission of any organization is its purpose, its reason for existence. As will become clear through this book, the legitimacy of any organization depends on whether or not its mission is positive and acceptable to the greater society. (See Chapter 2 for an expanded description of the mission of a healthcare organization.)

When a society deems the mission of an organization to be positive and legitimate, it is acknowledging that the service or product of that organization somehow benefits (or at least does not harm) society. Thus, society conveys, by accepting the legitimacy of the mission of the organization, a moral approval (or at least a moral neutrality) of that mission.

Because society welcomes the service mission of all healthcare organizations, and because this mission constitutes the basis for what healthcare organizations do or should do, the service mission is the foundation of any healthcare organization's moral core.

The moral core of the organization also depends on whether or not the organization and the individuals associated with it are prepared to fulfill its mission within the context of the values society associates with its mission. These values reflect the moral core of the organization. If the *values* of the organization are not appropriate to its mission, if they are not socially endorsed as being appropriate to the mission, the organization's moral core would be hard to identify, if it exists at all.

The moral core of any organization, even if its mission and values are acceptable to society, also depends on whether or not the organization and its stakeholders are committed to fulfilling its mission within the context of its values. If the organization and its stakeholders are not prepared to commit to the organization's mission and values, the organization's ability to fulfill its mission within the context of acceptable values is in doubt.

Thus, the preservation and enhancement of the moral core of any organization depends on three things: the mission of the organization, the values that reflect its mission, and the commitment of the organization and its stakeholders to fulfill its mission within the context of its values. This interplay is dynamic. Mission, values, and commitment affect each other as well as the moral core.

Moral core
The underlying explicit and implicit set of values that the organization or person holds, which drive the organization's or person's attitudes and behavior. Each healthcare organization and healthcare administrator will have a unique moral core, but common to all should be the mission to alleviate pain and suffering and to help restore the health of patients.

All healthcare organizations have the service mission. Therefore, part of the moral core of all healthcare organizations will be associated with this mission. But differing healthcare organizations have distinct missions, and they will have distinct moral cores and distinct values. For instance, a community hospital does not have a research mission and so need not have a moral core that reflects the values associated with research. Moreover, a commitment to a similar mission does not ensure that two healthcare organizations share the same values. For instance, two healthcare organizations can share a commitment to the health of the community as part of their moral core. But the values that drive this commitment can be different. One healthcare organization might prioritize the values associated with prevention through education. The other might prioritize the values associated with efficiency to maximize access. The important point is that the values reflected by the organization are socially acceptable and consistent. Thus, the **moral core** is the underlying explicit and implicit set of values that the organization or person holds, which drive the organization's or person's attitudes and behavior. Each healthcare organization and healthcare administrator will have a unique moral core, but common to all should be the mission to alleviate pain and suffering and to help restore the health of patients.

Individuals, including you, have a moral core as well. We said previously that the moral core of organizations is reflected through their values. This is true of individuals as well. Individuals reflect their moral core through the values they hold and espouse. And just as in organizations, these values are reflected in behavior, activities, and decision making. And therein lies the crux of many of the challenges you will face. You will be managing people who are passionately committed to the mission of the healthcare organization but who also believe that their values are the correct values and that these values should be reflected in the mission of the organization.

If the most important responsibility of the healthcare administrator or manager is to preserve and enhance the moral core of the organization, then you must be prepared to

1. continually measure the activities and decision making of your organization against the mission of your organization to ensure they are in alignment,
2. continually critique the activities and decision making of the organization and its stakeholders with the values your organization espouses in realizing its mission, and
3. ensure that the commitment of the organization and its stakeholders to its mission is consistent.

In this way you preserve and enhance the moral core of your institution.

You cannot assume that good people are aware of the moral core of your institution. You cannot assume that your people are aware of your organization's mission and values, have a firm commitment to them, and use them as the basis of their activities and decision making. Nor can you be sure that you are aware of your institution's moral core. You must always be open to appropriate changes in the mission of your organization. You must always be open to the possibility that values might change over time. Your colleagues may be right; their values may be the appropriate values. So you must listen to them. You must constantly critique yourself and your own values and question if they align with the organization's values. And you must question your own commitment to them.

These challenges require a perspective—the new perspective—that acknowledges their importance. They are not easy. Thus, our goal is to give you the conceptual and practical tools that you need to be positioned to preserve and enhance the moral core of your organization while meeting day-to-day and long-run challenges that threaten its operations and potentially compromise its viability. To achieve this goal, this book is grounded in the reality of healthcare administrators' experience.

This book is not a text for philosophers. We do not guide you to look for answers by appealing to ethical standards or norms (a belief of how we should behave) embedded in healthcare, such as autonomy (the right of a patient to make decisions about his care without controlling influences), beneficence (doing good and avoiding harm), nonmaleficence (avoiding harm), or justice (acting and making decisions fairly). These ethical standards or norms are important and in well-defined situations can provide guidance as to how you should behave and what decisions you should make. Knowledge about them is both important and helpful. But they do not and cannot provide answers to all the situations you will encounter. (See Chapter 14 for more discussion of the limitations of appealing to a standard or norm for an answer to a troublesome moral or ethical situation.)

This book exists to help you—the future administrators or managers of increasingly complex healthcare delivery organizations—understand that your decisions and activities have consequences that might challenge the moral core of the healthcare organization you serve.

This book is not a comprehensive guide to or catalog of the hard issues faced by healthcare administrators or managers. No such book could exist. Neither can hard issues be predicted; they are constantly changing. The way in which hard issues come to the individual and hospital vary with each situation. What will best serve you is not a cookbook that describes the hard issues—such as decisions made at the end of life—but a guide that focuses on *moral frameworks* that enable you to respond from your own clearly understood values in ways (not just one way) that you can live with comfortably, knowing that you have contributed positively to the outcome.

To respond to a hard issue or challenge, you need to recognize that it creates moral or ethical tension, or that it is a morally or ethically problematic issue or event, or that it creates moral distress in yourself or others. (Moral distress occurs when an individual knows or thinks he knows the right thing to do but is prevented or constrained from doing it. See Chapter 7 for more on this topic.) You cannot respond—you cannot begin the process of solving the issue or event by defining it, identifying what is at stake and for whom, determining the options for actions and their implications, and elucidating the values on which you will act—without first perceiving and acknowledging that the issue or problem exists. And importantly, you need to understand and measure your own response to these issues or problems. You will need to understand what enables you to perceive and acknowledge the issue or problem and to decide if your response is appropriate or not.

The primary objective of this book is to prepare healthcare administrators and managers to accept responsibility and accountability for a healthcare organization's moral core. To achieve this objective, this book will:

- explore the moral core of healthcare organizations and ask what this means in day-to-day operations and decisions;
- familiarize you with the ethical and legal frameworks currently relied on by healthcare organizations to preserve this moral core, and demonstrate 1) how these ethical and legal frameworks sometimes conflict; 2) why they are often inadequate to address many issues faced by healthcare organizations, especially in a period of rapid change; and 3) how these conflicts and inadequacies can weaken the moral core of the healthcare organization;
- present you with some of the concepts, resources, and tools you can use to prepare yourself to sustain and enhance the moral core of the healthcare organization you manage;
- remind you that unless you have a set of values that recognizes and accepts the moral core of healthcare organizations, you will be incapable of recognizing when the moral core of a healthcare organization might be threatened;
- explore the idea of organizational culture and ethical climate and examine what role they have in formulating and maintaining the moral core of a healthcare organization and how it can be influenced appropriately; and
- identify phenomena not commonly acknowledged, such as moral distress, and discuss their consequences.

We encourage you to incorporate this new perspective as you carry out your duties. We urge you to consider your decisions and activities in the context of the moral core of your institution—we believe you must if you are to fulfill the fundamental professional responsibility of your positions: to preserve and enhance the moral core of the organization you serve.

About the Book

The editors cannot claim expertise in all the different areas that affect the moral core of healthcare organizations. For instance, we are not business ethicists—and perceiving the healthcare organization as a business, albeit a unique business, is entirely reasonable. And, of course, the way in which a healthcare organization conducts its business reflects its moral core.

The contributors are a distinguished panel of experts who share the vision of a new perspective on healthcare managerial ethics. They have been carefully selected to enrich the reader's understanding of the scope of ethical challenges facing the field. Their efforts, expertise, and insights are an important and much appreciated contribution.

The editors have tried to bring consistency to the chapters, despite the various styles of the contributors. For example, each chapter begins with Learning Objectives and ends with Points to Remember. On the other hand, several chapters begin with definitions of stakeholders, but we have chosen not to edit these perceived redundancies for several reasons. First, each contributor needs planks on which to build her case. Second, these repetitions allow the reader to continue reading without going back and looking up the definition. And, more important, many of the presentations are nuanced such that the contributor may be relying on a part of the definition not emphasized in another chapter.

To ground the book in experience, most chapters include cases. Using cases to illustrate the sorts of moral and ethical dilemmas facing healthcare organizations and their administrators has potential limitations. Although specific issues and specific problems are embedded in the cases, the point is not to ask you to formulate a "right" or "wrong" answer to a specific issue or problem, but to encourage you to think about and question the underlying values represented and how decisions can impact the moral core of the healthcare organization.

Through the use of cases, we hope to embed in your mental model (a deeply held set of generalizations or beliefs about the world, the organization, or the microsystem) the idea that most actions, events, and decisions, whether large or small, whether ethically or morally troubling or not, arise from the underlying values of individuals and groups. Consequently, if you do not know your own values, you will not be able to identify the values of others, let alone recognize an ethical or moral conflict that might threaten the moral core of the organization.

Using This Book for Competency-Based Learning

At the beginning of each chapter of this book, you will see a list of competencies that are related to the content of that chapter. Each competency addresses an important point that you can reflect on as you read the chapter to expand your ethical managerial competence.

The competencies are clustered into five leadership and management domains:

1. Communication and Relationship Management
2. Leadership
3. Professionalism
4. Knowledge of the Healthcare Environment
5. Business Skills and Knowledge

These domains, and the competencies within each domain, have been identified as being valuable to executives, administrators, and managers by the Healthcare Leadership Alliance (HLA), which is composed of the American College of Healthcare Executives (ACHE), the American College of Physician Executives, the American Organization of Nurse Executives, the Healthcare Financial Management Association, the Healthcare Information and Management Systems Society, and the Medical Group Management Association (Stefl 2008).

ACHE publishes a Competencies Assessment Tool that is derived from the HLA competencies; it is updated annually and can be found at ache .org/career.cfm. The competencies in the assessment tool are relevant to management and leadership tasks typically performed by members of ACHE. The competencies listed at the beginning of each chapter in this book were chosen from the competencies in the ACHE Competencies Assessment Tool.

Ethics and Morality

We indicated earlier the importance of your having a moral framework. A moral framework is a set of questions designed to help a person work through an ethically or morally difficult situation or event. The moral frameworks presented in several chapters in this text are not meant to be comprehensive, nor are they meant to be set in stone. Circumstances will differ, and so different questions may need to be asked and answered. But the questions asked in moral frameworks often overlap. For instance, all moral frameworks should ask: What are the facts of the situation? Who is affected? How are they affected? What are the values embedded in the situation? What are the options? Again, moral frameworks are presented in the hope of embedding in your mental model the kinds of questions you should ask when you recognize an ethical or moral dilemma.

The terms *ethics* and *morality* are often used interchangeably, but they have subtle differences. Morality is generally considered an informal public or social system, different from convention, prudence, obedience to law, or etiquette. Morality governs the behavior that affects others and has as its goal the lessening of evil or harm. Morality generally refers to the accepted norms and standards of a society concerning what is right to do or wrong to do.

More narrowly, ethics is a branch of philosophy—philosophical thinking and questioning about morality, moral problems, and moral judgments. When we defend, justify, or try to explain to others our moral judgments—why we believe something is right or wrong—we are engaging in ethical analysis or discussion and may find ourselves using the language of ethics, speaking of obligation, of principles, or of values.

The content of particular moral judgments or issues may change over time. For instance, that euthanasia could be justified under any circumstances was once unthinkable. Physicians and the wider society considered euthanasia morally wrong. Now, society's views are changing, and there is active debate about when and under what circumstances euthanasia can be thought of as morally justifiable. And such debates necessarily reflect the concerns of people in different cultures, circumstances, or social roles. For instance, because of professional medical ethics, many physicians may feel that that their social role requires a certain position on euthanasia.

In discussions about euthanasia, we sometimes appeal to other widely accepted norms, such as the autonomy of a patient. This discussion is an ethical one. We are questioning, trying to search for common ground—a convergence of our shared values—to figure out how and under what circumstances euthanasia can be morally justifiable and what morally justifiable role (if any) physicians may have.

Because ethics is discussion, questioning, reasoning, or debate about morality (the right thing to do), the terms are often used interchangeably. While we recognize that we seldom differentiate the two terms in casual conversation, we have tried to maintain the distinction in the book. Some contributors use the terms interchangeably and some are explicit about how they are using the terms. If you understand that when a contributor is talking about ethics, he or she is generally referring to discussion of or questioning about widely accepted and stable norms and standards, and when a contributor is talking about morality, he or she is referring to our society's understanding of right and wrong, you will be able to differentiate the two.

Conclusion

Each of the health professions has its own code of ethics that prescribes the behavior of its professionals and articulates the goals to which its professionals should aspire. You will be a professional. You will be asked to think about and commit yourself to the goals of your profession.

You would hope that these codes of ethics, some of which have been around for hundreds of years, would make it easy to recognize and navigate your way through an ethical or moral dilemma. You would hope that the army of well-intentioned, highly educated, committed professionals, who are needed to ensure excellent care delivery, would guarantee that the moral core of a healthcare organization is protected. And sometimes these codes of ethics do help; sometimes a moral or ethical issue or decision is obvious and is either prohibited or sanctioned by one's specific code of professional ethics. Sometimes the decision and the way forward is, or should be, clear to the professional.

But more often, morally or ethically problematic situations or events are murky and have no unequivocal yes or no answer. No clear answer or defined way forward exists. Moreover, ethically or morally problematic situations or events are not always recognized as being ethically or morally problematic. These are the hard situations or events. These situations or events may end up compromising the moral core of your institution and preventing you from making the kind of positive contribution you want to make. For these reasons, we believe healthcare administrators and managers need a new perspective that they apply in their daily decision making and activities.

—Gary L. Filerman, Ann E. Mills, and Paul M. Schyve

Reference

Stefl, M. 2008. "Common Competencies for All Healthcare Managers: The Healthcare Leadership Alliance Model." *Journal of Healthcare Management* 53 (6): 360–73.

INTRODUCTION TO ETHICS

Mary V. Rorty

This chapter is relevant to the following competencies identified in the ACHE Competencies Assessment Tool (see p. xxv):

Communication and Relationship Management
- Identify stakeholder needs/expectations
- Sensitivity to what is correct behavior when communicating with diverse cultures, internal and external
- Facilitate conflict and alternative dispute resolution

Leadership
- Potential impacts and consequences of decision making in situations both internal and external
- Create an organizational culture that values and supports diversity
- Assess the organization including corporate values and culture, business processes, and impact of systems on operations
- Encourage a high level of commitment to the purpose and values of the organization
- Serve as the ethical guide for the organization

Professionalism
- Organizational business and personal ethics
- Professional norms and behaviors

Knowledge of the Healthcare Environment
- Socioeconomic environment in which the organization functions

Business Skills and Knowledge
- How an organization's culture impacts its effectiveness
- Organizational mission, vision, objectives, and priorities

Learning Objectives

After completing this chapter, the reader will

- understand the importance of mastering the language of and various perspectives on ethics for healthcare administration,
- gain a general appreciation of the variety of normative approaches and the possibility of conflict and uncertainty among them,
- be able to differentiate between various levels of ethical relevance (individual, organizational, social), and
- be introduced to various ethical resources for the organization.

Introduction

Talking about ethics for the leaders of healthcare organizations is a daunting task.

The literature of ethics, both in professional contexts and in ordinary language, presents a bewildering array of connotations and implications. This chapter is intended to introduce the language of ethics, give examples of different ways in which it can be relevant to the leaders of healthcare organizations, and contextualize and illustrate how it is relevant to both internal and external decision making—important for the individual members of the organization, the organization itself, and for the larger society. Later chapters will expand in greater detail on specific issues relevant to the administration of this important social institution.

Why This Audience?

The administrator's role is an important and difficult one.

You are not in medical practice per se—although many people most influential in healthcare administration do come from, or have experience of, clinical roles. But the organizations you serve are a crucial part of the chain by which healthcare is delivered to the members of the society in which you operate.

You may not deliver direct care to the patients who are the main reason for the existence for your organization, but the decisions you make affect that care, and you are often the person who is held responsible when things go awry. Your organization structures and coordinates the important social resource of care delivery and, like an individual, will be judged by the values it reflects.

You are required to master many skills and knowledge areas that are peripheral to the various professionals with whom you interact daily, while nonetheless required to discriminate between excellent and inadequate performance in a variety of specialized clinical and administrative areas.

You are a professional, influenced by your own code of ethics. But an important part of promoting excellent care and performance requires communication and negotiation with other professionals bound by their own codes. Finding or forming a common language in which to carry out those negotiations can be challenging and may require sensitive exploration of the moral foundations that underlie many disagreements.

Your role in the institution is critical for its success. Every decision you make has implications for your **stakeholders**, a wide variety of individuals, groups, or institutions, internal and external, who are immediately affected by the operations of your organization. (For a more complete discussion of stakeholder theory, see Chapter 4.) Stakeholders of healthcare organizations include the patients your institution serves, the professionals and other employees who labor within it, the board or owners who govern its operations, the community that houses your institution, the regulators that oversee its operations, the organizations that partner or interact with it, and the larger society by which you are constantly scrutinized—politicians, journalists, affected community members, fellow citizens.

Stakeholder
Any individual or group, including the community, that is affected by the activities of an organization.

For these reasons, an understanding of the language of ethics and the various (sometimes competing and contradictory) **ethical standards** and values by which you and your organization are judged is important to a healthcare administrator. Administrators make decisions on behalf of the organization, and three rules of thumb are important to keep in mind as you deal with the day-to-day issues that come to your attention:

Ethical standards
A belief about how we should behave.

1. Decisions made by individuals in the organization have ethical implications for organizational morale, reputation, and viability.
2. Decisions made and actions taken on the organizational level have ethical implications for individuals in the organization.
3. The operation of the organization has ethical implications for the social environment within which it operates.

Keeping this perspective on the role of leadership will help you strategize to maintain the integrity of your organization as you work to ensure its viability.

The Language of Ethics

Although the terms *ethics* and *morals* are often used interchangeably, the distinction is one of the degree of abstractness. Morality describes the norms, values, and beliefs embedded in social processes that define right and wrong for an individual or community; the language of ethics is how we talk about those norms and values (Crane and Matten 2007).

When we hear that someone has been accused of immoral or unethical behavior, we tend to understand the meaning in terms of the context of practice in which the accusation arises. In Congress, "ethics" often reduces to accepting bribes or doing the bidding of contributors. In the academy, it is frequently associated with plagiarism or falsifying research results. Corporations or charitable organizations are considered to have behaved unethically insofar as they are revealed to have carried out their operations in ways that damage or exploit workers or people living in their immediate environment or have pocketed or misapplied charitable contributions. Even nation-states are popularly condemned—for genocidal operations on subgroups of their own populations, for aggression beyond their borders, or for systematic failures to live up to their own espoused ideals.

Obviously, such a wide range of application of terms of ethical praise or condemnation makes it hard to pin down the specific content of ethics language. The very vagueness and versatility of the language of ethics are what make it so powerful. To paraphrase Justice Potter Stewart's famous quote, we may not be able to precisely define what we mean when we respond to something as unethical, but we know it when we see it. Spelling out why some decision or consequence in the context of healthcare can be considered ethical or unethical may involve recourse to a number of different principles or values.

Normative Uses of Ethical Language

The realm of ethical language is the realm of human choices and decisions. We have wishes, desires, and intentions toward specific results in the world, and we formulate strategies and embark upon courses of action to bring about those desired results. We find ourselves in situations that demand of us some course of action and must decide among alternatives how to "do the right thing" or act "for the best."

We use ethical language when we praise or blame, approve or disapprove of, the actions, intentions, or character of an agent. We speak of "the right thing to do," of our duties and obligations, our responsibilities, privileges, and rights. We worry about honesty, telling the truth, just (or unjust) rewards, treating people fairly. Another word for *ethical*, and one that is not as tightly tied to the level of individual action, is *normative*. Like ethics, normativity is associated with goals and values and with our choices of the means to attain them.

Non-Normative Uses of Ethical Language

Not all uses of those same terms are necessarily normative, but we can usually tell the difference. The "right" tie for this shirt is not the morally better tie but the one that looks best. A "bad" tomato is not evil or blameworthy, but it may be too ripe to be used in a salad. People who live in glass houses really shouldn't throw stones, but that may be more of a practical recommendation than a moral one. In addition to the moral implications of our actions, personal, political, economic, or (as in the case of a glass house) prudential considerations also play into the decisions we make.

Relation to Law

Breaking the law or disobeying or ignoring regulations is generally acknowledged to be unethical. But not all unethical behavior is illegal. Typically the law, in its permutations of regulations, standards, codes, statutes, and accreditation, is designed to enforce moral minimums. For instance, illegal behavior, breaching well-established and socially agreed legal boundaries, is almost universally considered unethical. The broader category of ethical behavior is a supplement and corrective to the narrower and more specific realm of illegal behavior. Often ethical breaches and the public disapproval following them have led to changes in regulations and codes to bring them more in line with the (changing but important) wider ethical standards. And the converse may also be true; sometimes obeying a given law can be argued to be unethical in terms of a competing moral obligation. In such cases we may see that laws or policies become more liberal to accommodate changing social mores. Conscientious objection, an appeal to moral considerations that are claimed to justify disobedience to socially sanctioned laws or regulations, represents a case in which it is claimed that legal behavior would be unethical. Organizations, as well as individuals, can appeal to conscientious objection. For example, some hospitals with religious connections are exempted from providing some healthcare services expected of other hospitals.

Three Poles of Ethical Judgment

Ethical judgments tend to fall into three categories, centered around the poles of agent, act, and effect. We formulate wishes, desires, and intentions toward specific goals or values—results we wish to bring about in the world around us. We formulate strategies and embark upon courses of action to bring about those ends, those desired results. We find ourselves in situations that demand of us some choice and try to figure out how to act for the best and do the right thing (Frankena 1973).

Typically we have justifications—reasons or grounds—for our use of ethical language, whether we articulate or examine them or not. Having ethical promptings, our moral intuitions, that are always clear and unequivocal would be nice. But how often does that happen in administration? Sometimes we have conflicting reactions or inclinations, stemming from different layers of our socialization as moral beings. (We learn from interaction with our social environment that some choices and behaviors are more acceptable than others. As we move from the narrow family circle into the extended social network, then into stages of schooling, eventually perhaps into socialization into the professional ethics of a specific social role, the internalized permissions and prohibitions from the various layers of our moral onion-self may reinforce each other or contradict, depending upon the homogeneity of the society in which we mature.)

Sometimes we have good reasons for wishing to choose both of two mutually exclusive courses of action. Sometimes we have reasons to regret actions or decisions we know are obligatory. These gut reactions are useful information, the data of our normative lives.

Meta-Ethics: Types of Ethical Theory

Philosophers have long dreamed of one simple ethical theory to explain and reconcile all our sometimes-competing moral judgments, and many have suggested candidates. The only problem is that the theory-candidates are all different, and none of the competitors has as yet won the field. Rather than routes to moral truth, the theoretical alternatives are something like "important but partial contributions to a comprehensive, although necessarily fragmented, moral vision" (Steinbock, Arras, and London 2009, 9).

These theories tend to fall into one of three categories, each taking as ethically primary one of the three poles of ethical judgment: the intentions or character of the agent, the nature of the action contemplated, or the ethical value of the goal or end of the action. To be really adequate, a theory must account for all three poles but may consider one of the poles to be determinative of the moral value of the other two. Because philosophers have been dreaming of "the ultimate theory" for so long, you will not be surprised to learn that the three major theory-types have Greek names.

Aretaic, or virtue-theories, take as the basic determinant of the moral value of a course of action the character of the agent from which the action stems. (*Arete* is Greek for excellence and is often translated as "virtue.") The primary ethical judgment, then, would be something like "His action was courageous." The virtuous man, according to Aristotle (350 BCE), would always do the right thing in the right way at the right time to the best effect, having been well raised and acting out of a fixed disposition to behave in an appropriate manner. (To give him credit, Aristotle did consider ethics properly a subdivision of politics and acknowledged that the excellence of the results of the actions of a virtuous man would be dependent upon the excellence of the society in which he was living. The plight of the moral man in immoral society has been a theme of books, plays, and poems ever since.) Benevolence and justice always appear among the list of virtues.

Deontological theories emphasize the moral value of the act itself. Some actions are obligatory or prohibited regardless of the motive or the consequences. (*Deon* is Greek for "duty.") Promise keeping and lying are examples of kinds of action that carry their own implicit moral value. "Do what is right, though the world should perish," Kant is purported to have said (Zwiers 2007). There are varieties of deontological, act-centered moral theories. Act-deontologists consider the basic judgments of obligation to be particular: "In this situation, I should do *x*." Rule-deontologists tend to prioritize rules or principles, of varying generality. "Don't be evil," the unofficial motto of Google, may be the commercial equivalent of the Hippocratic injunction "Do no harm." So-called situation ethics and bioethical principlism tend to be interpreted as deontological (Frankena 1973).

Teleological or consequentialist ethical theories (from the Greek *telos*, end or goal) focus on consequences, the effect or result of our choices and acts. The suggestion is that the moral end to be sought in all we do is the best possible balance of good over bad—with "good" and "bad" being interpreted non-normatively, in terms of natural preferences, such as pleasure or happiness, or nonmoral goods, such as efficiency or safety. For instance, acting in this way rather than that may produce a situation with a net balance of pleasure over pain. This fact about the *result* is what makes this act morally preferable, normatively "better," the right thing to do.

Consequentialist theories include ethical egoism (where the good to be considered accrues to the agent alone) and universal consequentialism, of which the agent is not the only intended beneficiary. Jeremy Bentham (1776), who termed his theory *utilitarianism*, expounded, "It is the greatest happiness to the greatest number of people that is the measure of right and wrong."

Like deontological theories, utilitarianism too has "act" and more general, or "rule," versions. Act-utilitarians ask, "What effect will my action in this situation have on the balance of good in general?" General or rule-utilitarians, as the name suggests, ask rather, "What effect would this action in this situation have on that balance if everyone in a similar situation acted similarly?" Or, considering the role of rules or principles central to moral action, they may decide that "in this situation, the rule that best applies tells me that I should (tell the truth, keep my promise, meet the contractual obligation)." The rules, for the universalistic consequentialist, are determined by considering what rules will best promote the general good.

The codes and standards of behavior for members of a given society have to do with the conditions of our lives together, and that renders salient issues of justice and care—including equitable distribution of resources, fairness, attention to the needs of the less advantaged, and relationships. Movements such as communitarian ethics, feminist care ethics, and contemporary

versions of contract theory address this need and apply the language of ethics beyond individual agency to larger social interactions. In this communal
context, the structures and processes of our social institutions are no less
important than the actions of individuals. The various approaches to ethical
theory we have described are attempts to systematize widely accepted common morality, and, as we can see even in the move from "act" to "rule" levels
of generality, are intended to be applied to the larger social context as well as
to the individual context.

Applied Ethics: From Theory to Rules of Thumb

Of course no one facing choices picks a theory and deduces from it the
proper way to behave. We operate on gut reactions, rules of thumb, or experience of results in analogous situations—we navigate through life on our
accumulated moral training, experience, and sensitivity. (See Chapter 7.) For
that reason, the term *applied ethics* is controversial, implying a kind of top-
down relation of ethics to actual situations. The situation itself prompts our
ethical reactions, and our responses are seldom systematized enough to count
as any one theory. Some approaches to ethics start from this level of particu-
larity and may work up to formulation of general principles (what Immanuel
Kant might have called "maxims") without ever attempting to formulate a
more universal rule.

In another sense of *applied*, what constitutes ethics in various professional or institutional fields has been explored considerably. Business ethics,
professional ethics, journalistic ethics, engineering ethics, and our area of
interest, healthcare managerial ethics, have all been the subject of considerable study in recent years. In those fields, the approach typically centers
on cases, an approach canonized in the literature as casuistry (Jonsen and
Toulmin 1990), with the cases often being discussed in terms of principles
or maxims drawn from all of the theories discussed here (Beauchamp and
Childress 2008). In the chapters that follow, reference to particular cases
will be helpful in calling attention to the ethical implications of the practical
decisions that are the bread and butter of healthcare administration. Seeking
out the values implicit in the conflicts represented by particular cases will
help you seek resolutions that best contribute to the ethical operation of your
organization.

Moving Beyond the Individual: Ethics and Organizations

This introductory chapter presents the healthcare organization as analogical
to the individual, as an agent with a particular character, acting toward goals
and values that are common to all such organizations but with individual

variation depending upon the specific history and self-definition of a particular institution. How the organization acts—the strategies and policies, the choices and decisions that operationalize these values and determine how they affect the day-to-day work of your institution—are to a great extent the responsibility of the leaders, the healthcare administrators.

In the twenty-first century clearly not all actions are the actions of individuals. Collectives act as well and are judged on the nature of their actions and their consequences. Ethical expressions—such as right and wrong, just and unjust, good and bad—are used to evaluate institutional and social values, decisions, and outcomes. We hold organizations and, as noted previously, even social systems and individuals morally responsible. We describe, analyze, and evaluate motivations, practices, and outcomes on at least three levels:

1. *Micro*: the level of the individual ethics, scrutinizing character, actions, choices, and results.

2. *Macro*: the level of political theory, where we apply moral criteria to the arrangements and ideologies of entire social systems or their institutions: "an unjust society," " a cruel penal system," "an irresponsible dictator." Although judgment of the acts of individuals and their consequences may be the origin of some of our normative language, there are obvious and common social uses as well. For instance, political theorist John Rawls (1971) refers to justice as "the first virtue of social institutions."

3. *Meso*: Between the micro and macro levels lie the collectives for which you are responsible as administrators, the level of organizations: corporations, clubs, unions, churches, businesses, and systems. Neither preprogrammed instruments of the larger society nor merely the sum of the interactions of the individuals that compose them, organizations are important agents in their own right. Proper appraisal of their goals, actions, and effects requires us to speak of them in ways that are borrowed not only from ethics but also from social and political norms.

For you as future leaders of organizations, appreciating this intermediary position is particularly important. Your institution is itself a collective; a member of a collective consisting of similar organizations, your peers, and contractors; and an individual constituent of the collective that is the larger society. Some of the things that most affect your organization are internal to it. Actions of individual members can affect the morale or reputation of the whole organization. Other important challenges for administration are external. Some changes in the larger society—changes in regulation, reimbursement, or health policy—will affect the operation of your organization.

Organizations are instruments designed to attain certain specified goals. In the case of healthcare organizations, the goal is provision of certain kinds of healthcare to specified populations, and the success—indeed, sometimes even the survival—of the organization depends on the extent to which the performance of the organization meets the expectations of the society that supports it. The structure and processes of the organization, of which you are custodians, are the means of delivering this care.

The Role of Ethics in Organizational Leadership

Readers should keep some important things in mind regarding the role of ethics in organizational leadership:

Normative judgments
Evaluations in moral terms.

- **Normative judgments**, evaluations in moral terms, can be made not only of individuals, but also of collectives—and indeed, they are constantly being made by all the stakeholders, internal and external, of your organization.
- Individuals accrue not only moral responsibilities to their own character, intentions, and choices but also responsibilities stemming from their role and the positions they occupy in various formal and informal social institutions: their families and friends, membership in cultural or social affinity groups, their job responsibilities, and their professions.
- Institutions, like individuals, occupy social roles and are held responsible for how they meet the obligations that their role determines.

Organizations as Ethical Agents: Values and Virtues

As agents, organizations act toward certain goals or ends—effects that they are designed to achieve and specific values that accompany those effects. As an institution in our society, a healthcare organization aims at sustaining and improving the health of the members of society, with particular subgroups designated by the kind of organization in question. Rehabilitation centers serve a specific purpose, as do psychiatric services. Hospitals are typically oriented toward acute care and can include emergency and trauma centers, operating rooms and surgical services, and intensive care units. Children's hospitals serve an age-limited population.

From the standpoint of teleological ethics, as instruments of policy directed toward goals or ends that are not themselves necessarily moral in nature, the moral excellence of an organization is a function of its success in reaching those goals. The Institute of Medicine (2001) has suggested specific values or goals to be pursued by any excellent healthcare system: Care should be safe, effective, patient-centered, timely, efficient, and equitable. Other sources express the values to be pursued by the healthcare organization in explicitly ethical terms. The Institute for Ethics of the American Medical Association (Ozar et al. 2000) suggests the following values to guide organizational decision making, noting that they are not listed in order of priority: patients' healthcare services; professionals' expertise; public health; unmet healthcare needs; advocacy for social policy reform; relationships with clinical staff, management, employees, and affiliated professionals; organizational solvency and survival; and benefit to the community. The Joint Commission (2011), responsible for accrediting healthcare organizations, makes the normative explicit: The leadership of the institutions subject to accreditation is charged to "carry out their patient care and business arrangements in an ethical manner."

Of course, any administrator—indeed, anyone familiar with the operations of any healthcare organization—can instantly see the strengths and the weaknesses of these universals. They are all worthy values for aspiration. But what happens when they conflict? If a patient desires care that is ineffective, which of the values takes priority? And what about your responsibility for the economic viability of your institution? What if the more effective medicine for a given syndrome costs ten times—or 100 times—more than the second most effective pharmaceutical? Resource management is the most important responsibility of the healthcare administrator and can present the greatest ethical challenges.

Hospitals and other healthcare organizations formulate mission statements and ethics codes that express the values they profess, tailored to their individual service area. The values included typically express responsibilities to both internal and external constituencies—fair treatment for employees, responsiveness to social expectations, and standards for internal operations. Determining those values, balancing and prioritizing in light of current needs, and frequently revisiting them are important for keeping the various parts of the organization moving in a unified way toward its goals.

When Values Conflict

Demands for the highest quality and quantity of excellent care likely must be balanced with the need for fiscal responsibility and the maintenance of the organization's survival and viability in a competitive environment. Think of the resulting problems in terms of value conflicts, and strategize to maximize the outcomes in ethical terms. Communication skills can become crucial in leadership. Listening to and talking with affected stakeholders can ensure that competing or conflicting values do not lead to an impasse or an adversarial situation. If you can articulate the situation in a way that acknowledges the values at stake, you can make the most of them and contribute to mutual understanding, even if consensus is not always attainable. Mutual understanding allows for mutual respect between individuals or departments, whose priorities may, for good reasons, differ in controversial situations.

Organizational Character: Culture and Climate

We speak of moral agents as having good or bad character, which often means their habitual patterns of action, their immediate response to typical or unusual situations, and the goals or values that they prioritize. A handy way to talk about these concepts for organizations is to speak of their culture and climate.

Organizational culture
The customary or traditional ways of thinking and doing things, which are shared to a greater or lesser extent by all members of the organization and which new members of the organization must learn and at least partially accept in order to be accepted into the service of the firm.

The mission, goals, and collective activities of an organization create its culture—"the customary or traditional ways of thinking and doing things which are shared to a greater or lesser extent by all members of an organization," according to Jaques (1951). For example, the culture of a tertiary medical center, capable of high-tech interventions and trauma care, is different from that of a small community hospital with no emergency room (Chapple 2010). Even different service units in the same hospital can have different minicultures; maternity wards and transplant services work toward their shared values with very different styles.

One component of **organizational culture** is of particular relevance to the administrator. The **ethical climate** is the functional analogue of the character of an individual, and it is defined by a shared perception of how ethical issues should be addressed and what constitutes ethically correct behavior for the organization (Victor and Cullen 1988). The character of a collective is something that the individuals in it can judge by their experience of what the ethical expectations are and whether they are expressed in the actions and atmosphere of the organization. How do the people in the organization feel about the extent to which the values espoused by the institution are actually implemented? Institutions are subject to normative judgments concerning the extent to which they accommodate the moral agency of the individuals within them. Morale is sure to suffer if too much of a gap exists between organizational behavior and the expectations of its members, especially with respect to values that affect working conditions. (See Chapter 7.) A number of organizations, including the Department of Veterans Affairs and the American Medical Association, have developed useful instruments for sampling institutional character, various "ethical climate" surveys (Fox et al. 2007; Wynia et al. 2010).

Ethical climate
Shared perceptions of how ethical issues should be addressed and what is ethically correct behavior for the organization.

Managing Structures and Processes

The healthcare organization is complex and hard to classify. Some of its functions—billing, inventory, supply chain management—require precision and tight quality control, quasi-mechanical operation. Other tasks intrinsic to the institution require flexibility and room for individual judgment. Compartmentalization, hierarchy, and strict role definition are among the strategies that allow this complex organization to fulfill its various functions. This need for simultaneous rigidity and flexibility makes it hard to apply the standard categories of organizational theory to healthcare organizations. As some observers have noted, the hospital is a setting where "leadership roles are shared, objectives are divergent, and power is diffuse" (Denis, Lamothe, and Langley 2000).

Is the healthcare organization best conceptualized as a rigid system with some flexible parts, or a flexible system with some compartmentalized areas where rigidity is important? How you think about your organization can make a difference in your managerial strategies and value priorities. One common way of thinking of some organizations is as analogous to organisms. Just as an injury in an appendage or an organ affects the total function of an animal, a signal event or a disruption in an administrative unit can affect the whole hospital. Another way of conceptualizing the healthcare organization, and one that is finding increasing resonance, is as a complex adaptive system (Mills, Rorty, and Werhane 2003; Plsek 2001). This way of thinking about the organization emphasizes the interdependence of the systems, subsystems of the whole, and emphasizes our dependence on, and vulnerability to, changes in our external environment.

The healthcare organization is structured in departments that operate according to varyingly rigid or flexible rules, standards, and procedures. Establishing and implementing the various processes and systems that move the work of the healthcare organization forward is a managerial responsibility, as much an art as a science. Integration, coordination, intercommunication, and cooperation of these different functions—business, clinical, professional—is the challenging task of the hospital administrator.

Although values may be shared, individuals with different responsibilities may prioritize them differently, and insofar as the values of different parts of the organization are out of alignment, its function is impaired. So in healthcare managerial ethics, as in clinical ethics, communication is crucial. Listening to the reasons for the choices and decisions of the leaders of different functional units is the best route for achieving a possible balance among competing needs. Open discussion and transparency within leadership, and between leaders and their constituent members, contribute to an organization's ability to move with mutual understanding toward shared goals. Alignment of values is important not only between leaders and within the organization but also between the organization and the community it serves (Denis, Lamothe, and Langley 2000).

The healthcare organization is interpenetrated on all levels by normative demands and influences of agents external to the organization. Not all the policies, regulations, standards, and laws that govern the operation of your organization are under your control: various regulators, accrediting agencies, evaluators, and legislators impose parameters on healthcare organizations within which they must operate. (See Chapter 11.) You do not have the option of ignoring these externally imposed requirements, and the challenge for leadership is to implement them in ways that maximize excellent patient care and minimize possible ethical conflicts and dilemmas for your professionals and staff. In this area managerial style is expressed. How the various positive and negative incentives associated with processes are implemented is important for morale, for community trust, and for excellent leadership.

Allies in Ethical Management

The healthcare organization has a number of normative loci devoted to various aspects of excellent organizational function. Compliance programs pay attention to legal and regulatory obligations. Quality assurance and risk management are important allies in defining and determining how to carry out the procedures that represent the organization's values. Institutional ethics committees, although often narrowly prescribed (see Chapter 6), can be useful for wider organizational ethics projects (see Chapter 5), and some have healthcare organizational ethics subcommittees specifically designated to deal with ethical issues that do not fall within the traditional clinical ethics areas. Some healthcare organizations have leadership ethics councils or operations committees. Some institutions associated with academic medical centers have relations with ethics centers. When ethics is recognized as important to the organization, it is less likely to be viewed as a compartmentalized silo and acknowledged to be a value distributed throughout the culture of the organization (Spencer et al. 2000). This understanding allows for the better integration of the contributions of each individual and functional unit to the whole.

Conclusion

The healthcare organization is a Hippocratic institution. In all its operations, it is directed toward the same ends and values as its professional members. The ethical conduct of those operations is as central a concern for the administrator as is their effectiveness and efficiency. This concern for the ethical aspects of its structures and processes pervades the institution and requires of you the fair and fitting distribution of its resources—time, labor, and money. Not only individuals, but individual components—departments and services—are value driven and subject to judgment about how their activities contribute to, or detract from, the ethical balance of the organization as a whole.

As a leader *in* your organization, your own character—your personal and professional integrity, honesty, empathy, and commitment—are under scrutiny. Your skills of communicating values and of listening to the responses and concerns of others are in constant demand. As a leader *of* your organization, your sensitivity to the ethical expectations of both the people with whom you work and the communities you serve is one of the basic requirements of your position.

This chapter has highlighted the importance of values for the daily operations of and the long-term viability of the organizations you serve, affecting both your team's morale and your organization's reputation. The values your organization espouses and furthers, and the structures and processes by which they are operationalized, are your responsibility as a leader.

Points to Remember

- Conflict and uncertainty about specific issues often involve underlying value differences or differences in priorities of shared values and can best be resolved by attention to those more basic issues.
- The efficiency and effectiveness of a healthcare organization depends in part on the alignment of values, among the leaders, between leaders and their constituency, and of the organization as a whole with the values of its partners and community.
- Reconciling competing needs and obligations requires a familiarity with different ethical approaches and sensitivity to the values they represent. Some familiarity with the language of ethics can provide one tool for this demanding task.
- A leadership role in a healthcare organization involves both individual and collective ethical responsibilities.
- Janus, the Roman guardian of doorways and city gates, had responsibility for both the people inside the house or city and those outside. For this task he was given two faces and elevated to the status of a god. Your role as leader and administrator is liminal in the same way—although the reward is seldom as great.

References

Aristotle. 350 BCE. *Nichomachean Ethics*. Translated by W. D. Ross. Accessed March 18. Constitution Society. www.constitution.org/ari/ethic_00.htm.

Beauchamp, J., and J. Childress. 2008. *Principles of Biomedical Ethics*, 6th ed. New York: Oxford University Press.

Bentham, J. 1776. *A Fragment on Government*. Accessed March 18. www.constitution.org/jb/frag_gov.htm.

Chapple, H. 2010. *No Place for Dying: Hospitals and the Ideology of Rescue*. Walnut Creek, CA: Left Coast Press.

Crane, A., and D. Matten. 2007. *Business Ethics*, 2nd ed. New York: Oxford University Press.

Denis, J. L., L. Lamothe, and A. Langley. 2000. "The Dynamics of Collective Leadership and Strategic Change in Pluralistic Organizations." *Academy of Management Journal* 44 (4): 809–37.

Fox, E., M. Bottrell, M. B. Foglia, and R. Stoeckle. 2007. "Preventive Ethics: Addressing Ethics Quality Gaps on a Systems Level." *Integrated Ethics*. Accessed March 18. www.ethics.va.gov/docs/integratedethics/Preventive_Ethics_Addressing_Ethics_Quality_Gaps_on_a_Systems_Level_20070808.pdf.

Frankena, W. K. 1973. *Ethics*, 2nd ed. Englewood Cliffs, NJ: Prentice Hall.

Institute of Medicine. 2001. *Crossing the Quality Chasm: A New Health System for the 21st Century*. Washington, DC: National Academies Press.

Jaques, E. 1951. *The Changing Culture of a Factory: A Study of Authority and Participation in an Industrial Setting*. London: Tavistock Publications.

Joint Commission. 2011. *Comprehensive Accreditation Manual for Hospitals: The Official Handbook*. Oakbrook Terrace, IL: Joint Commission Resources.

Jonsen, A. R., and S. Toulmin. 1990. *The Abuse of Casuistry: A History of Moral Reasoning*. Berkeley, CA: University of California Press.

Mills, A., M. V. Rorty, and P. H. Werhane. 2003. "Complexity and the Role of Ethics in Health Care." *Emergence* 5 (3): 6–21.

Ozar, D., J. Berg, P. H. Werhane, and L. Emanuel. 2000. "Organizational Ethics in Healthcare: Toward a Model for Ethical Decision Making for Provider Organizations." *Institute for Ethics National Working Group Report*. Chicago: American Medical Association.

Plsek, P. 2001. "Appendix B: Redesigning Health Care with Insights from the Science of Complex Adaptive Systems." In *Crossing the Quality Chasm: A New Health System for the 21st Century*, 309–22. Washington, DC: National Academies Press.

Rawls, J. 1971. *A Theory of Justice*. Cambridge, MA: Harvard University Press.

Spencer, E. M., A. E. Mills, M. V. Rorty, and P. H. Werhane. 2000. *Organization Ethics in Health Care*. New York: Oxford University Press.

Steinbock, B., J. D. Arras, and A. J. London. 2008. *Ethical Issues in Modern Medicine*, 7th ed. New York: McGraw-Hill.

Victor, B., and J. Cullen. 1988. "The Organizational Bases of Ethical Work Climates." *Administrative Science Quarterly* 33 (1): 101–25.

Wynia, M., M. Johnson, T. P. McCoy, L. P. Griffin, and C. Y. Osborn. 2010. "Validation of an Organizational Communication Climate Assessment Toolkit." *American Journal of Medical Quality* 25 (6): 436–43.

Zwiers, J. 2007. *Building Academic Language: Essential Practices for Content Classrooms, Grades 5–12*. Hoboken, NJ: Jossey-Bass.

ETHICS AND THE HEALTHCARE ORGANIZATION

Ann E. Mills

This chapter is relevant to the following competencies identified in the ACHE Competencies Assessment Tool (see p. xxv):

Communication and Relationship Management
- Identify stakeholder needs/expectations
- Facilitate conflict and alternative dispute resolution

Leadership
- Potential impacts and consequences of decision making in situations both internal and external
- Assess the organization, including corporate values and culture, business processes, and impact of systems on operations
- Encourage a high level of commitment to the purpose and values of the organization

Knowledge of the Healthcare Environment
- The interrelationships among access, quality, cost, resource allocation, accountability, and community
- The patient's perspective (e.g., cultural differences, expectations)

Business Skills and Knowledge
- How an organization's culture impacts its effectiveness
- Organizational mission, vision, objectives, and priorities
- Patients' rights, laws, and regulations

Learning Objectives

After completing this chapter, the reader will be able to

- discuss the purposes of a healthcare organization;
- demonstrate how ethical tensions might occur in the mission and values of the healthcare organization;
- demonstrate how ethical tensions, if not resolved, can damage the healthcare organization;
- discuss how ethical tensions might be resolved;
- discuss why the formation and maintenance of an appropriate culture and ethical climate is important to the performance of a healthcare organization; and
- discuss some controversial issues that generate ethical conflicts about the missions of healthcare organizations, particularly those of hospitals.

Introduction

Hospitals can be large or small, part of a large system or a stand-alone community hospital. They can be general or more specialized, for-profit or not-for-profit. Their missions may differ. Yet in spite of their differences, they share a similar purpose. They are organizations that provide some kind of healthcare to those in need by means of specialized staff and equipment. Because hospitals share a similar purpose, they have similar stakeholders.

A stakeholder is "any group or individual who can affect or is affected by the achievement of the organization's objectives" (Freeman 2010). From the perspective of the administrator, stakeholders of the hospital include patients and their families, healthcare financing organizations, buyers, community organizations, professional and nonprofessional staff and the professional associations and unions that represent them, regulatory organizations (including state and national organizations), accrediting organizations, trustees or the governing board, other administrators, suppliers, other hospitals and clinics, and the community in which the hospital resides (Griffith and White 2010). Each of these individuals or groups of individuals can affect or be affected by the achievement (or not) of the hospital's objectives, and by the decisions made on behalf of the hospital.

Hospitals are unique even though they share a similar purpose and similar stakeholders. They have different visions and prioritize different commitments. Understanding a specific hospital or healthcare organization requires understanding its specific purpose and how it achieves that purpose. One way an organization lets stakeholders know its purpose and how it achieves its purpose is through its public documents. Thus, we begin this chapter with an introduction to the sorts of documents that inform a hospital's stakeholders. These documents are meant to be statements of what the entity does and how it fulfills its promises; therefore, these documents also articulate the ethical standards and values that the organization says it espouses.

Public documents are meant to influence behavior internally in the hospital and externally as employees and healthcare providers interact with the hospital's environment. Because these documents affect behavior, they are intended to affect the organization's culture. This chapter explains what is meant by *culture,* and it identifies and explains an important part of organizational culture—the ethical climate.

Limited resources ensure that, at times, a healthcare organization's missions will compete or be in conflict. Moreover, limited resources ensure a healthcare organization's values will compete or be in conflict with the healthcare organization's missions. To be more specific, the actions that will best achieve one mission or one value may compete with the actions that would best achieve another mission or value.

The kinds of conflicts that might occur can be at either the micro or macro level. For instance, on the micro level, a busy nurse may think that because of understaffing, she is not delivering the kind of quality care promised by the hospital to its patients. She understands that revenue has shrunk over the past year and that the hospital must balance available resources among the hospital's priorities. Nevertheless, she believes quality care is being sacrificed to the value of stewardship—the value that the hospital monitors and uses its resources wisely. The nurse is confused about the priority of hospital values and the implementation of these values.

On the macro level, decisions can be made that compromise a healthcare organization's missions and values. For instance, a hospital has a long history and proud tradition of being committed to the well-being of the community. Leadership in the hospital knows that the hospital expanding some of its services would be in the community's interests. However, this expansion can be cost effective only if the hospital is allowed to buy the only park in town to build a new building. The board is split on the issue and uncertain how to proceed.

This chapter explores how these tensions can occur and offers a framework in which they can be discussed and resolved. The chapter concludes with a discussion of some of the issues that face today's hospitals and challenge their missions.

Organizational Statements

Mission Statements

The **mission statement** of any entity describes its reason for existence, its purpose, and its specific activities. It can guide management and staff when difficult decisions have to be made because it can serve to remind decision makers of the organization's purpose. While the real-life mission of the entity often differs from its professed mission, ideally decision makers should be able to justify their decisions within the context of the organization's stated mission statement.

The mission statement, particularly of a healthcare organization, also reflects societal expectations of the entity. Societal expectations of healthcare organizations, specifically hospitals, have formed and changed as the hospital grew from an almshouse catering to the "deserving" poor to the complex organization it is today (Rosenberg 1987; Starr 1982). If a hospital reflects current societal expectations, the existence of the hospital and its purposes are legitimized.

A mission statement also allows stakeholders to make judgments about the entity as to whether or not the entity is fulfilling its purpose. If a hospital promises to deliver quality care but a significant number of patients acquire preventable infections, stakeholders might question that promise.

Examples of Mission Statements

Massachusetts General Hospital is the third oldest hospital in the country. Founded by a group of wealthy philanthropists in 1811 to give relief to the poor and sick in Boston, the hospital is owned by General Hospital Corporation, a nonprofit. The mission statement of Massachusetts General (2013a) is as follows:

> Guided by the needs of our patients and their families, we aim to deliver the very best health care in a safe, compassionate environment; to advance that care through innovative research and education; and to improve the health and well-being of the diverse communities we serve.

Bon Secours Richmond Health System (Bon Secours RHS) was founded by the Sisters of Bon Secours with the opening of St. Mary's Hospital in Richmond, Virginia, in 1995 and the acquisition and opening of three other Richmond-area hospitals. The mission statement of Bon Secours RHS (2013a) is:

> to bring compassion to healthcare and to be good help to those in need, especially those who are poor and dying. As a System of caregivers, we commit ourselves to

help bring people and communities to health and wholeness as part of the healing ministry of Jesus Christ and the Catholic Church.

One of the largest for-profit (or investor-owned) healthcare delivery systems in the nation is Tenet Healthcare Corporation. As of April 2012, it owns 50 acute care hospitals and 99 outpatient centers in 11 states. Each hospital's mission statement reflects Tenet's (2013) mission:

At Tenet, our business is health care. Our mission is to improve the quality of life of every patient who enters our doors. Our approach makes us unique and defines our future.

These three mission statements overlap somewhat, reflecting the similar purpose of hospitals. All three statements focus on "bringing health," "improving health," or "improving the quality of life" for stakeholders. But several differences highlight the more specific purpose and activities of each organization. For instance, Massachusetts General emphasizes its commitment to advance care through innovative research and education, Bon Secours RHS says it is especially committed to those who are poor and dying, and Tenet's mission statement is focused on quality. These differences will be reflected in the specific activities associated with the goals of each hospital or groups of hospitals.

Note also that societal expectations are reflected in all three mission statements. Massachusetts General promises to deliver quality care. Tenet is also committed to quality. One aspect of quality in healthcare delivery is safety, and Bon Secours RHS promises to deliver safe care. We, as a society, expect to see the value of safety reflected in the day-to-day operations of a hospital.

All three mission statements also reflect the specific ownership of the hospital or system. Massachusetts General is a nonprofit with its roots in the community, Bon Secours RHS is a Catholic mission-driven health system, and Tenet is a for-profit healthcare system. Both Massachusetts General and Bon Secours RHS refer to compassion for those in need and both reference the communities served, while Tenet unapologetically states healthcare is its business.

Values Statements

A **values statement** articulates the **core values** of an organization. This statement is often referred to as the organization's "guiding principles." It lets stakeholders know how the organization intends to achieve its mission, so it articulates the values or ethical standards of the organization.

A values statement serves many of the same purposes as a mission statement. It can help guide decision makers and give internal and external

Values statement
A public statement describing the values endorsed by the entity. Because these statements are public, they allow judgments about the entity. They can also legitimize the entity if societal expectations are reflected.

Core values
Essential values of an organization; sometimes referred to as "guiding principles."

stakeholders a basis on which to make judgments about the organization. Moreover, values statements reflect society's expectations of the entity. The Institute of Medicine (IOM 2001) has articulated what it considers to be the most important values of healthcare organizations. Care should be:

- *Safe*—avoiding injuries to patients from the care that is intended to help them

- *Effective*—providing services based on scientific knowledge to all who could benefit and refraining from providing services to those not likely to benefit (avoiding underuse and overuse, respectively)

- *Patient-centered*—providing care that is respectful of and responsive to individual patient preferences, needs, and values and ensuring that patient values guide all clinical decisions

- *Timely*—reducing waits and sometimes harmful delays for both those who receive and those who give care

- *Efficient*—avoiding waste, including waste of equipment, supplies, ideas, and energy

- *Equitable*—providing care that does not vary in quality because of personal characteristics, such as gender, ethnicity, geographic location, and socioeconomic status

If a healthcare organization endorses safety as a core value, stakeholders will expect it in their interactions with the hospital, its professional staff, and employees, and will have a basis for judgment if they do not experience it. But just as the actual mission of an organization may not align with its stated mission, the professed or stated values may not align with the real-life values of an organization.

Examples of Values Statements

Values statements can be intertwined with mission statements or they can be stand-alone documents. For instance, the mission statements of both Massachusetts General and Bon Secours RHS endorse the value of compassion. They can be called something other than a "values statement." For instance, Massachusetts General (2013c) articulates its core values in a document called "Quality and Safety" (note the integration of the IOM values):

> Our approach to patient care encompasses our commitment to safety, effectiveness, patient centeredness, timeliness, efficiency and equity—an approach that is always evolving based on the latest research findings.

The values statement of Bon Secours RHS (2013b) can be found in its "Heritage" document, which states:

Providing "good help" to those in need has been the passion of the Sisters of Bon Secours since 1824. And while the ministry has evolved over the years, the values at the heart of Bon Secours remain the same—providing quality healthcare with an emphasis on respect, quality, justice, compassion, stewardship, integrity, growth and innovation.

Tenet (2013) combines its core values with its mission statement. Tenet's core values are:

As we seek to improve the quality of our patients' lives, to serve our communities, to provide an exceptional environment for our employees and affiliated physicians and provide an attractive return to our shareholders, we are guided by five core values:

Quality. Quality is at the core of everything we do and every decision we make.

Integrity. We manage our business with integrity and the highest ethical standards.

Service. We have a culture of service that values teamwork and focuses on the needs of others.

Innovation. We have a culture of innovation that creates new solutions for our patients, physicians and employees.

Transparency. We operate with transparency by measuring our results and sharing them with others.

These values are the reasons our patients and physicians choose us, and we seek relationships with those who share them.

These statements share many common values, as all three reference "service" and "innovation" in one way or another, yet note the differing values emphasized by the organizations. Tenet emphasizes transparency, which the other two do not mention it. Tenet emphasizes its commitment to patients, physicians and staff, and shareholders, while the values statements of Massachusetts General and Bon Secours are entirely patient and community focused.

Patient Rights and Responsibilities

The Joint Commission, which accredits and certifies more than 20,000 healthcare organizations and programs in the United States, has been concerned with patient rights for many years. The Joint Commission develops standards that hospitals and other healthcare organizations must meet to be accredited. Because accreditation entitles a hospital (and some other forms

The Joint Commission
An independent, not-for-profit organization that accredits and certifies more than 20,000 healthcare organizations and programs in the United States.

Case Study

A rural hospital mission statement says that the hospital endorses the values of integrity and transparency in its relationships with all stakeholders, including the community. A local paper reports that community leaders are concerned about the number of people in the area who do not have easy access to the hospital. Community leaders are considering the possibility of building a clinic that can help improve access. Hospital leaders are concerned that the clinic will ultimately be a source of competition and are not eager to support the effort. They are unsure how the hospital should publicly react to the report. You are a senior administrator. You have been asked for your advice. What do you say?

of healthcare organizations) to receive Medicare and Medicaid reimbursements, and because most hospitals and other healthcare organizations seek reimbursements from Medicare and Medicaid (AHA 2009), most are fairly assiduous in following The Joint Commission's standards.

Standards associated with patient rights are detailed in The Joint Commission's (2011) Standards on Patient Rights and Responsibilities. These standards are embedded in the following examples.

Examples of Statements on Patient Rights and Responsibilities

Massachusetts General's (2013b) statement on patient rights and responsibilities is as follows:

These Are Your Rights:

- You have the right to be treated in a caring and polite way.

- You have a right to know all the facts we have about your illness, treatments and possible outcomes. Your doctor or other health care giver will give these facts to you.

- You have the right to know the name and specialty of the doctor responsible for your care.

- You have the right to say yes to treatment. You also have the right to say no or refuse treatment.

- You have the right to agree to an advance directive, such as a health care proxy, which tells the hospital and doctor how you want to be treated and whom you want to make decisions for you if you cannot speak for yourself at the time. The person you choose in your proxy is your Health Care Agent.

- You have the right to be examined in private by your doctor or other health care giver, and you have the right to talk to your doctor in private.

- You have the right to look at your medical records and get a copy for a reasonable fee.

- You have the right to take part in a research study if you are asked. You also have the right to say no if you do not want to take part.

- You have the right to expect evaluation and treatment of pain.

- You have the right to expect that we will try to get back to you as quickly as possible when you ask us to do something.

- If you are a female rape victim of childbearing age, you have the right to be promptly offered emergency contraception upon request, and receive written information about emergency contraception.

- You have the right to receive written notice of how your health information will be used and shared in order for you to receive the highest quality of care. This is called our Privacy Notice and it contains patient rights and our legal duties regarding your health information. You may request a copy of this Privacy Notice from any staff member.

- You, your family, your significant other or your guardian have the right to report concerns about safety to your doctor, nurse or other health care giver or by calling our anonymous reporting line at 617–726–1446.

- You, your family, your significant other or your guardian have the right to tell us when something is wrong. This is called presenting a complaint. If you present a complaint, your care will not be affected in any way. If you have a problem that you cannot solve with your doctor, nurse or other caregiver, please call the Office of Patient Advocacy at 617–726–3370.

- If you send a complaint by fax, e-mail or written letter, OPA will acknowledge your communication within two business days.

    A representative from OPA will contact you, review your complaint, and make every effort to resolve your concerns at that time. If your complaint cannot be resolved in a timely manner it will become a grievance. OPA will review and resolve the grievance within 10 business days. If other departments are involved in the review, every effort will be made to resolve the issue within 30 days. An OPA representative will communicate with you if there is no resolution within the above time frames. A letter will be sent to you with the resolution. A letter will be sent to you that will include the name of the hospital contact, steps taken for the review, results of the review, and the completion date.

- You have the right to file a complaint with an outside agency. You can file a quality of care complaint to the Massachusetts Division of Healthcare Quality at 617–753–8150 or to The Joint Commission at 800–994–6610. If you think your civil rights have been violated, you can call the Massachusetts Attorney General's Office at 617–727–2200.

The following is a list of your responsibilities in helping us give you the best care while you are in the hospital.

These Are Your Responsibilities:

- Be honest with us and tell us all you know about your present illness, including other times you have been in the hospital, your health history, your current symptoms and anything else you know about your health that would help us treat you.

- Tell us the medicines you are taking, including the strength and how often you take them. Include over the counter medications, dietary supplements and herbal products you take and/or alternative medicines or treatments that you receive. Talk about any allergies or reactions you have had to any medications.

- Follow the treatment plan recommended by the practitioner primarily responsible for your care.

- Ask your doctor or nurse when and how you will get the results of tests and procedures.

- Tell us if you do not understand what our staff is saying to you or if you do not understand what they are telling you to do; also please tell us if you think you will not be able to do what is asked of you during your care.

- Make sure you understand what will happen if you need surgery. Tell the surgeon, anesthesiologist and nurses if you have allergies or ever had a bad reaction to anesthesia.

- Make sure that you, the practitioner primarily responsible for your care and your surgeon all agree on exactly what will be done during the operation.

- Accept the responsibility for your actions if you refuse treatment or do not follow your practitioner's instructions.

- Report unexpected changes in your condition to your doctor, nurse or other caregiver.

- Be considerate of the rights of other patients and hospital personnel and assist in the control of noise and the number of visitors.

- Follow hospital rules and regulations affecting patient care and conduct, including the no smoking policy.

- Respect the property of others and of the hospital.

- Give the hospital all of the information they will need about the payment of your medical care.

- Ask questions if you do not understand instructions given to you at discharge about the treatment plan that you will use at home, including the medications that you will take and the activities that you can do.

Bon Secours RHS's (2013c) statement on the rights and responsibilities of patients is as follows:

Patients at a Bon Secours facility have the right to:

- Receive care in a safe setting that is appropriate to their needs.

- Receive care that is both respectful of their personal beliefs and consistent with the Mission and values of the Bon Secours Health System.

- Have their pain assessed and treated in a manner respectful of their individual needs and wishes.

- Know the identity and professional status of the individuals directly responsible for their care.

- Receive clear and easy-to-understand information about diagnoses, treatment plans, prognoses and participation in investigational studies/clinical trials prior to any procedure or treatment.

- Participate in decisions regarding their care, including the right to accept or refuse treatment to the extent permitted by the law and the moral tradition of the Catholic Church.

- Be informed of the medical consequences related to their decisions; this includes the right to refuse or withdraw from life-sustaining treatments.

- Participate in the resolution of ethical questions that may arise during the course of their care.

- Make an advance directive (a living will), designate someone to make choices about their medical care for them, or include/exclude family members who would be able to make medical decisions.

- Review their medical records with their physician and have the information explained.

- Request a second opinion about their diagnosis or treatment plan.

- Change physicians during the course of their illness.

- Expect that communications and records concerning their care will be treated in a confidential manner.

- Know the hospital rules and regulations that affect their behavior and the behavior of their family and visitors.

- Know what resources exist if they have questions or concerns about their care or need prompt resolution of a grievance. They may contact Patient Advocacy for this information, or they may call the Virginia Department for Quality Healthcare Services and Consumer Protection.

- Access protective services as provided by law.

- Participate in their discharge planning.

- Have their bill explained to them regardless of the source of payment.

Patients at a Bon Secours facility have the responsibility to:

- Provide their caretakers with complete and accurate information about their illness, including information about past illnesses, hospitalizations and medications.

- Make known whether or not they understand the proposed procedures or treatment plans.

- Follow the agreed-upon treatment plan.

- Be considerate of other patients, the staff, hospital regulations and hospital property.

The following is the policy on patient rights and responsibilities of Ochsner Health System (2013), an eight-hospital system in Louisiana owned by Tenet.

Your Rights as a Patient

We consider you a partner in your hospital care. When you are well informed, participate in treatment decisions and communicate openly with your doctor and other healthcare professionals, you help make your care more effective. While you are in the hospital, your rights include the following:

You have a right to be provided services in a non-discriminatory manner in accordance with the provisions of Title VI of the Civil Rights Act of 1964, Section 504 of the Rehabilitation Act of 1973, the Age Discrimination Act of 1975, the Americans with Disabilities Act as well as any other applicable Federal and State laws and regulations.

You have the right to a reasonable, timely response to your request or need for care, as well as the right to considerate and respectful care including an environment that preserves dignity and contributes to a positive self-image. You are responsible for being considerate and respectful of hospital staff and property as well as other patients and their property.

You have a right to information regarding patient rights, advocacy services and complaint mechanisms, and the right to prompt resolution of any complaint. You or a designee has the right to participate in the resolution of ethical issues surrounding your care. You have a right to file a complaint if you feel that your rights have been infringed, without fear or penalty from Ochsner or the federal government. You may file a complaint with Patient Relations by calling (504) 842–3971. At any time, you may lodge a grievance with the LA Department of Health and Hospitals by calling (866) 280–7737, or the Joint Commission at (800) 994–6610.

You, or someone acting on your behalf, have the right to understandable information on your health status, treatment and progress in order to make decisions. You have the right to know the nature, risks and alternatives to treatment. You have the right to be informed, when appropriate, regarding the outcome of the care that has been provided. You have the right to refuse treatment to the extent permitted by law, and the right to be informed of the alternatives and consequences of refusing treatment.

You, in collaboration with your physician, have the right to make decisions regarding care and the right to participate in the development and implementation of the plan of care and effective pain management. You have the right to know the name and professional status of those responsible for the delivery of your care and treatment.

You have a right within legal guidelines to have a guardian, next-of-kin or legal designee exercise patient rights when you are unable to do so. You have the right for your wishes regarding end-of-life decisions to be addressed by the hospital through advance directives. You have the right to personal privacy and confidentiality and to expect confidentiality of all records and communications pertaining to your care. You have the right to request a paper copy of our complete Notice of Privacy Practices, which we are required to provide to you and follow.

You have the right to receive communications about your health information confidentially. You have the right to request restrictions on the uses and disclosures of your health information. You have the right to inspect, copy, request amendments and receive an accounting of to whom we have disclosed your health information.

You have the right to know if your physician wishes to include clinical investigation as part of your care or treatment. You have the right to refuse to participate in such research.

You have the right to information about the hospital charges and available payment methods before services are rendered; immediate and long-term financial implications of treatment choices, insofar as they are known. You have the right to request an explanation of your bill for hospital charges and to be given timely notice of non-coverage of services by your payor.

You have the right to be provided with interpretation services if you do not speak English; to alternative communication techniques if you are hearing or vision impaired; and to have any other resources taken on your behalf to ensure effective communication. These services are provided free of charge.

You have a right to personal safety (free from mental, physical, sexual and verbal abuse, neglect and exploitation). You have the right to access protective and advocacy services. You have the right to protection of personal possessions, entrusted to the hospital for safekeeping. If you have a safety concern, we encourage you to report it to a department manager or to Patient Relations.

You have the right to consent and rescind consent to recording or photographic, video, electronic or audio filming for purposes other than identification, diagnosis or treatment.

Your Responsibilities as a Patient

To the limit of capability, you are responsible for providing accurate and complete information relevant to the provision of services, including but not limited to present complaints, past illnesses, hospitalizations, medications, pain management and advance directives.

You are responsible for making a reasonable attempt to understand what is expected of you, including asking questions as needed. To the limit of capability, you are responsible for accepting the consequences for the outcomes if you do not follow the care, treatment and service plan.

You are responsible for entrusting valuables to the hospital for safekeeping, when other options are impractical. You are responsible for complying with hospital safety regulations, operational policies and financial policies, and for helping your caregiver provide a safe patient care environment.

The three documents closely follow Joint Commission standards. For instance, all three insist that patients be honest with their health history. All three provide information for patients wishing to make a complaint, as required by The Joint Commission. However, all organizations are different. Note that Bon Secours RHS, which adheres to the morals associated with the Catholic Church, delimits the right to accept or refuse treatment "to the extent permitted by the law and the moral tradition of the Catholic Church." Massachusetts General, however, explicitly grants rape victims of childbearing age the right to emergency contraception, while Ochsner Health System (owned by Tenet) does not mention the issue.

Other Statements

An organization can fashion other statements to help guide decision making. For instance, some healthcare organizations create vision statements. These statements are usually inspirational in that they articulate what the healthcare organization would like itself or the community it serves to

Case Study

A patient is recovering from surgery. Her husband has been feeding her ice chips because her mouth and throat are dry and she cannot easily swallow fluids. He asks one of the nurses to bring him more ice chips. After 40 minutes the husband leaves the patient to hunt for someone who can help him. Later, the husband complains to a patient representative who reports to you, a midlevel administrator. How should you respond after hearing the complaint?

become. Most hospitals and other healthcare organizations have codes of conduct that instruct employees on the type of behavior the organization wants to encourage and the type of behavior it will not tolerate. Ideally, these statements align with and are supportive of the healthcare organization's mission and values statements.

Genesis of Ethical Tension

Clearly, the mission of a healthcare organization can adjust with changes in ownership, physical location, resources, or environment. And while periodically reviewing its mission, values, and patient rights statements is a good idea for healthcare organizations, a significant change might necessitate a prompt review.

Conflicts might arise among these three statements for a number of reasons, especially limited resources. For example, most academic medical organizations have a trifold mission that represents the organizations' core values: a commitment to patient care, education, and research. Over the past few years many academic medical organizations have faced declines in revenues (operating revenue, grants, and investments) and have had to encourage their doctors to generate additional revenue through expanded clinical service. If doctors spend more time seeing patients, they have less time for research and teaching activities, and so over time the teaching and research mission of an academic medical organization might be compromised.

This example demonstrates an important aspect of conflicts between values, even when there is no disagreement about the values themselves. In this example, the core values of commitment to patient care, to teaching, and to research are affirmed by all. The conflict arises because the activities to be undertaken to better achieve one value (patient care) will compromise achievement of another value (research). This distinction about where the conflict lies becomes important in negotiating conflicts.

Conflicts might occur between values unrelated to the mission of the organization. For example, a hospital may endorse the values of quality care and stewardship. But conflict can occur between physicians and administrators when physicians believe providing quality care requires the acquisition of new and expensive technology, while administrators believe that acquiring this technology is not essential for quality and therefore is not good stewardship.

Ideally, values reflected in an organization's mission statement, values statements, and statement on patient rights are all aligned. But they may conflict in certain instances. For instance, the mission statement of most hospitals

Case Study

A large academic medical organization includes innovative research as one of its missions. But grants from the National Institutes of Health (NIH) are slowing and expected to decline further as the budget of the NIH has been cut. Several of the hospital's most promising young researchers are nearing the expiration of their grants. Hospital leadership knows that some of these researchers have begun looking for other positions because these grants partially or fully support their salaries. Administrators are looking for ways to support these researchers. How do you generate resources for these researchers without compromising the hospital's other missions?

includes some reference to delivering quality care to the communities they serve. Many hospitals are also interested in growing their organizations. Some may want to increase market share to be better positioned when negotiating with payers. Some may want to be better able to compete with other hospitals. Some might think that growth allows them to more easily accomplish their mission. Whatever the reason, some hospitals, like Bon Secours RHS, endorse growth as a value. But growth might require diverting resources from the community already served by the hospital. So the risk may be that a hospital's mission is diluted as it seeks to grow.

Inevitably, conflicts among the values in an organization's mission, values, and patient rights statements have ethical ramifications because they represent the articulated ethical standards that guide the organization. A later section in this chapter explores one way of untangling these ramifications.

Organizational Culture

Elliott Jaques (1951) defined organizational culture as the "customary or traditional ways of thinking and doing things, which are shared to a greater or lesser extent by all members of the organization and which new members of the organization must learn and at least partially accept in order to be accepted into the service of the firm."

This definition captures two important dimensions of culture. First, it captures the idea that culture is something shared to a greater or lesser degree by members of an organization. Second, because culture informs organization members how they should think and do things, culture is a mechanism that at least partially controls how people in an organization interact with each other and with others outside the organization. As such, culture affects the behavior of those in the organization. If culture promotes a common vision, and influences behavior, it can help the organization become more efficient and effective by promoting and reinforcing the way in which the business of the organization is conducted.

Most organizations have understood for some time that having a cohesive and shared culture is in their best interests (Peters and Waterman 1982). Organizations that have been successful in developing an appropriate culture have been shown to be more successful in realizing their goals than those that have not (Black 2012; Collins and Porras 1994).

The documents and statements of Massachusetts General, Bon Secours RHS, and Tenet Health Systems are intended to notify the wider society of what it can expect from their organizations, and they inform organization members of how they should behave. Ideally these documents influence and reflect organizational culture.

Of course, culture may not align with an organization's mission, values, and patient rights statements. This misalignment is most likely to occur when an organization's professed mission is different from its real-life mission or when its professed values are different from its real-life values.

Ethical Climate

The term **ethical climate** is a little confusing because it sometimes refers to organizational culture (Malloy et al. 2009). Indeed, ethical climate is one important component of organizational culture, one that helps guide the organization when it is facing a moral dilemma. Victor and Cullen (1987) distinguish ethical climate from organizational culture by defining *climate* as the shared perceptions of how ethical issues should be addressed and what is ethically correct behavior for the organization. So ethical climate contains both content—the shared perceptions of what is ethical behavior—and processes—how ethical issues will be handled. The ethical climate of an organization can be measured on two axes: the existence of appropriate ethical values within the organization's culture and the extent to which these values are manifested in the day-to-day operations of the organization.

Obviously, both culture and ethical climate can be positive or negative. But if ethical climate is truly one component of culture, then having a positive culture without a positive ethical climate would

> **Ethical climate**
> Shared perceptions of how ethical issues should be addressed and what is ethically correct behavior for the organization.

Case Study

A hospital prides itself on its commitment to safety. A newly hired nurse is working in a clinic where the attending physician has a reputation for arrogance. She notices that two of the patients have the same last name and the same first initial. She is concerned that treatment orders have been mixed up, with one patient getting prescriptions intended for the other patient. But she is afraid to say anything to the physician. Later, it is discovered that the prescriptions were indeed switched.

Although neither patient suffered any adverse effects from the switch, the nurse is horrified. You are the administrator responsible for the clinic. The nurse approaches you and asks for a transfer to another clinic. You ask her why. When she tells you, what do you do?

Case Study

A well-respected cardiologist affiliated with a nationally known hospital in the Mid-Atlantic region has been questioned as to whether all of the large number of stents he has been implanting in his patients are medically necessary. Without admitting guilt, the hospital has agreed to repay the federal government $22 million to settle a whistleblower lawsuit over the questionable implants. Top-level administrators, including you, have been tasked with reviewing the case and making recommendations so that questionable or unsafe activities are addressed sooner rather than later. What are some of your recommendations?

be difficult. Spencer and colleagues (2000) describe a positive ethical climate as having at least two important characteristics:

First, it is an organizational culture where the mission and vision are consistent with its expectations for professional and managerial performance, and consistent with the goals of the organization as they are actually practiced. Second, a positive ethical climate is one that embodies a set of values that reflect societal norms for what organizations should value, how they should prioritize their mission, vision and goals, and how they, and their professionals and managers, should behave.

In most organizations, no simple ways of prioritizing missions and values exist. However, as Werhane (2000) points out, the fundamental purpose of healthcare organizations is to provide quality care. Therefore, ensuring that quality care is delivered should be the first priority of all healthcare organizations.

A Culture of Safety

Culture of safety
A component of the organizational culture that focuses on ensuring safety for patients and their families, staff, and practitioners. It includes a just culture that recognizes the inevitability of human error and yet holds individuals accountable for irresponsible actions. Required by The Joint Commission in healthcare organizations.

Because safety is a universally accepted value for the healthcare organization, a healthcare facility's organizational culture must encompass a **culture of safety**.

The safety of patients in hospitals became a major issue after the IOM's landmark publication, *To Err Is Human: Building a Safer Health System* (1999), which estimated that as many as 98,000 people die in hospitals each year as the result of preventable medical errors. In the IOM's follow-up publication, *Crossing the Quality Chasm: A New Healthcare System for the 21st Century* (2001), hospitals were urged to create a "culture of safety" that would translate into a safe environment for patients. Moreover, The Joint Commission leadership standards insist that hospital leaders create and maintain a culture of safety and quality throughout the hospital (Joint Commission 2011).

According to one widely accepted definition, a culture of safety is "the product of individual and group values, attitudes, perceptions, competencies and patterns of behavior that determine the commitment to, and the style and proficiency of, an organization's health and safety management" (Advisory Committee on the Safety of Nuclear Installations 1993).

Pointing to the characteristics of a safety culture is much more difficult for hospital leadership than is describing a safety culture.

In response to the need for hospital leadership to be able to describe the characteristics of a safety culture, Sammer and colleagues (2010) undertook a review of the literature in which they identified and critically examined studies that address the "important beliefs, attitudes, and behaviors that are integral to a culture of safety within hospitals." They found seven characteristics of a safety culture:

1. *Leadership*. Leaders acknowledge the healthcare environment is a high-risk environment and seek to align vision/mission, staff competency, and fiscal and human resources from the boardroom to the frontline.

2. *Teamwork*. A spirit of collegiality, collaboration, and cooperation exists among executives, staff, and independent practitioners. Relationships are open, safe, respectful, and flexible.

3. *Evidence-based*. Patient care practices are based on evidence. Standardization to reduce variation occurs at every opportunity. Processes are designed to achieve high reliability.

4. *Communication*. An environment exists where an individual staff member, no matter what his or her job description, has the right and the responsibility to speak up on behalf of a patient.

5. *Learning*. The hospital learns from its mistakes and seeks new opportunities for performance improvement. Learning is valued among all staff, including the medical staff.

6. *Just*. A culture that recognizes errors as system fail-

Case Study

You are a senior administrator. You have been told to build a culture of safety in the hospital. You have rewritten the mission and values statements to reflect a new commitment to safety, which the CEO and governing board have approved. You have told nursing supervisors to develop plans to ensure that the environment is safe. You are quite pleased with some of the results. For instance, one person is now delegated during shift changes to ensure that medical information is correctly communicated. Moreover, nursing supervisors have urged you to develop a process in which mistakes can be investigated. You have agreed to this.

One night a patient is given the wrong medication. What is your reaction?

ures rather than individual failures and, at the same time, does not shrink from holding individuals accountable for their actions.

7. *Patient-centered.* Patient care is centered around the patient and family. The patient is not only an active participant in his own care, but also acts as a liaison between the hospital and the community.

These characteristics of a culture of safety are similar to the characteristics of an organizational culture that has a positive ethical climate.

Barriers to Building Organizational Culture and Ethical Climate

In a complex organization, many barriers to building and maintaining an appropriate organizational culture and ethical climate exist. These barriers include:

1. Hospitals employ or are affiliated with a large number of various professionals, including administrators, physicians, nurses, physical therapists, social workers, chaplains, and others. Different professional groups often have their own subculture.

2. The external environment of the hospital is complex. Hospitals must respond to a number of legislative and regulatory bodies at the state and national level. Moreover, hospitals must work with various and diverse public and private payers who generally have their own requirements hospitals must meet to be reimbursed. Hospitals must consider the needs of their respective communities when they make decisions.

3. Hospitals often both serve and employ members of diverse cultural, religious, and ethnic populations. Behavior that is acceptable in one culture may not be acceptable in another culture.

4. Cost-containment pressures have stretched hospital resources. As hospitals try to do more with less, professionals, including administrators, might experience the phenomenon known as "moral distress." Moral distress has been defined as the anguish a person may experience when faced with a situation in which she knows the right thing to do but is prevented from doing it by institutional constraints (Jameton 1984). Moral distress can cause burnout, anger, confusion, and insecurity and can lead to feelings of hopelessness and worthlessness. (Moral distress will be more fully examined in Chapter 7.)

5. Stakeholders in a healthcare organization can be confused and uncertain if the organization's missions and values are not clear and prioritized.

6. In patient safety, hazardous situations and even adverse events are often not recognized by staff, practitioners, or patients. For that reason, Sammer and colleagues (2010) list acknowledging the high-risk nature of the healthcare environment as the first characteristic of a culture of safety. A culture of safety requires a constant attitude that "something could go wrong" and vigilance to spot unwanted variation. The same issues arise in the ethical realm. Often, the fact that an intended action may compromise an organization value is simply not recognized. This lack of sensitivity to or lack of recognition of an ethical conflict—or the denial of it—is the greatest risk to individual and organization ethical behavior. The ethical issue must be recognized to be resolved.

> **Case Study**
>
> A case manager works for a hospital that says it places the highest priority on patient care. She notes that the decisions of a particular insurance company appear arbitrary. While the insurance company has paid the bill of one patient, it has denied the stay of another who has a similar diagnosis. She is told by her supervisor that she must tell her patient that the hospital must discharge him. She is told to tell him that he is ready to go home.
>
> You are responsible for the clinic in which the case manager works. The case manager comes to you and asks for help. What is your reaction?

Complexity; subcultures; diverse religious, cultural, and ethnic populations; moral distress; conflict or confusion among missions and values and their priority; lack of sensitivity to, lack of recognition of, or denial of an ethical conflict—any of these issues might complicate the formation of a shared culture.

A Process for Resolving Ethical Conflict

The Joint Commission recognizes that ethical conflict can occur among staff or between patients and staff in hospitals and other healthcare organizations. Standard LD.04.02.03 for hospitals requires that "ethical principles guide the hospital's business practices" (Joint Commission 2011). The first performance element associated with this standard is that "the hospital has a process that allows staff, patients, and families to address ethical issues or issues prone to conflict" (Joint Commission 2011).

This requirement acknowledges that a potential ethical conflict may be recognized by any stakeholder in the organization's processes and that the individual concerns should seriously be considered rather than dismissed by others. Remember, a frequent cause of failure to manage an ethical conflict appropriately is to not recognize the potential conflict before acting.

The second performance element associated with this standard requires a hospital to use this process: "The hospital uses its process to address ethical issues or issues prone to conflict" (Joint Commission 2011).

The Joint Commission also recognizes that conflict can occur among leadership groups, particularly between physicians and administrators. Standard LD.02.04.01 requires that "the hospital manages conflict between leadership groups to protect the quality and safety of care" (Joint Commission 2011). One performance element associated with this standard is: "Senior managers and leaders of the organized medical staff work with the governing body to develop an ongoing process for managing conflict among leadership groups" (Joint Commission 2011).

The Joint Commission gives no hint of what the process that allows staff, patients, and families to address ethical issues or issues prone to conflict should look like, preferring to leave it up to the individual hospital. The Joint Commission provides only general guidance for processes meant to manage conflict among leadership groups.

The conflict management process includes the following (Joint Commission 2011):

- Meeting with the involved parties as early as possible to identify the conflict
- Gathering information regarding the conflict
- Working with the parties to manage and, when possible, resolve the conflict
- Protecting the safety and quality of care

Organization ethics processes
Processes designed to help leadership, staff, and professionals think through ethical uncertainty or conflicts that can occur when missions and values conflict. They are distinct from clinical ethics processes. Required by The Joint Commission.

Processes designed to manage the sorts of ethical conflicts that have been described in this chapter are often called **organization ethics processes** (Spencer et al. 2000). This terminology distinguishes them from processes designed to manage ethical conflicts at the bedside and those associated with clinical ethics. (See Chapter 6.)

Hospitals meeting these requirements have wide latitude in how they design and implement processes to manage ethical conflict. Once an ethical conflict or uncertainty has been identified—which is often the weakest link in the chain—a series of steps can be used to manage the conflict or uncertainty.

William Nelson (2005) developed a straightforward, eight-step process for ethical decision making:

1. Clarify the ethical conflict. Make sure it is clearly articulated.
2. Identify all of the affected stakeholders and their values.

3. Understand the circumstances surrounding the ethical conflict. Identify any relevant facts or relevant outcomes.

4. Identify the ethical perspectives relevant to the conflict. Ask what kind of conflict this is. Is this a conflict associated the various professions in the hospital? Is this a conflict between the missions or values of the hospital?

5. Identify different options for action.

6. Select among the options. Justify the choice within the context of the organization's mission and values.

> **Case Study**
>
> A nonprofit healthcare system in a southeastern state began more than 100 years ago as a 25-bed "retreat for the sick." The system's charitable mission is to provide innovative services to treat illness and to promote the improvement of personal health.
>
> The CEO has been successful in acquiring and consolidating market share in the area, which includes several affluent communities, towns, and one small city.
>
> The system now owns four of the five acute care hospitals in the area, 25 other sites of care, and many of the significant physician practices. The CEO has been advised by his executive team that the time is right to raise prices. The CEO knows that most of the payers in the area will go along with price hikes because they will not have a choice. The CEO also knows that many of the system's patients, particularly from the city, self-pay and certainly will not be able to absorb price hikes.
>
> You are a senior administrator. The CEO asks you for advice. What are some of the issues you tell the CEO he should consider before he makes his decision?

7. Share and implement the decision. Make sure stakeholders know how they will be affected.

8. Review the decision to ensure it achieved the desired goal.

Controversial Issues and the Healthcare Organization

The following two sections provide an overview of two issues that generate conflicts among values in healthcare organizations, particularly hospitals. Both of these issues challenge the hospital's mission of providing quality care. Both issues are complex and have no easy resolutions. Moreover, they will continue to be of concern into the foreseeable future.

Racial and Ethnic Disparities in the Provision of Care

The IOM (2003) detailed the stark facts of disparities in *Unequal Treatment: Confronting Racial and Ethnic Disparities in Health Care*. The report reviewed myriad studies and found that racial and ethnic minorities tend to receive lower-quality healthcare than do whites, even when insurance status, income, age, education, and severity of conditions are comparable. More recently, Mead and colleagues (2008) reviewed the disparities in health status and mortality, access to care, health insurance coverage, and quality of care. A few examples of these findings, from these and other sources, should suffice to illustrate the magnitude of the problem.

In regard to general health status, Mead and colleagues (2008) report that minorities (except Asians) generally rate their health as poorer than whites. For instance, African Americans are more likely to have a chronic illness or disability than whites, with almost half reporting such a condition (Mead et al. 2008). In regard to health status and mortality, if infant mortality is used as an indicator of the health and well-being of a population, African Americans are by far the worst off among all the races or ethnicities examined. The infant mortality rate for non-Hispanic African Americans in 2003 was almost two and a half times greater than that for whites (Harper et al. 2007). Another example is the prevalence of AIDS. The case rate for African American adults and adolescents is ten times greater than for white adults and adolescents. Yet African American HIV patients are less likely to receive antiretroviral therapy, even after controlling for access to care. The Agency for Healthcare Research and Quality (AHRQ) reports, in terms of quality, minorities suffer more of the consequences of unsafe care. For example, Asians and Hispanics are more likely to die from complications during hospitalization than non-Hispanic whites (AHRQ 2006). Given how diverse the United States is and considering it will grow more diverse over the next several decades, if these disparities are not addressed adequately, many more Americans will find themselves at risk for disease and poor quality of healthcare.

Addressing this issue is daunting. The various causes of healthcare disparities include location, environmental conditions, culture, income, education, lack of usual provider, lack of insurance, and provider stereotyping. Each of these barriers to quality care is complex. Intervention is difficult and can be expensive.

One goal of the Patient Protection and Affordable Care Act (ACA) is to eliminate most discrepancies related to access by expanding coverage (Kocher, Emanuel, and Deparle 2010). In addition, the ACA contains provisions that would fund community health centers and provisions whose goal is to increase the number of providers in underserved communities, particularly in the areas of general medicine, pediatrics, and geriatrics. Some disparities-specific provisions in the ACA would provide for data collection on race, ethnicity, geographical area, primary language, disability, and cultural competence of providers. (See Chapter 13.)

More specifically for hospitals, the American Hospital Association (AHA 2013) has issued a number of recommendations that parallel the recommendations issued by the IOM and the Commonwealth Fund. These recommendations center on the hospital knowing the community it serves, collecting valid data from patients, developing targeted interventions, providing culturally competent care, and communicating with staff, patients, and community leaders on the barriers to care. The AHA also encourages hospitals to tie the elimination of healthcare disparities to the hospital's mission (Umbdenstock and Lofton 2009). Because one part of a hospital's mission is to serve its community, and because the hospital's community undoubtedly includes racially and ethnically diverse members, some of the responsibility for reducing these discrepancies lies with the hospital; therefore, eliminating them should be part of a hospital's mission.

> ### Case Study
>
> A small hospital services a community with a large elderly patient population that is predominately on Medicare. The mission statement describes the hospital's "passion" for serving the community. But the geriatric clinic consistently loses money, and making up the shortfall is stressing the hospital and preventing it from offering other services. A large state-funded hospital three hours away offers geriatric services. The CEO is thinking of closing the clinic.
>
> You are part of the executive team. What is your reaction when the CEO tells you about his plan?

The Role of For-Profits in the Healthcare System

The debate concerning the role and influence of for-profit hospitals in the healthcare system has been vociferous and impassioned, with one side claiming for-profit hospitals are "evil," while the other side claims that profits have no influence on the provision of quality care. Among the issues are the ethical dilemmas that might arise from resource management, particularly cost-cutting:

- What role should stockholders or other investors play in leadership decisions concerning for-profits?
- Can nonprofits remain stable and still achieve their community service mission?
- Who pays for care for the poor and how?
- The question that lies at the root of the many controversies in healthcare—Is healthcare a business or is it something else?

These questions are good but not easy to answer. Some believe that the sheer size of hospital chains, whether for-profit or nonprofit, will prevent the delivery of locally focused care because control might move away from the community. For instance, Tenet's (2013) mission statement applies to every hospital that it owns. Tenet owns hospitals in 11 states and not every locality has the same needs—differing missions might be appropriate.

Others will argue that size promotes efficiency; therefore, large chains should be able to deliver lower-cost quality care. This argument may be one reason Bon Secours RHS (2013a), a nonprofit chain committed to the poor and dying, values "growth."

Stability has been considered a characteristic of nonprofits in that they are "owned" by the community. But stability is not a function of type of ownership. Both nonprofits and for-profits have seen their revenues fall over the past few years. Many nonprofits have been forced to sell themselves to for-profit chains (Gold 2010). A study exploring factors associated with bankrupt hospitals found that bankrupt hospitals are smaller than their competitors, less likely to be associated with a system, and more likely to be investor owned (Landry and Landry 2009). Regardless of ownership type, communities might look with gratitude on the for-profit or nonprofit that enabled the community to keep its hospital. Both for-profits and nonprofits can give back equally to the communities they serve. For instance, for-profits and nonprofits alike sponsor educational outreach activities. For-profits and nonprofits can both provide uncompensated care. And although for-profits are obliged to generate returns for investors, nonprofits are required to not default on their bonds. Both can be seen as similar pressures.

Moreover, the evidence on whether status or ownership causes variations in cost, quality, and access differs greatly across studies. And critics argue that the studies that have been done are flawed. For example, Schlesinger and Gray (2006) argue, "Much apparent inconsistency in the effects of ownership emerges when scholars carelessly combine findings based on different health services or performance measures. By contrast, meta-analyses that aggregate studies involving a single service and a single well-defined outcome find consistent ownership-related differences." Their study concludes that nonprofits provide higher-quality, less expensive care and more uncompensated care than do for-profits (Schlesinger and Gray 2006).

Case Study

Two for-profit healthcare systems compete in a small state. Both are large systems, and each owns a number of hospitals, outpatient care campuses, nursing homes, and local physician practices. Both are vying for the purchase of a small community hospital, which is strategically located and which has been financially weakened over the past few years. This small community hospital has been in existence for more than 100 years and is well regarded by the community it serves. However, it is seen as a "prize" because whichever system acquires it will be able to block the growth of the other. Because of this competition, each organization has offered more than the market price of the hospital.

You are the CEO of this small hospital. Both rivals have asked you to stay on and help with the consolidation process. Both have offered you a substantial package to help with the transition.

The board is considering accepting one of the offers. One board member asks you what the community hospital will look like if it is acquired by one of the two competitors. How do you respond?

Because the Schlesinger and Gray study had major policy implications, it evoked a firestorm. The Center for Regulatory Effectiveness examined the study to determine whether or not it met the requirements of the Data Quality Act (DQA) for use of its findings by federal agencies (Kelly 2008). The review found "substantial data quality deficiencies," with conclusions that relied on out-of-date and irrelevant studies, declaring the Schlesinger and Gray study does not "meet DQA standards and would have to be rejected for use by a federal agency" (Kelly 2008). The question of whether ownership type has implications for cost, quality, and access has not been definitively answered.

The distinction between for-profit and nonprofits, including mission-driven hospitals, is beginning to blur. For instance, Ascension Health, the nation's largest nonprofit, nonfederal health system by revenue, announced in February 2011 a partnership with a private equity firm, Oak Hill Capital Partners (Carlson 2011). Their intent was to form a new for-profit, Ascension Health Care Network, which would buy ailing Catholic hospitals. The new network's mission would remain the same as that of the nonprofit system, but dividends would be produced and distributed to Oak Hill's shareholders (Carlson 2011). As of early 2012, Ascension Health Care Network was in talks with a number of Catholic hospitals (Popovici 2012).

How hybrids such as Ascension Health Care Network, which has caused unease among those who believe that healthcare should not enrich shareholders, will fare is anyone's guess. However, given the severe shortage of capital accessible to many nonprofits, we will likely see the emergence of other hybrid business models in the future.

Regardless of whether a hospital has a for-profit,

Case Study

You are the CEO of a well-known children's hospital that competes for physicians and leadership with some of the foremost children's institutions in the country. Your hospital is a proven leader in the development and application of innovative technology in treating children's illnesses and injuries.

Your hospital endorses the values of stewardship, honesty, and integrity in all its relationships, among other values.

To date, you have been responsible for the compensation packages of your top performers. You send pay and performance metrics for leadership to the compensation committee for approval; those metrics are then sent to the board to ratify. You have tried to be fair and impartial in your recommendations, and you have tried to benchmark your recommendations with outside information.

Yesterday, a board member approached you about the possibility of making the compensation committee more independent. The committee would be charged with looking into various aspects of the hospital, including operations, IT, finance, patient services, and other areas, with the intent of setting goals for hospital leadership and ensuring they are real and measurable. Compensation would be tied to the achievement of these goals for middle management and above but not before the board is satisfied that goals have been met.

(continued)

(continued from previous page)

You have met with your senior leadership team. Many of them have strong feelings about the plan. Some oppose the idea because they are afraid of arbitrary goals being set—goals that are unrealistic and therefore unattainable—by people unfamiliar with the work of a specific area. Some are in favor of the plan because it would force the board to become more knowledgeable about the hospital and its business practices. Others believe that a number of mechanisms are in place already that are designed to familiarize the board with the problems and achievements of the hospital. You are still undecided about the plan as you leave the meeting.

That night, you continue to think about the plan and its implications. You ask yourself:

1. Is there an ethical conflict in the plan or a potential ethical conflict? What is it?
2. Which stakeholders would be affected by the plan? How would they be affected? What are their values?
3. What are the facts around the situation?
4. What are the various ethical perspectives?
5. What are your options?
6. How will you select the best option?
7. How will you keep the results of the decision under review?

nonprofit, or hybrid structure, the more relevant ethical questions for a hospital are:

- Does the hospital have an open and transparent relationship with the community it serves?
- Does the hospital have an appropriate mission for the community it serves?
- Does the mission align with community expectations?
- Does the hospital endorse appropriate values for the community it serves?
- Do these values align with community expectations?
- Does the hospital live up to its public pronouncements?
- Does the hospital have mechanisms to ensure that its culture and ethical climate support its mission and values?
- Does the hospital have appropriate mechanisms to address the ethical conflicts it will certainly encounter at both the micro and the macro level?

Conclusion

Most people in the United States believe that the delivery of healthcare has a moral core. The responsibility for framing this moral core and seeing that it is implemented in the day-to-day business of a hospital or any healthcare organization is the responsibility of all hospital stakeholders, particularly the administrators who serve in leadership positions.

The governing board of a hospital establishes the mission, values, and vision of a hospital. The board selects a chief executive officer (CEO), who then selects a leadership team, whose responsibilities include helping the CEO implement the mission, values, and vision developed by the governing board. And leadership has a moral component (Griffith and White 2010). Leadership is highly visible, sets standards for behavior, serves as examples, makes resource decisions, advises the board, and helps make the board's decisions regarding the future direction of a hospital—all of which influence and are influenced by the organizational culture and ethical climate of the hospital.

Points to Remember

- The mission or purpose of individual healthcare organizations will differ, but all healthcare organizations share the common mission of helping to alleviate pain and suffering and promoting health.
- The values of healthcare organizations describe how the healthcare organization will achieve its mission or purposes. The values statement can help guide decision makers and give stakeholders a basis on which to make judgments about the organization. The values statement also reflects society's expectations of the organization.
- Ethical tension can occur if a hospital's mission conflicts with its practices or if its values conflict with each other. Ethical tension can affect a healthcare organization's culture and ethical climate. Organizational ethical processes can be helpful in resolving ethical tension.
- A healthcare organization faces numerous barriers in developing an appropriate culture and ethical climate.
- Because safety is a universally accepted value for the healthcare organization, a healthcare facility's organizational culture must encompass a culture of safety. Characteristics closely associated with a safety culture include learning, communication, teamwork, leadership, and patient-centeredness, among others.
- Controversial issues—such as disparities of care—can generate conflicts among values in healthcare organizations, particularly hospitals. These issues challenge the hospital's mission of providing quality care.

References

Advisory Committee on the Safety of Nuclear Installations. 1993. *Organizing for Safety: Third Report of the ACSNI Study Group on Human Factors.* Health and Safety Commission of Great Britain. Sudbury, England: HSE Books.

Agency for Healthcare Research and Quality (AHRQ). 2006. *National Healthcare Disparities Report*. Rockville, MD: US Department of Health and Human Services.

American Hospital Association (AHA). 2013. "Eliminating Racial and Ethnic Disparities." Accessed March 10. www.aha.org/advocacy-issues/disparities /index.shtml.

———. 2009. "Underpayment by Medicare and Medicaid and Medicare Fact Sheet." Accessed March 9. www.aha.org/aha/content/2009/pdf /09medicunderpayment.pdf.

Black, A. 2012. "CEOs Link Workplace Culture to Business Success." *Minneapolis/St. Paul Business Journal*. Published October 12. www.bizjournals .com/twincities/news/2012/10/12/the-importance-of-corporate-culture .html?page=all.

Bon Secours Richmond Health Systems. 2013a. "'Good Help' to Those in Need." Accessed March 6. www.bonsecours.com/about-us-mission-and-outreach .html.

———. 2013b. "Heritage." Accessed March 6. www.bonsecours.com/about-us-about-bon-secours-values-and-heritage.html.

———. 2013c. "Your Rights and Responsibilities." Accessed March 7. http://richmond.bonsecours.com/patients-and-visitors-patient-rights-and-responsibilities.html.

Carlson, J. 2011. "All Eyes on Ascension: New For-Profit System Is Called Workable Model." *Modern Healthcare* 41 (9): 14.

Collins, J., and J. Porras. 1994. *Built to Last: Successful Habits of Visionary Companies*. New York: Harper Collins Publishers.

Freeman, R. E. 2010. *Strategic Management: A Stakeholder Approach*. New York: Cambridge University Press.

Griffith, J. R., and K. R. White. 2010. *The Well-Managed Healthcare Organization*, 7th ed. Chicago: Health Administration Press.

Gold, J. 2010. "Mergers of For-Profit, Non-Profit Hospitals: Who Does It Help?" Published July 13. *USA Today*. http://usatoday30.usatoday.com/money /industries/health/2010-07-13-hospitalmergers13_CV_N.htm.

Harper, S., J. Lynch, S. Burris, and G. D. Smith. 2007. "Trends in the Black–White Life Expectancy Gap in the United States, 1983–2003." *Journal of the American Medical Association* 297 (11): 1224–32.

Institute of Medicine (IOM). 2003. *Unequal Treatment: Confronting Racial and Ethnic Disparities in Health Care*. Washington, DC: National Academy of Sciences.

———. 2001. *Crossing the Quality Chasm: A New Health System for the 21st Century*. Washington, DC: National Academies Press.

———. 1999. *To Err Is Human: Building a Safer Health System*. Washington, DC: National Academies Press.

Jameton, A. 1984. *Nursing Practice: The Ethical Issues.* Englewood Cliffs, NJ: Prentice Hall.

Jaques, E. 1951. *The Changing Culture of a Factory: A Study of Authority and Participation in an Industrial Setting.* London: Tavistock Publications.

Joint Commission. 2011. *Hospital Accreditation Standards.* Oakbrook Terrace, IL: The Joint Commission.

Kelly, W. 2008. "Problems with Some Studies on the Benefits of Nonprofit Hospitals." *Health Affairs* Accessed March 29. http://content.healthaffairs.org/content/25/4/W287.abstract/reply#healthaff_el_3349.

Kocher, R., E. Emanuel, and N. M. Deparle. 2010. "The Affordable Care Act and the Future of Clinical Medicine: The Opportunities and Challenges." *Annals of Internal Medicine* 153 (8): 536–39.

Landry, A. Y., and R. J. Landry. 2009. "Factors Associated with Hospital Bankruptcies: A Political and Economic Framework." *Journal of Healthcare Management* 54 (4): 252–71.

Malloy, D. C., T. Hadjistavropoulos, E. F. McCarthy, R. J. Evans, D. H. Zakus, I. Park, L. Yongho, and J. Williams. 2009. "Culture and Organizational Climate: Nurses' Insights into Their Relationship with Physicians." *Nursing Ethics* 16 (6): 719–33.

Massachusetts General Hospital. 2013a. "Hospital Overview." Accessed March 6. www.massgeneral.org/about/overview.aspx.

———. 2013b. "Office of Patient Advocacy." Accessed March 7. www.massgeneral.org/advocacy/rights/default.aspx.

———. 2013c. "Quality and Safety." Accessed March 6. www.mgh.harvard.edu/about/qualityandsafety.aspx.

Mead, H., L. Cartwright-Smith, K. Jones, C. Ramos, K. Woods, and B. Siegel. 2008. "Racial and Ethnic Disparities in U.S. Health Care: A Chartbook." *The Commonwealth Fund.* Accessed March 9. www.commonwealthfund.org/Publications/Chartbooks/2008/Mar/Racial-and-Ethnic-Disparities-in-U-S--Health-Care--A-Chartbook.aspx.

Nelson, W. A. 2005. "An Organizational Ethics Decision Making Process." *Healthcare Executive* 20 (4): 9–14.

Ochsner Health System. 2013. "Your Rights as a Patient." Accessed March 7. www.ochsner.org/patients_visitors/patient_services_patient_rights_and_responsibilities.

Peters, T. J., and R. H. Waterman. 1982. *In Search of Excellence: Lessons from America's Best-Run Companies.* New York: Harper and Row Publishers.

Popovici, A. 2012. "A Catholic Foray into For-Profit Health." *National Catholic Reporter.* Published May 29. http://ncronline.org/news/people/catholic-foray-profit-health.

Schlesinger, M., and B. H. Gray. 2006. "How Nonprofits Matter in American Medicine, and What to Do About It." *Health Affairs* 25 (4): W287–W303.

Rosenberg, C. 1987. *The Care of Strangers*. New York: Basic Books Publishing.

Sammer, C. E., K. Lykens, K. P. Singh, D. Mains, and N. A. Lackan. 2010. "What Is Patient Safety Culture? A Review of the Literature." *Journal of Nursing Scholarship* 42 (2): 156–65.

Spencer E., A. Mills, M. Rorty, and P. Werhane. 2000. *Organization Ethics in Health Care*. New York: Oxford University Press.

Starr, P. 1982. *The Social Transformation of American Medicine*. New York: Basic Books Publishing.

Tenet Healthcare Corporation. 2013. "Mission and Values." Accessed March 6. www.tenethealth.com/about/pages/missionandvalues.aspx.

Umbdenstock, R., and K. E. Lofton. 2009. "Hospitals Must Take the Lead in Eliminating Disparities in Care." *AHA News* 45 (13): 1.

Victor, B., and J. B. Cullen. 1987. "A Theory and Measure of Ethical Climate in Organizations." In *Business Ethics: Research Issues and Empirical Studies*, edited by W. C. Frederick, 51–71. Greenwich, CT: JAI Press.

Werhane, P. H. 2000. "Business Ethics, Stakeholder Theory, and the Ethics of Healthcare Organizations." *Cambridge Quarterly of Healthcare Ethics* 9 (2): 169–81.

ETHICS AND GOVERNANCE

John F. Wallenhorst

This chapter is relevant to the following competencies identified in the ACHE Competencies Assessment Tool (see p. xxv):

Leadership
- Potential impact and consequences of decision making in situations both internal and external
- Adhere to legal and regulatory standards
- Establish a compelling organizational vision and goals

Business Skills and Knowledge
- Governance theory
- Governance structure

Learning Objectives

After completing this chapter, the reader will be able to

- discuss how the ethical governance of a healthcare organization is informed by the nature and purpose of healthcare,
- outline the leadership roles and ethical duties of healthcare board members,
- highlight some ethical responsibilities and challenges of healthcare managers in relationship to healthcare boards,
- outline the key characteristics of board membership,
- discuss some areas of ethical focus and challenge for healthcare boards, and
- outline key elements of board effectiveness and evaluation.

Introduction

Healthcare organizations have unique responsibilities to individuals and communities. With significant advances in medical technology, widespread availability of medical information, formation of large health systems, and social challenges in providing equitably available and responsibly financed health services, the role of healthcare boards is critically important. Most healthcare organizations are governed by boards of **directors** or **trustees**, although for many organizations (especially not-for-profit hospitals) the terms are interchangeable. These boards have wide-ranging responsibilities for ensuring that health systems, hospitals, skilled nursing facilities, and other related organizations are operating in a manner that is consistent with organizational mission and an array of ethical, legal, and regulatory obligations.

The principal objective of this chapter is to define the ethical responsibilities of healthcare boards and to suggest methods for evaluating board effectiveness in fulfilling those responsibilities. The chapter will also highlight some special ethical responsibilities and challenges of healthcare managers in relationship to boards. To accomplish these objectives, the chapter will address five areas: healthcare as a service, governance leadership and duties, board composition, areas of focus, and effectiveness and evaluation. While many laws and regulations relate to the governance of healthcare organizations, this chapter will focus on the more fundamental ethical obligations of boards. Except to the extent that it supports these obligations, legal and regulatory compliance will not be addressed.

Although healthcare organizations vary greatly in size, services, demographics, and foundations, this chapter focuses primarily on not-for-profit, community-based organizations. Most dimensions of ethical board leadership described here, however, will apply to any healthcare organization. Special ethical issues related to for-profit organizations and academic medical centers will not be covered in detail.

Healthcare as a Service

To outline the leadership role and ethical duties of healthcare boards, discussing the nature and purpose of healthcare itself is important. The medical profession is, at heart, committed to caring for persons. This foundational commitment has been played out for centuries in a variety of ways. Doctors, nurses, midwives, social workers, and other healthcare professionals have cared for persons in need of care in homes and offices, hospices and clinics. Over the past 100 years or so, hospitals and nursing homes have been widely established to address healthcare needs in particular communities. In contemporary healthcare, an increased, and sometimes renewed, focus on the importance of primary care, health promotion, preventative care, and treatment of chronic illnesses exists.

Although provided in a variety of ways and by a variety of healthcare professionals, the primary goal of medicine is to care for persons. Medicine, from this point of view, "is a not a trade to be learned, but a profession to be entered" (ACP 2012). This classical understanding of the medical profession clearly applies to physicians; this view is advanced and protected by the structures of medical education, professional association, and law. Without compromising this special dimension of medical professionalism, the complex nature of healthcare delivery today means that the duty of service and a commitment to care for persons are applicable to all in the healthcare field, including doctors and nurses, managers and board members.

This goal of caring for persons is not simply a practical aim. It is a commitment at the heart of the healthcare professions, and it is the guide by which we may assess the ethical compass of healthcare professionals and organizations (Hall 2004).

Based on this age-old commitment, healthcare is first and foremost a necessary human service (Taylor 2002). Healthcare leaders, then, have an ethical obligation to carry out their responsibilities in a way that is consistent with this central mission. This obligation is in contrast to organizations that simply sell products.

Most product-focused organizations legitimately focus their work on producing and marketing items for sale. Often these are items that, while desirable, are not absolutely necessary for human life and health. In our day, healthcare organizations have acquired some of the characteristics of conventional businesses—even product-focused businesses. However, because of its essential nature, healthcare is a special type of business. Such service is not optional—people need healthcare services to maintain health, fight disease, and live satisfying, productive, and happy human lives.

A healthcare organization's ethical foundation is rooted in the commitment to provide care, and its ethical practice is evaluated by how well its actions align with that core commitment.

But if healthcare is focused on persons, persons are always members of larger communities. Most hospitals were established precisely to address the health needs of specific communities. In city neighborhoods, in remote rural settings, in expanding suburbs, and often in collaboration with physicians, universities, and faith communities, hospitals came to life to advance community health and welfare.

Therefore, the ethical commitments of healthcare organizations clearly extend to the communities in which they are a part. And in our increasingly interconnected national and world community, these responsibilities extend well beyond the local community served.

Community benefit
A wide array of activities non-profit hospitals are required to provide and account for—and for-profit hospitals may provide—to benefit their community, such as delivering free and discounted services to persons in need, conducting community needs assessments, collaborating with other organizations to improve community health and well-being, providing health promotion programs and information, and engaging in community building activities.

Healthcare then is both a necessary, person-centered service and a social and community good (Galarneau 2002). The ethical responsibilities of healthcare organizations extend beyond the bedside to the home, community center, school, and legislative chamber. **Community benefit** is one important dimension of this commitment (Bilton 2005). Providing resources aimed at improving the health of the community and addressing some of the social, environmental, and cultural determinants of health is an important responsibility. Local and national advocacy is another dimension of this social obligation. Advocating for and practically supporting an equitable, accessible, and effective healthcare system is a contribution to community good.

Finally, healthcare organizations are also communities of practice. They bring together physicians, nurses, social workers, pharmacists, support persons, administrators, and a variety of business professionals. Health services are now usually provided through a highly complex community of care. Healthcare ethics consequently has a bearing on the healthcare organization as a community of care and employer. These organizations have a responsibility to cultivate a work environment in which person-centered quality care is delivered, in which community members are both stakeholders and beneficiaries, and in which the community of work is just, respectful, and mission-driven.

The ethical compass of a healthcare organization, and of its leaders and governing board, should be focused on its responsibilities as a provider of care, a community member and citizen, and an employer (ACHE 2011; Weber 2001).

Healthcare ethics is rooted in the assumptions that (1) healthcare is a necessary human service and a social good, and (2) healthcare organizations and healthcare leaders and boards have an obligation to understand and act in accordance with their special responsibilities as caregivers, community members, and employers. Healthcare boards have a unique role in addressing these commitments. During a time of great change and evolution in the provision of healthcare services, clearly defining the role of boards is both a practical good and an ethical priority.

Governance Leadership and Duties

Historically hospitals have been managed by a team of healthcare professionals and governed by a volunteer board of community members (Jennings et al. 2002). Traditionally these board members were called trustees. Trustees were "entrusted" with the responsibility of ensuring that hospitals stayed true to their purpose. Boards of trustees focused on the quality of healthcare services, on alignment of services with community needs, and on strategic direction and financial performance. The trustees were the responsible stewards of an important community resource.

Stewardship here was understood broadly. The goods and services of the hospital were held in trust for the community. Hospital managers were asked to oversee day-to-day operations. Trustees were asked to ensure hospital goods and resources were used to provide care and to support community health and well-being.

As healthcare delivery became more complex, and hospitals increased in number and size, large integrated health systems were created. And with the advent of large health systems, the role of trustees changed and expanded. The rise of integrated health systems brought many benefits and some ethical dilemmas. Increasingly these systems—and their hospitals, skilled nursing facilities, and other institutions—were led by persons from a wide array of business backgrounds. The discipline of forming complex systems, which requires strategic thinking, strong financial management, and legal and regulatory skills, often called for new forms of management. Healthcare leadership was increasingly influenced by the culture, methods, and polices of for-profit and non-healthcare organizations.

As these large systems formed, the role of governing boards evolved. Board members were frequently responsible not only for thinking about the quality of care and community benefit but also about strategic alignment and advantage, local and regional competition, and allocation of limited financial resources. During this time, some of "boards of trustees" became known as "boards of directors." While in some ways this change was just in terminology, in other ways it suggested an important and noteworthy change in emphasis. Trustees are entrusted with protecting and advancing a specific community resource. Directors, on the other hand, are responsible for the ultimate oversight and direction of often large and complex organizations and systems of care (Jennings et al. 2002). The term *director* is in many respects apt. It represents an expanded role for board members. But it is also a term borrowed from for-profit and publicly traded businesses.

The formation of large health systems required some of the disciplines and strengths of the for-profit world. But the benefits also came with some ethical burdens. Health systems began to think and operate in a more strategic manner and with greater operational discipline. At the same time, some of these systems began to lose sight of their community roots and charitable mission.

However, healthcare boards today, whether they are hospital- or system-focused, and whether they use the term *trustee* or *director*, continue to have important ethical responsibilities and duties. The following section examines three leadership roles and two legal and ethical duties of healthcare directors.

Stewardship
An understanding that all of the resources of the organization, including financial resources and real property, are held in trust by the organization for the good of others.

Leadership Roles

Healthcare boards today operate in a challenging environment. While retaining many of the classic dimensions of trusteeship, one framework for understanding the contemporary ethical obligations of boards suggests that healthcare directors exercise three forms of leadership: fiduciary, strategic, and generative (Chait, Ryan, and Taylor 2005).

As fiduciary leaders, board members oversee the use of the organization's assets. This role involves the stewardship of goods that are designated for a particular purpose. As strategic leaders, board members contribute to, refine, and approve organizational direction, ensuring that the healthcare organization is pursuing a plan that is clear, actionable, and consistent with its mission. As generative leaders, board members contribute to organizational learning by reflecting on past successes and failures, envisioning future possibilities, and creatively engaging managers in the process of creating a values-based future.

This dynamic way of viewing healthcare boards suggests that directors have an obligation not simply to conserve the past and past promises, but to guide the organization toward the future while maintaining a commitment to mission and core values. Organizational integrity here is animated by the past but always reaching toward the future. Directors, as leaders, help to create, support, and advance that compelling vision.

Healthcare managers have an important ethical responsibility to support the board's leadership by providing accurate, timely information; encouraging candid and creative discussions; and acknowledging the important distinction between management's responsibility for day-to-day operations and the board's fiduciary responsibilities.

The interplay of board and management is often one of ethical complexity. For boards to exercise their role fully, management must support legitimate direction from the governing body and must be careful not to stifle board input and engagement. Likewise, the board must respect the role of managers in managing operations and collaborate with managers in setting direction and supporting a vibrant and ethical corporate culture. In short, management has an ethical responsibility to manage, and the board has ethical responsibility to govern.

Duties

The specific duties of directors are typically spelled out in the organization's bylaws. Bylaws are legal documents and clearly express precise legal obligations, but they also suggest obligations of a fundamentally ethical nature. Law and ethics here are not at odds. Rather they express in different ways, and with different and complementary implications, the significant obligations of healthcare directors.

The first legal and ethical duty is the **duty of loyalty**. The duty of loyalty requires that directors exercise their responsibilities in the best interest of the organization and in accordance with its mission and not in their own interest or the interest of other persons or entities. In a not-for-profit system, this obligation entails protecting and advancing the organization's charitable mission and purpose (Independent Sector 2007; Jennings et al. 2002). And because of the nature of healthcare as an essential service, the duty of loyalty also suggests that directors in for-profit healthcare organizations must promote care for persons and communities as a primary ethical responsibility.

The duty of loyalty also includes an obligation to maintain in confidence organizational information that is not already known. Failure to act in the best interest of the organization and to maintain confidence may be considered, in extreme cases, an abuse of power.

As part of this duty, directors are required to disclose actual or potential conflicts of interest or activities or associations that may give the appearance of a conflict. Directors with a clear material conflict of interest are required by law to recuse themselves from discussions or decision making related to the conflict (Independent Sector 2007). Healthcare organizations should have formal policies and procedures for handling the disclosure of conflicts and a method for ensuring that the process is effective (Jennings et al. 2002).

The second legal and ethical duty is the **duty of care**. The duty of care requires that directors exercise independent judgment in the exercise of their responsibilities on behalf of the organization and that they be reasonably well informed. The duty of care suggests that directors take the time needed to study, understand, and discuss matters that are brought to their attention. Directors are required to act in good faith and to exercise sound and informed judgment in making organizational decisions. Failure to act in this matter may in some cases be considered negligence.

Although both the duty of loyalty and the duty of care have important legal dimensions, they also reflect the profound ethical responsibilities of healthcare boards. To protect and extend a healthcare organization's charitable mission in a selfless manner (loyalty) and to participate in informed and thoughtful decision making (care) are clearly characteristics of ethical directors. While these principles are supported by law, they also reflect a higher moral commitment.

Once again, healthcare managers have an important ethical obligation to support the board by respecting the independent judgment of directors and creating an environment in which decision making is carried out through challenging discussion and careful deliberation. Management has an obligation to contribute to this process by providing sound information and analysis and, in many cases, by suggesting a recommended course of action. In doing this, however, management must not co-opt the board's legitimate

Duty of loyalty
Requirement that directors exercise their responsibilities in the best interest of the organization, not in their own interest or the interest of other persons or entities.

Duty of care
Requirement that directors use independent judgment in the exercise of their responsibilities on behalf of the organization and that they be reasonably well informed.

duties. Finally, management has an ethical obligation to follow the board's direction and faithfully implement its policies.

Personal Example

In carrying out their responsibilities, healthcare directors also lead by personal example. Moral leadership in an organization is a function of many factors. But one of the key markers of an ethically sound organization is the tone set by executive leaders and board members. The American College of Healthcare Executives (ACHE) Code of Ethics affirms that healthcare executives contribute significantly to the moral life of an organization. Although they need to demonstrate ethical leadership in the exercise of their responsibilities, they also "should lead lives that embody an exemplary system of values and ethics" (ACHE 2011).

Moral climate
Shared perceptions of how ethical issues should be addressed and what is ethically correct behavior for the organization.

By personal and professional example, directors also contribute to the **moral climate** of an organization. They help that organization to act "habitually in a manner consistent with moral integrity" (Taylor 2002) and to communicate expectations regarding high ethical standards. Effective health system boards motivate executives and managers to define ethical competencies and to resolve difficult ethical cases thoughtfully (Hanson 2008).

Although fulfilling the duties of loyalty and care is critically important, a healthcare director will also be an individual who personally models ethical behavior (Smallman, McDonald, and Mueller 2010). Modeling ethical behavior includes at least two dimensions: maintaining a reflective stance and demonstrating relational skills that are not only respectful, but also are rooted in the belief that the moral life takes place in community. By personal example, directors have an opportunity to demonstrate how to deal with moral ambiguity reflectively, responsibly, and calmly in an increasingly complex and pluralistic world (Goldstein 2000). Directors also have the opportunity to demonstrate what some have a called a "covenantal ethic" (see page 69) in which self-interest is subordinated to service and "business" is a matter of pursuing multiple "bottom lines," not just financial success or personal gain (Dallas 2004; Nash 1993).

Board Makeup

The historical role of board members as trustees, as overseers and caretakers, of an important community asset has in some cases become overshadowed by other pressing board responsibilities. Boards need to guide strategic direction, monitor safety and quality, oversee physician relationships, approve budgets, and ensure financial stability and a mission-focused use of assets. As multifaceted health systems have become more complex, so have the responsibilities of healthcare boards.

Because of this complexity, board membership is critically important. Effective, ethically sound governance depends, at least in part, on the commitments, expertise, and abilities of directors. Recruiting, selecting, educating, and retaining good board members is one of the ethical responsibilities of a healthcare organization.

At least five considerations should be taken into account in the formation of sound governance structures and the selection of board members:

1. Personal commitment
2. Mission commitment
3. Expertise and ability
4. Diversity and inclusion
5. Independence

Case Study

You have recently been appointed to the board of a local hospital system. The system has a 150-bed hospital, a small skilled nursing facility, and a home care agency. You bring much-needed expertise to the board in the areas of human resources, compensation, and benefits. You have been in the community for five years and are delighted with the opportunity to provide this service.

Unfortunately your work and personal schedules have recently become complicated. You have been promoted in your own organization and are now required to travel at least three times each month. In addition, you are the only child of an aging and increasingly frail mother who lives in a neighboring state. It takes you approximately four hours to reach her by car.

Since your appointment to the board nine months ago, you have missed one board meeting, participated in one meeting by phone, and attended two board meetings in person. You have found it difficult to make time to prepare thoroughly for the meetings. However, you have made a number of helpful suggestions related to compensation strategy, and you successfully assisted in the search process for a new vice president of human resources. You are concerned that you may not be living up to your responsibilities as a good board member.

- From your perspective, what key ethical issues are at stake here?
- What alternatives are open to you?
- How might you be able to assess your performance in an objective and thoughtful way?
- What do you think you would ultimately do?

Personal Commitment

Board members must demonstrate personal commitment. This requirement is both ethical and practical. Prospective directors need to express—credibly—their desire to be on the board. As with many human undertakings, motivations here may be complex. However, part of this personal commitment should include a desire to help the community and advance the work of the organization. The recruitment of new directors should include a process for assessing a candidate's personal commitment to the work of a healthcare board. This assessment should take into account commitments to both the tasks of board membership and to stewardship of a significant community asset.

Mission Commitment

Because the nature and purpose of healthcare is to provide a necessary human service, and not to create and market a commercial product, healthcare directors need to demonstrate commitment to the organization's mission. Because of the significant ethical importance of this commitment, the assessment should not be taken for granted. Because "healthcare is a uniquely personal and value-laden service" (Hall 2004), a healthcare organization and its leaders and directors must demonstrate an abiding, personal commitment to the mission of caring. Board candidates should be able to articulate a vision of healthcare as service and the alignment of that vision with the mission of the organization as it is lived out on a daily basis. Board members must be able to translate the "philosophy" of mission into practical terms. Care for sick and vulnerable persons, commitment to the community, and fairness for employees, when expressed through decisions and actions, are examples of this sort of translation.

Expertise and Ability

An organization has an ethical obligation to ensure that its board has appropriate expertise in most of the major disciplines that are needed to lead an effective health system, such as planning, quality of care, community benefit, marketing, human resources, healthcare financing, investment, and philanthropy. While technical expertise and skill are important, personal experience is also significant (Independent Sector 2007). Directors need to have technical skills and the ability, through practical experience, to apply those skills in supporting the organization.

Healthcare boards should also likely include appropriate representation from the medical and healthcare provider community. Physicians and nurses in particular bring unique forms of education, preparation, and clinical experience that might add an important perspective to board deliberations. Because of complex legal requirements and important considerations related to conflicts of interest and independence, a healthcare board should carefully balance the potential benefits and concerns related to inviting the organization's physicians to serve on the board.

Because of their unique professional responsibilities and code of ethics, physicians and nurses on boards must be careful to exercise their board duties with a clear understanding that they are not representatives of a stakeholder group but trustees of an important community asset. Managers have an obligation to support and respect the judgment of the entire board and not to focus primarily on the perspectives of clinically trained directors.

In addition to bringing important technical skills and experience, directors also need sufficient time to prepare for board meetings, attend and participate in meetings, and share in the evaluation of board and organizational effectiveness. Having personal commitment and professional expertise is not sufficient. Board members also need to have the time to be engaged in the work of the board and in the life of the organization.

Diversity and Inclusion

Effective boards need directors with diverse professional skills and backgrounds and with diverse personal backgrounds. Gender, racial, ethnic, and age diversity are dimensions that should be taken into account in establishing sound governance structures. Credible efforts should be made to build healthcare boards that include persons of diverse backgrounds.

Historically, hospital boards were made up either exclusively or primarily of community members. Although this practice continues to have some merit, as health systems become larger and may include multiple communities, it has also become more difficult. Nonetheless, community demographics and the persons served by a health system should be taken into account in creating diverse boards.

A board that has a mix of women and men from different racial, ethnic, and cultural backgrounds may have an enhanced ability to deal more responsibly, justly, and sensitively with matters related to quality of care, community involvement, and employee relations and voice. In addition, a board that reflects diverse points of view and perspectives may set the stage for richer discussions, creative thinking and problem solving, and practically supporting an organizational culture of inclusion (Boyle et al. 2001).

Independence

Taking the duty of loyalty into account, healthcare boards should be composed primarily of independent directors. Because the mission and interests of the organization need to be placed above personal interests, at least two-thirds of the board members should have no financial or professional ties to the organization (Independent Sector 2007). For healthcare boards to have some members who have financial or professional ties to the organization is not uncommon. To ensure a good mix of skills and community representation, these relationships may make good sense. But appropriate limits should be set on the number of such directors to ensure that decision making is objective and free from potential personal influences.

All board members have an ethical obligation to exercise their responsibilities in a way that they, thoughtfully and independently, believe advances the mission of the organization. Board members are not representatives of constituent groups, and they do not exercise their duties on behalf of others (Jennings et al. 2002). A board requires the personal good judgment of its members. Directors, it is true, should reasonably consider the legitimate rights and claims of key stakeholders—patients, community members, physicians, and employees. But in making decisions, directors are called upon to exercise independent judgment for the good of the organization's mission.

Areas of Focus

While the responsibilities of a healthcare board, and the rights that are reserved to it, are outlined in organizational bylaws, certain responsibilities should be areas of key attention and focus. Although not intended to be an exhaustive list, among these areas of focus are: organizational strategy, patient care, community benefit, workplace justice, financial stewardship, and ethical culture.

In each area, the mission of the organization should be employed as the primary ethical guide for taking action and assessing effectiveness. "The mission of the organization governed by a trustee is central to the ethics of the trustee role because it is the cornerstone of all of the trustee's other responsibilities. The board exists to direct the organization, but the organization exists to pursue and fulfill a mission, a moral and social objective. Without the mission, there would be no trustee role in the first place" (Jennings et al. 2002).

And because of the unique challenges of healthcare delivery today, boards must approach these areas of mission focus from the perspective of transformational leadership (Joshi and Horak 2009). Maintaining the status quo is not likely to support a vibrant, contemporary expression of mission.

Case Study

A major tobacco company has proposed that its new CEO be nominated to the board of directors of a three-hospital regional health system. The CEO lives and works in the community.

In addition to suggesting participation on the board, the tobacco firm has indicated a willingness to sponsor or cosponsor a variety of health promotion activities in the community, with special outreach to children and persons who are economically disadvantaged.

The health system's senior management team is divided about whether to proceed with the nomination. Some believe that because the CEO brings needed expertise in the areas of finance and investment, he is a good candidate for the board. Others believe that, despite these qualifications, such a nomination might be viewed as supporting the tobacco company's product and interests. Some on the management team are concerned about the company's motives in making the proposal. Still others are attracted by the possibility of advancing health promotion activities.

You are on the senior management team and are responsible for bringing this nomination to the board for consideration.

- From your perspective, what key ethical issues are at stake here?
- What values and principles will guide your approach?
- Are any of these values and principles in tension or conflict with one another?
- What course of action would you recommend?

Organizational Strategy

Historically, hospital boards were established to ensure that important community resources were run responsibly and used solely for the good of the persons and communities served. In today's more complex healthcare environment, this commitment to mission and purpose remains, but it requires greater attention to alternative forms of care delivery and partnership, relationships with neighboring healthcare organizations, variations in healthcare financing, and emerging community needs.

Today, healthcare boards are typically involved in advancing organization mission through the strategic planning process. The governing role here is not simply to endorse a strategy that is proposed by management but to participate in a complex and interdisciplinary process of setting strategy (Chait, Ryan, and Taylor 2005). It appears that most health system boards spend approximately a quarter of their time contributing to and monitoring organizational strategy (Prybil 2008). This work of the board is not tangential to its ethical obligations—it is central to them.

The obligation of boards to be integrally involved in the strategic planning process is rooted in the responsibility to advance and protect organizational mission. A board must assist management in responding to the new world of healthcare delivery and financing. Health systems and providers are being asked to deliver care in ways that have not been the norm over the past 50 years. Good primary care, preventative care, proactive treatment of chronic illness, care in outpatient settings, and care at home are all dimensions of this new world. In addition, systems and providers are being reimbursed in ways that may not support older, acute care–focused models.

Because of these changes, strategic plans need to be creative in seeking new, cost-effective ways of delivering care and health services. New partnerships, physician alignments, primary care strategies, and risk-sharing models are all part of the mix. Boards need to contribute to these new ways of thinking and operating. Directors must be both creative partners and mission stewards. Boards should keep organizations from creating a strategic plan, or pursuing strategic opportunities, that might have some financial benefit but that would ultimately compromise care for persons and communities.

Finally, an important subset of strategy relates to marketing and advertising. Healthcare boards have a responsibility to ensure that marketing and advertising activities are truthful, focused, and not aimed at increasing inappropriate utilization of services (Weber 2001). And because of a core commitment to care, marketing and advertising should not mislead patients and families regarding potential clinical outcomes.

Boards should question the uncritical use of awards, quality data, and other forms of self-promotion in advertising. This does not mean that healthcare organizations should not engage in marketing efforts. Marketing, however, should be demonstrably and credibly aligned with organizational mission, with the commitment to build human relationships, and with persons and communities. Marketing in healthcare should always reflect the core goals of healthcare and be held by board, management, and the community to high standards of honesty and integrity.

Patient Care

Healthcare boards are entrusted with ensuring the delivery of high-quality care. In fact, directors have a responsibility to oversee every dimension of care delivery, including protection of patients' rights, promoting a culture of safety, monitoring key quality measures, ensuring sound structures for clinical research, and approving all forms of physician relationships (Jennings et al. 2002; Joshi and Horak 2009).

Because this work is so vast and so important, board committees typically oversee various dimensions. The quality committee of the board reviews quality measures and safety and patient satisfaction data. The committee also works with management to advance the adoption of best practices and systems of control and continuous improvement. Other responsibilities of this committee include ensuring that services are provided in a way that reflects patient wishes and choice in a manner that genuinely improves health and reducing the risk of adverse outcomes. The review of measures related to infection control; standards of care for heart attack, heart failure, surgical care, and pneumonia;

hospital readmissions; and preventable deaths should be a routine part of this committee's agenda.

The audit and compliance committee (or a subcommittee, sometimes referred to as the intermediate sanctions committee) reviews and approves all physician employment relationships and other related financial transactions. This body is responsible for carefully reviewing recommendations from management. Special attention is given to the professional suitability of physicians who may be employed and to the financial and quality terms of a proposed agreement. This obligation is based on clear legal and regulatory requirements. However, it is also rooted in the board's broader ethical duty to ensure that healthcare resources are used wisely, fairly, and in the service of persons and communities.

Although these committees oversee detailed work related to quality of care and physician relationships, they must report to the full board about their activities. And on matters of greatest significance they must obtain input and approval from the full board. Annual quality and safety plans, for example, need to be reviewed at the full board level.

Finally, the board also has the important responsibility for monitoring the credentialing of physicians, and for granting physicians the privileges to admit and care for patients. The credentialing and privileging process is complex and governed by a variety of laws and regulations (Greene 2008). Credentialing entails gathering all relevant information about the physician, including education and licensure, and a careful review by the executive committee of the medical staff, a nonboard body composed of the hospital's physicians. The board works with management and the medical staff executive committee to ensure that the credentialing process is well run and thorough.

Based on recommendations from this committee, and the full board's own careful review, the board then has responsibility for granting or declining to grant privileges. This process applies to all physicians newly seeking a relationship with a hospital organization. In addition, on a periodic basis, physicians who have already been granted privileges must go through a similar process and apply for renewal.

Community Benefit

By tradition, law, and organizational mission, not-for-profit hospitals must provide and account for community benefit services (CHA 2008; Jennings et al. 2002). Because healthcare is rooted in a fundamental commitment to addressing the needs of persons and communities, the board has an ethical obligation to ensure the organization has a robust community benefit process. Community benefit includes a wide array of activities, including providing free and discounted services to persons in need, conducting community needs assessments, collaborating with other organizations to improve community health and well-being, providing health promotion programs and information, and engaging in community building activities (Bilton 2005).

The board's role in this process is important. A healthcare board has two obligations here: to provide input into the collaborative creation of a community benefit plan and to monitor progress and outcomes. The board demonstrates the duty of care by ensuring that a community benefit plan is created in a thoughtful and timely manner. The *process* itself is an important dimension of the board's ethical responsibility (Magill and Prybil 2011, 2004).

Such a plan should be created in a manner that ensures collaboration with members of the community. The plan should not be an imposition, however well intentioned, of the organization's own ideas. Secondly, the plan should be well integrated into the structures and processes of the organization as a whole. Community benefit should not be an "add-on."

In addition to the creation of a plan, the board also has a responsibility to monitor implementation and results. This monitoring activity will include a review, prior to submission, of the annual report to communities and the Internal Revenue Service Tax Form 990, Schedule H. Form 990 demonstrates the ways in which charitable organizations operate and the manner in which they contribute to the communities they serve (Dean, Robertson, and Trocchio 2007; Independent Sector 2007). Because of concerns regarding the legitimacy of not-for-profit status for many healthcare organizations, this requirement is both a legal necessity and a way in which health systems and their boards critically examine their own charitable performance and commitment (Magill and Prybil 2011).

Notwithstanding important legal and communication requirements, community benefit is, at heart, not a plan, program, or process. Rather, it fulfills a promise. For organizations dedicated to caring for persons and communities, and, in the case of not-for-profit systems, having a charitable mission and purpose, community benefit is a core commitment. As trustees of an important community resource, board members need to oversee this commitment.

Workplace Justice

A healthcare organization has ethical obligations as a provider, employer, and citizen (Weber 2001). Therefore, the board has a fiduciary responsibility to guide and oversee all dimensions of workplace justice and human resources. This requires review of the organization's policies and performance with regard to employee relations and satisfaction, labor relations, compensation and benefits, training and development, and evaluation methods. Evaluating the CEO's performance is a subset of this responsibility and also an ethical responsibility of the board.

Although all aspects of workplace justice are important, this chapter focuses on three: employee relations, compensation, and CEO evaluation. Employee relations involve creating an environment in which employees may responsibly exercise their duties and reasonably contribute to decisions related to their areas of expertise and their work conditions. Many laws relate to this obligation. But in addition to legal compliance, the board is ethically bound to promote a workplace that supports organizational mission and the care ethos of all healthcare services (ACHE 2011).

The board should periodically review data related to employee satisfaction, turnover and retention rates, exit interviews, and employee complaints. This information will guide the board in assessing the success of the organization in creating an environment of respect, accountability, and mission focus. From time to time board members may reasonably expect to have contact with frontline management and staff, such as through presentations or recognition opportunities during board meetings and occasional rounding through hospitals and other facilities.

An important dimension of employee relations and workplace justice is honoring employee voices (Jennings et al. 2002). The board should encourage management to adopt practices that allow employees to express their perspectives about care delivery, community needs, and day-to-day operations. This can be accomplished in part through annual employee surveys, routine department meetings, town hall forums, and open-door access to human resources staff and senior managers.

The board should also require just compensation practices. Business practices related to accepted compensation benchmarks are part of the justice analysis. But the board might also reasonably require adoption of a broad, justice-focused organizational policy on compensation. Such a policy might include requirements that go beyond conventional market analysis and competitiveness, include clear provisions related to the compensation of lower-paid employees, and establish an organizational just minimum wage (Magill 2001; Weber 2001).

Because of the significant and growing disparity of compensation and benefits between the lowest- and highest-paid employees in a healthcare organization, executive compensation should be carefully reviewed by the board. Without compromising the recruitment of committed and effective leaders, principles for executive compensation that are consistent with compensation for all other employees should be adopted (Weber 2001).

Professional preparation and expertise, related experience, demonstrated results from work in other organizations, and mission fit should all be considered. Market benchmarks should also be reviewed and taken into account. Those benchmarks, however, should not be the exclusive or even the key driver for executive compensation. And while the board may employ the assistance of outside compensation consultants, directors bear full ethical responsibility for the compensation of executive leaders. With increased public and political scrutiny of the tax-exempt privileges of many healthcare organizations, executive compensation is an area for critical ethical review and practical concern.

Finally, the board has an important fiduciary responsibility to evaluate the organization's CEO on an annual basis. This performance review is similar to that expected for any employee. However, because of the CEO's role in advancing organizational mission, ensuring the provision of quality care and community services, and enriching organizational culture, this responsibility is ethically complex and sensitive.

The selection, supervision, and compensation of the CEO typically fall to the board (Independent Sector 2007). The board should have a formal process for collecting and sharing feedback on all key dimensions of the CEO's performance. Often this process involves a written survey that is completed by directors individually and then, on the basis of combined data, discussed in an executive session that includes only board members without the CEO present. Once the board members have discussed their perspectives, the board chair invites the CEO in for a formal review. This activity should not be pro forma. By exercising the duty of loyalty and their own independence, directors should thoughtfully evaluate how the CEO has advanced organizational mission in all of its critical components.

Financial Stewardship

The board also has a responsibility to ensure that the organization has sound financial practices and controls and that it expends resources in ways that are consistent with its charitable mission and purpose. Often this responsibility is referred to as exercising financial stewardship. The important notion of stewardship is based on an understanding that all of the organization's resources, including financial resources and real property, are held in trust by the organization for the good of others. *Stewardship* here does not simply mean employing sound financial practices. It means responsibly caring for goods that are not one's own (Magill and Prybil 2004).

The board's ethical duty here is to ensure that the organization has up-to-date policies and procedures for managing and accounting for financial resources, for record keeping, and for independent auditing (Independent Sector 2007). The board should have mechanisms for monitoring these activities and providing feedback to management.

In addition, the board should be involved in the development of an organization's annual budget. This task should include an opportunity to review budget assumptions with management and provide feedback on the allocation of resources, including capital expenditures. Part of the board's responsibility here is to ensure that the budget is aligned with the mission of delivering needed healthcare services, advancing community health, and cultivating an engaged workforce. Expenditures that do not have a bearing on these obligations should be questioned. The board should also review financial performance on a regular basis and should oversee activities aimed at aligning actual revenues and expenditures with those that have been budgeted.

Finally, healthcare boards should be involved in policy setting and oversight of the organization's investment practices and fundraising activities. Even not-for-profit organizations expect to generate sufficient revenue to reinvest in programs, services, and infrastructure and to invest in new mission-aligned activities. Therefore, healthcare organizations will need to establish a policy and strategy for investing surplus funds. The board should approve and oversee all matters related to investment. Because of their core commitments, healthcare organizations should consider adopting socially responsible investment practices that advance community and global health (UNEP 2006).

The manner in which the organization undertakes fundraising should also be based on board guidance and approval (Independent Sector 2007). Responsible fundraising must be aligned with the charitable mission of the organization, and funds raised should be designated for uses that advance the care of persons and community health and well-being. Requests or requirements by donors for the allocation of funds may be honored if consistent with these aims and if approved by the appropriate organizational authority. The board has an ethical obligation to ensure that the acceptance and use of donated funds is legal and consistent with the organization's mission, desired culture, and reputation. Board members themselves should be expected to support the organization's philanthropic activities.

Ethical Culture

The final area of focus is on advancing an ethical organizational culture. While an ethical culture can be more difficult to define than the other areas, it is critically important to the vitality and sustainability of an organization. The board has at least three roles: promoting a **covenantal workplace**, providing leadership by example, and establishing related accountability and reward structures. (An organization cannot have an ethical culture without an ethical climate. But the two are intertwined—each promoting and enhancing or weakening the other. Chapter 2 differentiates between ethical climate and culture and provides a description of each. This section focuses on the types of relationships, values, and mechanisms necessary to promote an ethical climate and hence an ethical culture.)

The board has an obligation to ensure that the healthcare workplace promotes respect for all persons, fairness, openness, and inclusivity. This obligation is rooted in the nature of healthcare itself. Some refer to this sort

Covenantal workplace
A working environment in which relationships are based on mutual trust, engagement, and care; contrasted with a *transactional* workplace, in which employee skills are applied in order to advance organizational objectives and obtain a return benefit.

of workplace as covenantal (Dallas 2004; Nash 1993). Covenantal workplace relationships are based on mutual trust, engagement, and care, in contrast to *transactional* work relationships, in which employee skills are applied in order to advance organizational objectives and obtain a return benefit.

Advancing a covenantal approach is one way that the board can support an ethical organizational culture. "Research shows that employees' perceptions of covenantal relationships are associated with benevolent (caring) and principled climates, not self-interested climates" (Dallas 2004). Human resources and care delivery policies and practices that encourage openness and dialogue, and that reasonably include employees in organizational decision making, are ways for creating such an environment.

The board also leads by example. The tone of board meetings, including the manner in which questions are asked and recommendations are given, is important. Board members themselves demonstrate a covenantal approach when they view themselves as part of a larger community of care. This does not mean that board members refrain from asking difficult questions or shy away from difficult decisions. On the contrary, it suggests that they embrace such challenges in a collaborative and person-centered way.

Finally, the board supports an ethical culture by setting clear and specific expectations. Maintaining a vibrant culture requires articulating values and standards (Hall 2004; Spencer et al. 2000). Being clear about how organizational identity, commitments, and services relate to expected behaviors is part of the board's ethical requirement. This responsibility is not a static one. The board should periodically review and, if possible, assess the organization's alignment of practice with mission.

Management has a special obligation to provide the board with information related to organizational culture, engage the board in reflection and candid conversations supporting best ethical practices, and respectfully implement board policies aimed at cultural enhancement.

In addition to setting expectations, the board should see that accountability and reward structures are aligned with the creation of an ethical culture. Ethical behavior should be rewarded, and unethical or ethically questionable behavior should be handled directly and corrected (Dallas 2004). The board can assist here in defining ethical and unethical behaviors and the manner of assessing them.

Examples of ethical behaviors include promoting use of an ethical decision-making process, establishing respectful relationships, and handling problems, such as declining revenues, operational inefficiencies, and employee complaints, in a proactive, thoughtful, and nonpunitive way. To support such a culture, compensation and bonus structures should be aligned to specific behaviors and not just to financial or quality outcomes (Dallas 2004; Spencer et al. 2000).

Board Effectiveness and Evaluation

Because its ethical responsibilities are significant, a healthcare board should adopt practices that advance its effectiveness. It should also periodically evaluate its operational and ethical performance. Among the practices that the board should consider are preparing new members, establishing committee structures, having processes for making decisions, modeling transparency, and creating a process and timeline for board self-evaluation (Independent Sector 2007).

Preparation of New Members

New board members should participate in an orientation process that engages them in an understanding of the organization's history, mission, values, culture, healthcare services, and the nature, assets, and needs of the communities served. The orientation should also include details about management structure, medical staff, finance, and human resources. An overview of current market conditions is also appropriate. For this preparation to be most effective, new members should have ample opportunity for questions and dialogue and access to a variety of organizational leaders and employees. An opportunity to visit the organization's facilities and to round with employees would enrich the experience.

An important dimension of orientation is a review of the responsibilities of board members, including the duties of loyalty and care, board structures, and cultural and operational expectations. Special attention should be given to the duty of board members to exercise their responsibilities in an independent manner.

Committee Structures

Healthcare boards typically have supporting board committees. These committees assist the full board in overseeing its many tasks and ethical responsibilities. Committees are generally composed of members from the main board but may, as permitted by state law, also include outside members who bring important technical expertise. Governance structures often include a quality committee, audit and compliance committee, and governance committee. Larger regional or national systems may also have special committees for finance, human resources, compensation, and investments.

All committees are charged with reviewing, in detail, matters related to their charter and areas of responsibility. They report back to the full board on their activities, and, as appropriate, make recommendations to the full board for action.

Decision-Making Processes

An effective board will also take the time to engage in deliberative decision-making processes. Having sufficient information, time, and opportunity to discuss matters of importance are hallmarks of good governance. Employing a genuinely deliberative process for ethical decision making is the critical link between the foundation ethical question—Who are we?—and the practical ethical question—What do we do? (Magill and Prybil 2011). Process here mediates the ethical dimensions of identity and action. Effective boards will take the time to review information, ask questions, engage in dialogue, and make decisions.

An important process element of good governance also includes holding executive sessions. An executive session is time set aside during meetings for the board to meet without any members of management or staff, or to meet with only select persons, such as the CEO, compliance officer, or internal or external auditors. Executive sessions allow board members an opportunity to explore issues of great importance or sensitivity more deeply. On a more mundane level, executive sessions also provide board members with an opportunity to build community and share perspectives in a more private setting.

Transparency

In carrying out its ethical responsibilities, and in advancing a vibrant organizational culture, boards must be attentive not only to what they do but also to how they act. Acting with openness and transparency is characteristic of ethically sound organizations.

Clearly the written record of board meetings supports transparency. But this standard is just a threshold. The board will also need to regularly hear from members of the management team and engage them in conversation regarding important matters. This dialogue promotes a creative and open exchange of ideas regarding quality of care, strategic direction, and finances.

Having access to important information is critical for ethical decision making (Joshi and Horak 2009). Management supports transparency by providing accurate information to the board. And providing critical information and direction is necessary for effective operations. The board supports transparency by ensuring that information and direction is shared with the staff and community.

Transparency in governance provides a model to the entire organization for transparency in quality of care, patient relations, finance, and human resources. Transparency is an ethical value because it promotes truth-telling and trust and because it calls persons and organizations to accountability.

Board Evaluation

Effective boards will also typically engage in self-evaluation on a periodic and scheduled basis (Independent Sector 2007). This process provides feedback to the board chair and members regarding strengths and opportunities for improvement. The evaluation will typically focus on the effectiveness of board structures, meeting agenda and materials, and use of time. The evaluation should also solicit input on the effectiveness of board discussions, time to deliberate important matters, and areas for ongoing board education and development.

By employing a spirit of continuous improvement, the board may refine its structures and processes on the basis of self-evaluation. To be most effective, this evaluation should include both a written survey and ample time for discussion about results. The aim of evaluative reflection is to assist healthcare boards in carrying out their important ethical responsibilities.

Management has an important role in providing administrative support for effective board practices. Preparing board materials, scheduling and organizing board and committee meetings, supporting ongoing board education, and assisting with the recruitment of new board members are among management's tasks. In providing these important services, managers serve as staff support. They should be careful to exercise their role responsibly and in a way that does not overshadow, dominate, or unduly sway the board.

Case Study

You are the CEO of a large urban medical center. Your not-for-profit organization has a long and respected history of high-quality care and community presence and involvement.

A union organizing campaign is being conducted in your center. Most other healthcare organizations in your area have at least some union employees. Your hospital does not. The board just approved a sizeable capital investment plan for building a state-of-the-art heart center. This project is a complex strategic priority. It will require a significant amount of management time and oversight; it will take approximately two years to complete.

You have discussed the organizing campaign with your management team and new vice president of human resources. You have also had one-on-one conversations with your board chair and the chair of the board's quality committee. Both of them have strong roots in the community and have served the medical center for many years. They are recommending a cautious approach to this campaign.

Your vice president of human resources, who has little experience with unions, and one of your board members, who has expertise in finance, are advocating for the swift deployment of consultants and labor lawyers in order to address potential unionization.

- From your perspective, what key ethical issues are at stake here?
- What values and principles will guide your approach?
- Are any of these values and principles in tension or conflict with one another?
- What impact does the heart center plan have on your decision making?
- What course of action will you pursue?

Conclusion

Healthcare is rooted in a basic commitment to care for persons in need. This commitment comes to life in the context of community. Although healthcare today is a complex business, it is also the expression of a fundamental human capacity. Those who provide healthcare services are responding to a basic human need. Precisely because of this, the ethical obligations of healthcare organizations and healthcare boards are significant and profoundly human.

The governance of healthcare organizations is entrusted to boards of directors. Because of the nature of healthcare, and because of a commitment to care for and steward an important community resource, boards are responsible for ensuring that healthcare organizations authentically carry out their mission. This task is not easy. The ethics of governance require attention to multiple bottom lines and to the movement from organizational identity to values-based action.

Sharing in the human desire to care for persons in need, board members fulfill their ethical responsibility by bringing themselves—as persons, community members, technical experts, and professionals—fully to the task. With core ethical commitments, and with thoughtfully employed structures and processes, boards oversee healthcare organizations in carrying for persons, in advancing community health and well-being, and in being just and collaborative employers.

Points to Remember

- Boards have wide-ranging responsibilities for ensuring that healthcare organizations are operating in a manner that is consistent with organizational mission and ethical, legal, and regulatory obligations. Although some boards call their members "directors" and others "trustees," the underlying ethical responsibility is the same.
- Healthcare board members practice three kinds of leadership: fiduciary (the stewardship of resources that are designated for a particular purpose), strategic (contributing to and refining organizational direction), and generative (reflecting on performance, envisioning future possibilities, and engaging management in the process of creating a future based on a commitment to mission and core values).
- Managers have an ethical responsibility to support board leadership by providing accurate, timely information; encouraging candid and creative discussions; and acknowledging the distinction between management's responsibility for operations and the board's fiduciary

responsibilities. The interplay of the board and management is often ethically complex. Management must support the independent judgment of, and direction from, the board, and not stifle board input and engagement.

- The duty of loyalty requires board members to exercise their responsibilities in the best interest of the organization, maintain confidentiality, and disclose actual or potential conflicts of interest. The duty of care requires the exercise of independent well-informed judgment.

- Organizations should consider the following five elements in the formation of sound governance structures and the selection of board members: personal commitment, mission commitment, expertise and ability, diversity, and independence.

- Effective boards include members from diverse backgrounds to enhance rich discussions, creative thinking, problem solving, and an organizational culture of inclusion.

- The board has an ethical responsibility to participate in the development of a community benefit plan and monitoring the plan's progress and outcomes.

- The board supports an ethical culture by ensuring that the organization promotes respect for all persons, fairness, openness, and inclusivity. Management's obligation is to provide information related to organizational culture, engage the board in reflection and candid conversations supporting the best ethical practices, and respectfully implement board policies aimed at cultural enhancement.

- The board should periodically evaluate its operational and ethical performance, including consideration of not only what they do but also how they act. Openness and transparency are characteristics of sound organizations. Management has an ethical responsibility to provide accurate information about quality of care, patient relations, finance, and human resources.

References

American College of Healthcare Executives (ACHE). 2011. *Code of Ethics.* Chicago: American College of Healthcare Executives.

American College of Physicians (ACP). 2012. *Ethics Manual.* 6th ed. Philadelphia, PA: American College of Physicians.

Bilton, M. 2005. "Seeing Community Benefit Broadly: Everybody Wins When Hospitals Collaborate with Others to Serve Their Communities." *Health Progress* 85 (4): 39–43.

Boyle, P. J., E. R. DuBose, S. J. Ellingson, D. E. Guinn, and D. B. McCurdy. 2001. *Organizational Ethics in Health Care*. San Francisco: Jossey-Bass.

Catholic Health Association (CHA). 2008. *A Guide for Planning and Reporting Community Benefit*. St. Louis, MO: Catholic Health Association.

Chait, R. P., W. P. Ryan, and B. E. Taylor. 2005. *Governance as Leadership: Reframing the Work of Nonprofit Boards*. Hoboken, NJ: John Wiley & Sons, Inc.

Dallas, L. L. 2004. "Corporate Ethics in the Health Care Marketplace." *Seattle Journal for Social Justice* 3 (1): 213–27.

Dean, N., N. C. Robertson, and J. Trocchio. 2007. "What Counts? An Ongoing Question." *Health Progress* 88 (2): 4–5.

Galarneau, C. A. 2002. "Health Care as a Community Good: Many Dimensions, Many Communities, Many Views of Justice." *The Hastings Center Report* 32 (5): 33–40.

Goldstein, J. D. 2000. "Moral Compromise and Personal Integrity." *Business Ethics Quarterly* 10 (4): 805–19.

Greene, J. 2008. "It's a Privilege: The Board's Role in Physician Credentialing and Privileging." *Trustee* 63 (3): 8–11.

Hall, M. A. 2004. "A Corporate Ethic of 'Care' in Health Care." *Seattle Journal for Social Justice* 3 (1): 417–28.

Hanson, K. O. 2008. "Ethics and the Middle Manager: Creating 'Tone in the Middle.'" *Markkula Center for Applied Ethics*. Accessed February 8, 2013. www.scu.edu/ethics/practicing/focusareas/business/middle-managers.html.

Independent Sector. 2007. *Principles for Good Governance and Ethical Practice*. Washington, DC: Independent Sector.

Jennings, B., B. H. Gray, V. A. Sharpe, L. Weiss, and A. R. Fleischman. 2002. "Ethics and Trusteeship for Health Care." *Hastings Center Report* Special Supplement 32 (4): 2–27.

Joshi, M. S., and B. J. Horak. 2009. *Healthcare Transformation: A Guide for the Hospital Board Member*. Boca Raton, FL: CRC Press.

Magill, G. 2001. "Organizational Ethics in Catholic Health Care: Honoring Stewardship and the Work Environment." *Christian Bioethics* 7 (1): 69–93.

Magill, G., and L. D. Prybil. 2011. "Board Oversight of Community Benefit: An Ethical Imperative." *Kennedy Institute of Ethics Journal* 21 (1): 25–50.

———. 2004. "Stewardship and Integrity in Health Care: A Role for Organizational Ethics." *Journal of Business Ethics* 50 (3): 225–38.

Nash, L. L. 1993. *Good Intentions Aside*. Boston: Harvard Business School Press.

Prybil, L. D. 2008. "What's Your Board's Culture?" *Trustee* 61 (6): 16–18.

Smallman, C., G. McDonald, and J. Mueller. 2010. "Governing the Corporation: Structure, Process and Behavior." *Journal of Management and Organization* 16 (2): 194–98.

Spencer, E., A. Mills, M. Rorty, and P. Werhane. 2000. *Organization Ethics in Health Care.* New York: Oxford University Press.

Taylor, C. 2002. "The Buck Stops Here." *Health Progress* 82 (5): 37–40.

United Nations Environment Programme Finance Initiative (UNEP). 2006. *Principles for Responsible Investment.* New York: United Nations.

Weber, L. J. 2001. *Business Ethics in Healthcare.* Bloomington, IN: Indiana University Press.

4

THE HEALTHCARE ORGANIZATION, BUSINESS ETHICS, AND STAKEHOLDER THEORY

Patricia H. Werhane

This chapter is relevant to the following competencies identified in the ACHE Competencies Assessment Tool (see p. xxv):

Communication and Relationship Management
- Identify stakeholder needs/expectations

Leadership
- Potential impacts and consequences of decision making in situations both internal and external
- Adhere to legal and regulatory standards
- Assess the organization, including corporate values and culture, business processes, and impact of systems on operations
- Hold self and others accountable for organizational goal attainment

Professionalism
- Organizational business and personal ethics
- Professional roles, responsibility, and accountability
- Uphold and act upon ethical and professional standards
- Adhere to ethical business principles

Knowledge of the Healthcare Environment
- Corporate compliance laws and regulations

(continued)

(continued from previous page)

Business Skills and Knowledge
- Potential impacts and consequences of financial decision making on operations, healthcare, human resources, and quality of care
- Principles and practices of management and organizational behavior
- Build trust and cooperation between/among stakeholders
- Marketing principles and tools

Learning Objectives

After reading this chapter, the reader should be able to understand

- why business ethics is important to a healthcare administrator,
- how stakeholder theory is applicable to an administrator's evaluation of ethical issues in her organization, and
- how to prioritize stakeholders in a healthcare organization.

Introduction

This book is about ethical issues for healthcare administrators, so at first glance the reader may wonder why it has a chapter on *business* ethics. Business ethics often focuses on for-profit organizations, and many healthcare organizations (HCOs) are charitable, public, or nonprofit organizations. Yet this topic's importance in healthcare is obvious. Administrators work in HCOs. The first priority for an HCO is the effective delivery of healthcare and the well-being of patients and patient populations the organization serves. HCOs cannot function without competent healthcare professionals. Otherwise the organization is not a *health*care organization. HCOs must run efficiently and effectively in healthcare delivery and must be fiscally viable. So whether they are for-profit, not-for-profit, or publicly funded organizations, they must be solvent, at least in the long term. No HCO can survive for long if it consistently loses money. Running the organization efficiently without unethical activities in its administration, its human resource management, patient admissions, billing, discharges, and finances is critical, as critical as in for-profit companies. So business ethics becomes an important component of the ethics of HCOs and healthcare administrators.

Applied business ethics, as an area of **applied ethics**, is the study of ethics and economics, the analysis of individual and organizational decision making, and the examination of codes, rules, and principles that govern business conduct. Business ethics also seeks to understand, describe, and evaluate business practices, institutions, and managerial actions in light of some concept of human good or human rights.

Business is usually identified with certain utilitarian ends, such as profitability, economic sustainability, productivity, innovation, growth, or economic well-being, and ordinarily these goals also increase human satisfaction. A business that was unprofitable, engaged in risky choices that undermined its survivability, did not grow, or lost jobs for its employees is judged as poorly managed and as detrimental to human good. Similarly, while profitability is not or should not be a primary goal of HCOs, an HCO has similar goals: to be effective in healthcare delivery and efficient in managing and delivering healthcare. A poorly managed HCO that does not treat its patients, professionals, and employees with dignity and is fiscally unsound will not survive either.

In addition to utility, we appeal to other values in evaluating business decision making, actions, and outcomes: those of commonly accepted morality. An organization—including an HCO—that consistently mistreats or does not respect its employees, engages in unfair business practices, cheats its suppliers or customers, wantonly pollutes, or misrepresents its assets and liabilities is judged to be a bad company. Administrators that perpetuate these practices, even if they are within the letter of current law, are judged to be morally bad managers. On the other hand, organizations that do more than what is minimally required by law or morality, companies that promote human rights, institute equal opportunity in the workplace, develop environmentally sustainable and safe products and processes, promote competition, and advertise honestly, are judged to be excellent organizations by business ethics standards.

Business ethics is also **descriptive**. It analyzes the moral development of managers and how they behave. It describes and compares organizations, organizational cultures, the integration of ethics into administrative decision making, the role of codes and other authorities, and the effect of corporate sentencing guidelines and other government regulations on organizational activities. Descriptive business ethics also investigates causal relationships between individual moral beliefs or organizational mission statements.

As **normative applied business ethics**, business ethics evaluates business practice and decision making in light of standards and codes, it develops rules and codes appropriate to the context of management and administration, and it offers a framework of moral reasoning to think through recommendations and solutions to ethical dilemmas in business. Business ethics

Applied business ethics
The study of an organization's behavior through the lens of ethical or moral principles and values.

Applied ethics
The philosophical evaluation of controversial moral issues or practices.

Descriptive business ethics
Analyzes the moral development of managers; describes and compares organizations, organizational cultures, the integration of ethics into administrative decision making, the role of codes and other authorities, and the effect of government regulations on organizational activities. Investigates causal relationships between individual moral beliefs and organizational mission statements.

Normative applied business ethics Evaluates business practices and decision making in light of standards and codes, develops rules and codes appropriate to the context of management and administration, and offers a framework of moral reasoning to evaluate and solve ethical dilemmas. Seeks to develop and use sets of normative rules of conducts, codes, standards, or principles that govern what one ought to do when well-being, rights, or integrity are at stake.

seeks to develop and use sets of normative rules of conduct, codes, standards, or principles that govern what one ought to do in contexts where well-being, rights, or integrity are at stake.

This chapter focuses primarily on normative business ethics. Descriptive studies do play an important role in describing relationships among administrators, professionals, organizations, governments, cultures, and even the environment, however, as well as in describing how these relationships affect individual and organizational choices and actions. Cleanly separating normative and descriptive content is usually difficult because descriptive studies provide the information necessary for proper normative judgments.

Non-healthcare for-profit corporations and HCOs have many parallels. HCOs, whether they are nonprofit or for-profit concerns, increasingly operate in a competitive business environment and are subject to demands for economic sustainability (if not profitability), productivity, efficiency, innovation, customer satisfaction, growth, and economic stability, the same demands that drive businesses. HCOs are ordinarily more complex than many businesses, however, in that the economic criteria that determine the success of many businesses—while also necessary for HCOs to meet—are never sufficient tests for the excellence of an HCO. Other criteria, both internal and external to the HCO itself, are equally or more relevant. A profitable, productive, growing HCO may still fail, morally, if the professionals it employs do not meet high standards of competence, if its actual level of healthcare service does not match the expectations created by its projected standards, if it does not serve the community population adequately, or if it redefines its obligations without community consensus.

Although HCOs are not identical to other non-health-related businesses, the work done in business ethics on the nature of the corporation, on analyzing the nature of systems, on various kinds of evaluation, and on management practices constitutes a trove of knowledge that can be mined for the tasks of healthcare ethics. Business ethics provides us with various models for understanding decision processes in business. This chapter focuses on stakeholder theory as a useful model for understanding the HCO.

Stakeholder Theory

Sometimes neglected when considering the description of a manager's fiduciary responsibility to shareholders is an organization's obligations to other stakeholders, in particular, in business, to employees, managers, customers or clients, and the community. One could not run a business without employees, could not stay in business for long without customers, nor exist at all unless the community accepted commercial activity. These stakeholders are important, not merely because one could not exist or achieve profits without them, but also because they are individuals or groups of individuals— human beings with rights and interests.

An approach to business ethics that takes into account the rights and interests of the broad range of individuals and organizations that interact with and are affected by business decision making is **stakeholder theory**. Stakeholder theory is a promising model for healthcare ethics because it acknowledges a plurality of values and moral agency on different levels. By calling attention to the variety of roles that can be occupied by individuals, all of whom have a moral stake in the organization, stakeholder theory can help provide a framework for understanding and explicating the possibility of conflicts of value, loyalty, commitment, and interests. The complexity of an organization, and the difficulty as well as the importance of establishing an excellent organizational culture and ethical climate within an organization, can be understood on the basis of this theory.

Widely defined, stakeholders are "groups or individuals who benefit from or are harmed by, and whose rights are violated or respected by, corporate actions" (Freeman 1999). In a modern business corporation the primary or most important stakeholders commonly include employees, management, owners and shareholders, customers, suppliers, and the community. Focusing more narrowly, a stakeholder is any individual or group whose role relationship with an organization

> **Case Study**
>
> In an effort to balance its budget, the local community hospital has decided to charge uninsured patients more than insured patients. The local newspaper has criticized the hospital for this new policy, which it claims discriminates against poor people in the community. This hospital is located in a rural community and is the only healthcare facility within 150 miles. The administrator has been asked to draft a series of talking points to the CEO so that the CEO can explain her decision to the community. As the administrator, what reasons would you give for justifying this decision?

Stakeholder theory
The theory that the goal of any organization and its management is, or should be, the flourishing of the organization and all of the individuals or groups that affect or are affected by the organization.

1. "is vital to the survival and success [or well-being] of the corporation" (Freeman 1999, 250); or
2. helps to define the organization, its mission, purpose, or goals; or
3. is most affected by the organization and its activities.

In the first instance, stakeholder theory appears to be primarily descriptive; stakeholder relationships outline organizational role relationships within and outside the firm. Under the narrowly defined version, stakeholders appear to be those who are instrumental, one way or another, to the firm and its well-being (Donaldson and Preston 1995). Prioritizing stakeholders helps to sort out and clarify organizational priorities so that not every person, group, or other organization affecting or affected by the organization in question is equally important as a stakeholder. Otherwise the theory is vacuous. To prioritize stakeholder claims one examines an organization's purpose and mission, ranking stakeholders in terms of who has legitimate or appropriate claims, and who is essential to that mission and to the survival and flourishing of the organization.

The instrumentality of the prioritization, however, deals only with part of what is important in stakeholder relationships. It does not take away from the intrinsic value of each stakeholder's interests, according to proponents of stakeholder theory, and the intent of stakeholder theory is largely normative. "The descriptive accuracy of the theory presumes the truth of the core normative conception, insofar as it presumes that managers and others act [*or should act*] as if all stakeholders' interests have intrinsic value. In turn, recognition of these ultimate moral values and obligations gives stakeholder management its fundamental normative base" (Donaldson and Preston 1995).

Some time ago, Nobel Prize–winning economist Milton Friedman (1970) declared: "There is one and only one social responsibility of business—to use its resources and engage in activities designed to increase its profits so long as it stays within the rules of the game, which is to say, engages in open and free competition without deception or fraud."

This often misquoted statement does not advocate that "anything goes" in commerce. Law and common morality should guide our actions in the marketplace just as they guide our actions elsewhere. Nevertheless, given that important qualification, Friedman places primary importance on profit maximization as the role of business. Challenging the position that a manager's primary responsibility is to maximize profits or that the primary purpose of a firm is to maximize the welfare of its shareholders, stakeholder theory argues that the goal of any firm and its management, is, *or should be,* the flourishing of the firm and *all* its primary stakeholders. "The very purpose of a firm [and thus its managers] is to serve as a vehicle for coordinating stakeholder interests. It is through the firm [and its managers] that each stakeholder group makes itself better off through voluntary exchange. The corporation serves at the pleasure of its stakeholders, and none may be used as a means to the ends of another without full rights of participation of that decision. . . . Management bears a fiduciary relationship to its stakeholders and to the corporation as an abstract entity" (Evans and Freeman 1988).

Let us assume for our purposes that all stakeholders in question are individuals or groups made up of individuals. If stakeholder interests have intrinsic value, then, according to **R. Edward Freeman** (1999), the father of stakeholder theory, in every stakeholder relationship, the "stakes [that is, what is expected and due to each party] of each are reciprocal [although not identical], since each can affect the other in terms of harms and benefits as

R. Edward Freeman
Philosopher and professor of business administration who first conceptualized the firm as a vehicle whose purpose is to coordinate stakeholder interests.

well as rights and duties." Therefore stakeholder accountability relationships are reciprocal relationships.

Obligations between stakeholders and stakeholder accountability notions are derived on two grounds. First and obviously, stakeholder relationships are relationships between persons or groups of persons. So one is reciprocally morally accountable to various stakeholders just because they are people—for example, to treat individuals with respect, play fairly, avoid gratuitous harm, and so on. What is distinctive about stakeholder relationships, however, is that these relationships entail additional obligations because of the unique and specific organizationally defined and role-defined relationships between the firm and its stakeholders. For example, an organization has obligations to its employees because they are human beings *and* because they are employees of the organization. Conversely, because of their organizationally defined roles, employees have role obligations to the organization that employs them and its other stakeholders *as well as* ordinary moral obligations to that organization and its other stakeholders.

In HCOs these obligations become more complex. For example, an HCO has obligations to its employee-professionals

1. because they are moral agents,
2. because they are employees, and
3. because they are professionals and hired *as professionals.*

Conversely, healthcare professionals have role obligations to the HCO that employs them and role obligations to patients, to their profession, and to its associations. They may also have role obligations to the communities they serve and to healthcare payers, *and* they have ordinary moral obligations to all of these populations as well.

How does one evaluate various stakeholder claims with each other and with the profitability criterion Friedman and other economists advocate? Even not-for-profit HCOs must survive, and in the increasingly competitive healthcare climate, economic survival even for the most successful HCOs has become a critical issue. How, then, does one measure the importance of economic sustainability in HCOs against other claims—in particular, those defined by the mission to patient and population health?

In evaluating stakeholder claims, Evans and Freeman (1988) initially took a Kantian approach, arguing that because stakeholder relationships are relationships between individuals or groups of individuals, any decision must be one that affords equal respect to persons and their rights, valued for their own sake. A decision or action that uses people as means for other objectives would not meet this Kantian criterion. Similarly, even though respect for property, and thus profits, are important objectives for business, one must be careful not to prioritize property as equal to respect for persons, according to this line of reasoning. Such prioritization leads to judgments that value corporate material goals over persons, a valuation that would violate this kind of stakeholder approach. In addition to autonomy and respect for individuals, procedural fairness, informed consent, and respect for contractual agreements are means tests for stakeholder relationships. And in a properly constructed stakeholder arrangement, stakeholders should have viable avenues for self-governance and recourse.

Some thinkers, such as Robert Phillips (1997), develop a standard of fairness as the normative basis for stakeholder relationships. This principle argues, "Whenever persons or groups of persons voluntarily accept the benefits of a mutually beneficial scheme of co-operation requiring sacrifice or conurbation on the parts of the participants and there exists the possibility of free-riding, obligations of fairness are created among the participants in the co-operative scheme in proportion to the benefits accepted."

Moral minimums
The idea that although people cannot always agree about what is "good," they have almost universal agreement about what is "bad."

These formal considerations of such a fairness standard should provide a set of externally derived minimum guidelines or **moral minimums** for evaluating stakeholder decisions: for judging some of them morally acceptable or morally problematic. Decisions that affect various stakeholders must meet these minimum standards of respect for individuals, fairness of procedures and outcomes, informed consent, and availability of recourse.

Business Ethics and Healthcare Ethics

In the past, business issues in the HCO were relatively insulated from clinical issues for several reasons. First, the hospital at earlier stages of its development operated on a combination of charitable and equitable premises, often allowing for providing care to be separated from financial support. Second, the physicians, who were primarily responsible for clinical care, constituted an independent power nexus within the hospital and were governed by their own professional codes of ethics. In exchange for a great deal of control over their conditions of practice, they took almost complete responsibility for patient care. Thus clinical and professional ethics could to some extent be compartmentalized from the business issues—a much easier feat when, as in much of the past few decades, virtually all care was reimbursed from some source or other. Third, HCOs were not categorized as or treated as businesses, although they were presumed to be governed by the same expectation for good management as any other organization.

Today this separation of powers and of issues is less possible. Still, in HCOs there exists a temptation to separate business issues from clinical or professional issues. Ethical issues in the management of the HCO are often distinguished from those that face its clinical practice, and those, in turn, are distinguished from the challenges experienced by the professionals who carry out that practice. In the current climate, economic goals and exigencies often seem to override other considerations. In business too, where the business is not healthcare, the process of integrating and applying ethical standards to management practices can appear to be difficult because economic goals and exigencies often seem to override other considerations. But this is a misperception. Ethical issues are as much an integral part of economics and commerce as accounting, finance, marketing, and management. Business decisions are choices in which the decision makers could have done otherwise. Every such decision or action affects people or relationships between people in such a way that an alternative action or inaction would affect them differently, and every economic decision or set of decisions is embedded in a belief system that presupposes some basic values or their abrogation. Similarly, in the contemporary HCO, financial, clinical, and professional issues are all so interrelated that one cannot neatly separate, say, the cost of an MRI from a patient's need for it, the amount her insurer will cover, or from the professional expertise that determines the desirability of that protocol.

Case Study

A community hospital is located in a small coal mining town in West Virginia. It is a fine community hospital, and its board represents leaders in the community and management from the coal mine. While the hospital was thriving, rumors spread that some of the local mines might have to be closed. The result if this occurred would be a higher number of uninsured patients for the hospital. Recently the hospital was faced with another challenge: the need to modernize its heating system, which consisted of three coal-fired boilers. While the system could be replaced with a similar but more modern coal-fired system, a consultant recommended that the system be scrapped for a more efficient, environmentally cleaner gas-electric system. How should the administrator deal with the loss of insured patients? How should she deal with the community outcry against using non-coal-operated heating system? How does she balance the needs of the community, patient priorities, and predicted hospital financial challenges? (Adapted from Spencer 2001.)

Stakeholder theory provides an understanding of organizations and organizational accountability that best integrates financial issues with other considerations. The theory assumes that the organization and all its stakeholders form a shared moral community; it appeals to moral minimums or principles of fairness when evaluating organizational decisions. But even this finely differentiated account, in its original formulation, may also prove inadequate when applied to healthcare organizations without attention to several problems.

Exhibit 4.1 defines and illustrates stakeholders. A hypothetical corporation may well include a wide and diverse range of stakeholders as individuals or groups affecting or affected by its operations. However, this diagram does not capture the intricate and complex stakeholder accountability relationships in a typical HCO, nor does it adequately prioritize patients and populations as primary stakeholders.

While economic survival (if not profitability) is obviously a necessary consideration for the modern HCO in the present economic climate in the United States, important differences between HCOs and other business organizations remain. HCOs are engaged in more important value-creating activities, including the professional excellence of their medical staff, long-term organizational viability, community access, and, most important, patient and public health. What is strange is not that an HCO is concerned with efficiency, profitability, or at least sustainability. But the trouble begins when an HCO realigns its mission or creates an organizational culture in which efficiency, productivity, and profitability become the first priorities.

The overriding mission and rationale for the existence of healthcare organizations is, or should be, the provision of health services to individuals and populations. This constitutive goal stands in uneasy relation to economic ends. In a for-profit business organization, producing and selling a product or service yields a fee that normally results in a profit to the organization, and that profit ensures organization survival, new capital for research and expansion, and other benefits. In theory (although not in practice), the more the organization produces and sells, the more profit it enjoys. But the HCO has no such tight relationship between the rationale of the organization's existence and the condition for its economic survival. Indeed, in some instances an HCO is rewarded for providing fewer services, if it denies service to very ill or elderly people.

Exhibit 4.2 illustrates the complex stakeholder interrelationships and accountability links in a typical HCO, with the patient as the primary stakeholder. Exhibit 4.2 suggests that while garden variety stakeholder theory

EXHIBIT 4.1
Stakeholders

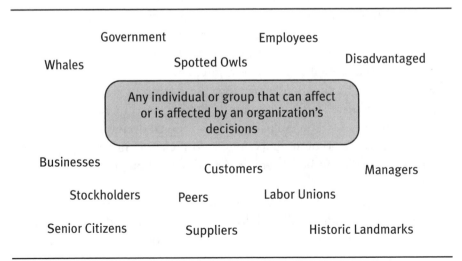

(as illustrated in Exhibit 4.1) does not capture the intricacies of HCO stakeholder relationships, a more complex version helps us think through these intricacies and better understand relationships and how they should be reciprocated. These various relationships often come into conflict with each other so that what in fact takes place belies our nice diagram. Still, setting out normative parameters for these relationships gives us a starting place to think about the ethics of HCOs.

The correlation between consumers and payers is very different in HCOs than in the usual business, and the stakeholder role of "customer" is ambiguous. Various forms of insurance, employer-sponsored health plans, or government agencies purchase health coverage for the individuals and patient groups who are the actual and potential patients for a given HCO. This three-way relationship complicates accountability between the parties affected in healthcare delivery. Unlike the typical customer, the patient may have no choice to go elsewhere or to change providers. Even in those cases where the recipient is also the payer, the consumer/patient is often ill and vulnerable. So unlike ordinary customers, patients are not always able to exercise their choices coherently. Worse, the complexity of the rapidly changing healthcare system is often not explained or clearly understood. The vulnerable patient may have no prior knowledge of what to expect and has little or reduced capacity to complain or to affect her own care delivery.

Healthcare professionals—physicians, nurses, members of other allied health professions—play key roles in the capacity of an HCO to deliver the services central to its definition and mission. The healthcare professional,

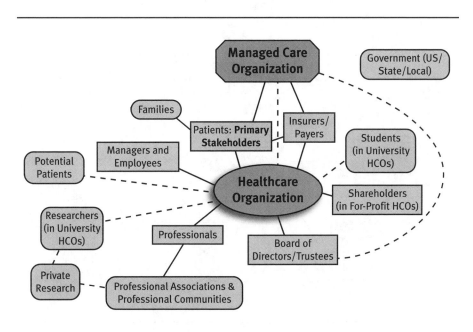

EXHIBIT 4.2
Healthcare
Organization
Stakeholder
Map

not the manager, is responsible for delivering care. One cannot gloss over, trade off, or subordinate professional commitments to patient health. Not only is this morally irresponsible for obvious reasons, it imperils the mission of any HCO, if an HCO is by definition a healthcare organization. Typically, healthcare professionals belong to, and are accredited by, independent professional associations. Many if not all professionals consider themselves primarily bound by the ethical prescriptions of their profession, preeminent among which are their duties to their patients. The necessity of professionals in HCOs complicates stakeholder relationships, particularly when the professional is also an employee of the HCO. Exhibit 4.3 illustrates stakeholder relationships from the point of view of the healthcare professional.

The complex accountability relationships between managers, professionals, and HCOs are not unlike managerial professional relationships in engineering firms—engineers are also specially trained professionals who belong to independent engineering associations. In both cases the presence of professionals complicates the organizational culture; in some instances it may even challenge the professional to choose between her professional obligations and those owed to the organization. This conflict is exacerbated in HCOs with an uncertain role for profitability or economic survival in the face of the overriding commitment to health.

EXHIBIT 4.3
Accountability
of the
Healthcare
Professional

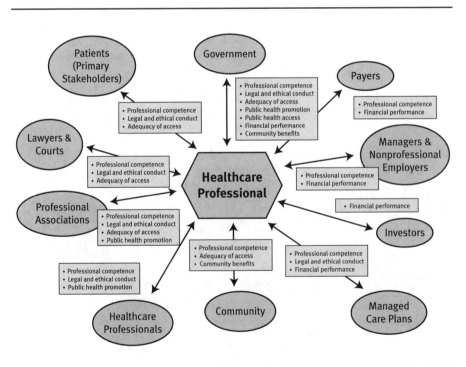

The contractual agreements an HCO enters with managed care organizations and health maintenance organizations; with other HCOs, insurance companies, and affiliated professionals; and its Medicare and Medicaid arrangements are increasingly important for the ability of the HCO to protect clinical and professional ethics. Today, HCOs are expected to provide care to defined populations at reasonable rates and as efficiently as possible. HCOs have fiduciary obligations to the contractual payers for their services; at the same time, they have primary role obligations to patients and populations. Moreover, if an HCO does not protect the integrity of its healthcare professionals, it will fail in its mission to provide adequate healthcare and thus fail in its obligations to patients and payers.

Case Study

A Catholic healthcare system in the Midwest has had to downsize 10 percent of its employees because of economic exigencies. The administrator is charged with developing criteria for dismissing each employee that will respect the mission of the system to be fair to each employee while taking into account the priority of providing excellent professional care for its patients. Possible criteria might include the following:

- Skill level
- Formal education and professional status
- Performance evaluations
- Seniority
- Current salary
- Ability to learn new skills and new roles
- Ability to work in teams
- Adaptability of each employee to the mission and values of the organization
- Employee financial needs

Should the administrator add other criteria? How might she prioritize these? What are her recommendations to management? (Adapted from O'Toole 2001.)

Conclusion

Theories of business ethics, although originally developed to analyze for-profit business organizations, are helpful in getting at ethical issues in HCOs as well. Stakeholder theory elaborates on the complex relationships between various stakeholders in HCOs, relationships that are sometimes oversimplified in some delineations of HCOs. Stakeholder theory reminds us that stakeholder relationships are normatively reciprocal accountability relationships prioritized by the organizational mission, roles and role obligations, organizational culture and ethical climate, professional interests and obligations, moral minimums, and societal expectations.

In other respects, issues that business ethics raise are important to HCOs, particularly as they function as managed organizational providers

Case Study

Mountain Children's Health System (MCHS) has three important proposed programs that need funding. In its present economic circumstances it can only fund one. The administrator is asked to make a recommendation to the board, keeping in mind the system's mission to provide high-quality comprehensive healthcare to children in the communities the hospital system serves as well as to retain its leadership in pediatric medical education. Each project will cost approximately $1 million per year. The projects include:

- State-of-the-art oxygenation: technology for supporting patients with cardiac problems who cannot be managed on a ventilator. Approximately eight to ten patients per year need this treatment after surgery, and if this technology were available, approximately 50 percent of those patients would survive. Without the new technology, young patients either die or are transferred to a university healthcare facility. MCHS will recover about 80 percent of the cost.

- Kidney transplant service: Currently MCHS has no such service. Approximately ten patients per year are in need of this service and go to university health centers for this operation. MCHS will recover about 70 percent of the cost.

- Rural pediatric healthcare services: In rural areas around MCHS facilities, ill children are not served adequately. A rural clinic would serve around 10,000 patients per year, and the critically ill children would be transported to a hospital in the MCHS system. MCHS would recover about 50 percent of the cost of this clinic and the transportation services.

You are the CEO. Which project would you choose? What are your reasons? (Adapted from Wells 2001.)

trying to offer good healthcare as efficiently and productively as possible for their patient populations. Profitability is not always the only priority even in businesses unrelated to health and healthcare. There is no reason, then, to imagine that profitability should be the first order of business even in a for-profit HCO. The most exemplary for-profit corporations think about profitability as, at best, only part of their mission. Conversely, however, separating business issues from those raised by clinical ethics or from the responsibilities of healthcare professionals may be detrimental to the HCO, to patients, and to the long-term professional commitment of healthcare specialists. Economic issues play a role in providing healthcare in every setting. Even in the "good old days" before managed care, healthcare professionals had to earn a living, and hospitals and clinics had to survive economically even on charity or governmental support. Therefore, bracketing economic issues as if economic survival or viability had no role in healthcare is not helpful because those issues affect, and have always affected, the quantity, quality, and kind of healthcare that can be provided. What is important for the ethics of HCOs is not to imagine that economic concerns are the only concerns or that profitability is the first priority, although these concerns are not irrelevant altogether.

Business ethics also reminds us that organizational accountability is as important as individual accountability. As it turns out, the HCO is a much more explicitly defined organization (in its mission and clientele) and often a more complex organization (in stakeholder accountability relationships, healthcare delivery, consumer and customer distinctions, service delivery, and reimbursement) than many garden-variety corporations. How the healthcare administrator deals with the uniqueness and complexity of an HCO remains the ongoing challenge.

Points to Remember

- Because most healthcare is now delivered in HCOs, and because HCO administrators must run solvent and efficient HCOs, business ethics is important to healthcare ethics.
- Stakeholder theory: a stakeholder is any individual or group whose role-relationship with an organization
  1. "is vital to the survival, and success [or well-being] of the corporation" (Freeman 1999); or
  2. helps to define the organization, its mission, purpose, or goals; or
  3. is most affected by the organization and its activities.
- Challenging the position that the primary purpose of a firm is to maximize the welfare of its stockholders, stakeholder theory argues that the goal of any firm and its management, is, *or should be,* the flourishing of the firm and *all* its primary stakeholders.
- In a healthcare organization the overlapping accountability relationships between the organization and its various stakeholders preclude separating medicine from professionalism and from the business dimensions of the organization.
- Still, this accountability does not preclude prioritizing patients as the most important stakeholder in any HCO. Profitability or even fiscal viability is fourth or fifth in priority.

References

Donaldson, T., and L. E. Preston. 1995. "The Stakeholder Theory of the Corporation: Concepts, Evidence, and Implications." *Academy of Management Review* 20 (1): 65–91.

Evans, W., and R. E. Freeman. 1988. "A Stakeholder Theory of the Modern Corporation: Kantian Capitalism." In *Ethical Theory and Business*, 3rd ed., edited by T. Beauchamp and N. Bowie, 101–105. Englewood Cliffs, NJ: Prentice Hall.

Freeman, R. E. 1999. "Stakeholder Theory and the Modern Corporation." Reprinted in *Ethical Issues in Business,* 6th ed., edited by T. Donaldson and P. H. Werhane, 247–57. Upper Saddle River, NJ: Prentice Hall.

Friedman, M. 1970. "The Social Responsibility of Business Is to Increase Its Profits." *New York Times Magazine* September 13, 122–26.

O'Toole, B. 2001. "Treatment of Employees During Downsizing." In *Developing Organization Ethics in Healthcare, A Case-Based Approach*, edited by A. E. Mills, E. M. Spencer, and P. H. Werhane. Hagerstown, MD: University Publishing Group.

Phillips, R. 1997. "Stakeholder Theory and a Principle of Fairness." *Business Ethics Quarterly* 7 (1): 51–66.

Spencer, E. M. 2001. "What Kind of Furnace?" In *Developing Organization Ethics in Healthcare, A Case-Based Approach*, edited by A. E. Mills, E. M. Spencer, and P. H. Werhane. Hagerstown, MD: University Publishing Group.

Spencer, E. M., A. E. Mills, M. V. Rorty, and P. H. Werhane. 2000. *Organization Ethics in Health Care*. New York: Oxford University Press.

Wells, R. D. 2001. "Hospital Planning Scenario." In *Developing Organization Ethics in Healthcare, A Case-Based Approach*, edited by A. E. Mills, E. M. Spencer, and P. H. Werhane, 33–35. Hagerstown, MD: University Publishing Group.

Parts of this chapter originally appeared in Spencer et al. 2000, 49–68. Reprinted by permission of the authors.

PROFESSIONAL ETHICS

Edward M. Spencer

This chapter is relevant to the following competencies identified in the ACHE Competencies Assessment Tool (see p. xxv):

Leadership
- Foster an environment of mutual trust

Professionalism
- Professional roles, responsibility, and accountability
- Professional standards and codes of ethical behavior
- Uphold and act upon ethical and professional standards
- Professional norms and behaviors

Business Skills and Knowledge
- Patients' rights, laws, and regulations

Learning Objectives

After completing this chapter the reader will

- understand the difference between morality and ethics,
- understand the components associated with professionalism,
- be familiar with various professional codes of ethics,
- be familiar with the development of the ethics of patient care,
- understand the importance of professionalism to healthcare organizations,
- be familiar with healthcare system development and recent changes as related to professional ethics, and
- understand the practical importance of professional ethics and how it can be maintained.

Introduction

Throughout history, the ethics of medical care has been defined primarily by the professional morality of medical practitioners, particularly physicians. As more attention is now being paid to healthcare organizations (HCOs), such as hospitals and nursing homes, and to the overall system of healthcare delivery, additional moral perspectives are being developed and introduced as appropriate sources for resolution of healthcare ethical issues. For instance, increasing attention has been paid to ethics associated with the operations of HCOs and the systems defined by these institutions. This perspective has been defined as "organizational ethics" (Spencer et al. 2000). Indeed, organizational ethics, which has focused on the healthcare organization developing an appropriate institutional culture and climate, has now been mandated a "leadership function" by The Joint Commission (2013). (See Chapter 14 for more discussion.)

But as these expanded ethical viewpoints receive greater attention in the consideration of ethical dilemmas and problems, there are underlying concerns that we are missing something important, that we should not lose sight of the traditional perspective or allow it to be unnecessarily trumped by other concerns.

Medical ethicist Albert Jonsen (1990) has written: "At a time when the genuine nobility of medicine is compromised and threatened from within and without, at a time when many of medicine's younger practitioners either have forgotten or have never learned the ethos of noblesse oblige, the challenge is the choice of an ethos—or rather the renewed commitment to an ethos." Although Jonsen was warning physicians not to lose sight or forget their commitment to an ethos, the same warning applies to all professions associated with healthcare delivery.

Numerous polls have demonstrated that a large percentage of the population wants a doctor they can trust—in other words, a physician with a moral compass to direct the care for his patient. Moreover, they also want to trust their hospitals to share the same commitment, based on the underlying ethics of healthcare.

But what is ethics, and what is its relationship to the healthcare system? All of us acknowledge and understand the traditional responsibility of healthcare professionals, such as doctors and nurses, but what of the "system"? Is the healthcare system governed by ethical guidelines and codes? If so, do these guidelines enhance the system, or are they constraining when other, sometimes more practical, guidelines could be used? And if not, should greater attention to ethics be encouraged or even mandated? These questions and similar issues are the focus of this chapter. By asking these questions, students should have a better understanding of the impact ethical issues have on the delivery of healthcare. This chapter should encourage future healthcare executives and administrators to pay attention to the role of the physician and other healthcare professionals and seek to advance and maintain some of the time-honored traditions related to medical decision making.

This chapter begins by defining the terms used in the discussion, then traces the development of medical ethics, nursing ethics, and healthcare administrative ethics. Professions and their associated codes of ethics often change in response to changing societal influence, including changes in the delivery system. However, these changes might be missing or ignoring the traditional perspective of medical ethics, and this perspective is vital to achieving the kind of care that society has endorsed. By the end of the chapter it should be obvious that the various professions associated with medicine will be well served by revisiting their codes of ethics and rewriting them in a way that promotes the traditional perspective of medical ethics while simultaneously recognizing the realities of modern life.

Defining the Terms

Morality focuses on the "good" or "right" answer to a problem or dilemma arising from a conflict involving fundamental human values. **Ethics** refers to the study and analysis of morality. Ethics is concerned with questions such as:

- Why is one course of action the right course?
- Do alternatives exist? If so, why were they not chosen?
- Is this course of action such that all similar cases will be decided the same, or will a change in circumstances change the ethical answer?

Although these two terms are frequently used interchangeably, notice that morality focuses on *what* should be done in a particular situation while ethics focuses on *why* a particular course of action is the right one.

Medical ethics is the study and analysis of moral issues (issues of right and wrong) as applied to the fields of medical treatment and research.

No single definition of a *professional* or **professionalism** exists. However, professionalism may be defined generally by these four essential attributes (Barber 1988):

1. A high degree of generalized and systematic knowledge
2. Primary orientation to community interests rather than to individual self-interest

Morality
Focuses on the "good" or "right" answer to a problem or dilemma arising from a conflict involving fundamental human values.

Ethics
The study and analysis of morality.

Medical ethics
The study and analysis of moral issues (issues of right and wrong) as applied to the fields of medical treatment and research.

Professionalism
Behavior characterized by traits that include a high degree of generalized and systematic knowledge; placing community interests over self-interest; self-control through codes of ethics and voluntary associations organized and operated by specialists in the same field; and a system of rewards that is primarily a set of symbols of work achievement rather than ends in themselves.

3. A high degree of self-control of behavior through codes of ethics internalized in the process of work socialization and through voluntary associations organized and operated by the work specialists themselves

4. A system of rewards (monetary and honorary) that is primarily a set of symbols of work achievement rather than ends in themselves

Professional ethics
Ethics as applied to questions concerning a particular profession.

Professional ethics refers to a code of ethics as applied to questions concerning a particular profession. Often accepted ethical tenets of the profession in question are kept by professional groups in ethical codes, ethical guidelines, or ethical statements. The American Medical Association's (AMA's) *Principles of Medical Ethics* (1958) focuses on the integrity of the physician as a moral agent. Underlying this focus is the question, "What kind of person should I be to fulfill my obligations as a physician?" rather than on answers to specific ethical questions.

But even though the professions associated with healthcare have similar core commitments to provide quality care, the codes of ethics of these professions differ. For instance, the code of ethics of the American College of Healthcare Executives (ACHE) insists that healthcare executives should be moral advocates and lead lives that embody an exemplary system of values and ethics. This general exhortation parallels the AMA's principles in that ACHE has a vision of the kind of person an executive or administrator must be to fulfill her obligations. But the code also focuses on the responsibilities the healthcare executive has to the hospital's stakeholders, including her responsibilities to the profession of healthcare management (ACHE 2011a).

Development of Ethical Codes and Guidelines

Medical Ethics

Code of Hammurabi
The first recorded set of laws in human history (circa 1772 BCE). These laws included acceptable standards for the practice of medicine.

The first attempt at defining medical ethics began about 4,000 years ago when the ruler of Babylonia created the **Code of Hammurabi**, the first recorded set of laws in human history. These laws included acceptable standards for the practice of medicine and were specific to their time and culture. For example, if a surgeon saved a patient's eye from a tumor, he received 10 shekels. In contrast, the doctor's hand would be chopped off if the patient died. Thus, the physicians of the time erred on the side of caution. The specificity of the Code of Hammurabi as related to time and culture probably precluded it from being of much value in the further development of meaningful ethical standards that could stand the scrutiny of time, so its value today is mainly historical.

Approximately 1,500 years later, the Greek physician Hippocrates and his followers wrote the **Hippocratic Oath,** which defined the ethical standard for practicing physicians and spelled out a number of virtues necessary for one to enter the profession. Most scholars consider the writings of Hippocrates, particularly the Hippocratic Oath, the most important early statements of the obligations of a physician (Areen et al. 1984).

Hippocratic Oath: Original Version

I swear by Apollo the physician, and Asclepius, and Hygieia and Panacea and all the gods and goddesses as my witnesses, that, according to my ability and judgment, I will keep this Oath and this contract:

To hold him who taught me this art equally dear to me as my parents, to be a partner in life with him, and to fulfill his needs when required; to look upon his offspring as equals to my own siblings, and to teach them this art, if they shall wish to learn it, without fee or contract; and that by the set rules, lectures, and every other mode of instruction, I will impart a knowledge of the art to my own sons, and those of my teachers, and to students bound by this contract and having sworn this Oath to the law of medicine, but to no others.

I will use those dietary regimens which will benefit my patients according to my greatest ability and judgment, and I will do no harm or injustice to them.

I will not give a lethal drug to anyone if I am asked, nor will I advise such a plan; and similarly I will not give a woman a pessary to cause an abortion.

In purity and according to divine law will I carry out my life and my art.

I will not use the knife, even upon those suffering from stones, but I will leave this to those who are trained in this craft.

Into whatever homes I go, I will enter them for the benefit of the sick, avoiding any voluntary act of impropriety or corruption, including the seduction of women or men, whether they are free men or slaves.

Whatever I see or hear in the lives of my patients, whether in connection with my professional practice or not, which ought not to be spoken of outside, I will keep secret, as considering all such things to be private.

So long as I maintain this Oath faithfully and without corruption, may it be granted to me to partake of life fully and the practice of my art, gaining the respect of all men for all time. However, should I transgress this Oath and violate it, may the opposite be my fate.

From the time of Hippocrates to the present, other cultures have developed written principles concerning the practice of medicine, but the Hippocratic Oath has remained as an example of ideal conduct for physicians, in particular the emphasis on nonmaleficence (do no harm) and beneficence (obligation to help the patient to the extent possible) as defining the duty of physicians toward the individual patient.

Hippocratic Oath
Written by Hippocrates and his followers in the fifth century BCE; defined the ethical standard for practicing physicians and spelled out a number of virtues necessary for one to enter the profession. It emphasized the principles of nonmaleficence (do no harm) and beneficence (obligation to help the patient to the extent possible) as defining the duty of physicians toward the individual patient.

From Hippocrates to the early nineteenth century, some movement occurred toward incorporating the values of the Christian, Jewish, and Islamic religions into the Hippocratic tradition. Adherence to religious values in practice was generally accepted, but the initial Hippocratic focus on the duty of the physician to work for the benefit of his individual patient remained (Burns 1977).

John Gregory, a Scottish physician in the late eighteenth century, advanced a more modern, secular, virtue-based concept of professional obligations. He has influenced many thoughtful physicians to consider what it means to be a physician and the character necessary to fulfill the obligations associated with the profession. Gregory's writings did not contradict the Hippocratic Oath but clarified what it should mean for physicians of his time (McCullough 1998).

Percival's *Code of Medical Ethics*
Published in 1803 by Thomas Percival. The code emphasized the Hippocratic tradition and professional etiquette and was written for physicians practicing in hospitals or other medical institutions, thus adding institutional considerations to the patient focus.

An addition to Gregory's influence was **Percival's *Code of Medical Ethics***, published in 1803 (Leake 1927). This book was a "scheme of professional conduct relative to hospitals and other charities" that emphasized the Hippocratic tradition and professional etiquette. But it was written for physicians practicing in hospitals or other medical institutions, thus adding institutional considerations to the patient focus.

In recent years, many physicians and medical schools have questioned the relevancy of the Hippocratic Oath, feeling that it is inadequate to answer or provide guidance in a world that has seen so many scientific, economic, political, and social changes (Orr et al. 1997). For example, note the absolute prohibition of euthanasia and abortion. Furthermore, note that physicians are strictly forbidden to "use the knife," a prohibition that can hardly accommodate modern-day practice. In addition, some physicians and medical schools think the oath does not represent the shared moral values held by Christians, Jews, and Muslims (Orr et al. 1997). For these reasons and others, most graduating medical students take a modern version of the oath. An updated version was written in 1964 by Louis Lasagna, academic dean of the School of Medicine at Tufts University.

Hippocratic Oath: Modern Version

I swear to fulfill, to the best of my ability and judgment, this covenant:

I will respect the hard-won scientific gains of those physicians in whose steps I walk, and gladly share such knowledge as is mine with those who are to follow.

I will apply, for the benefit of the sick, all measures [that] are required, avoiding those twin traps of overtreatment and therapeutic nihilism.

I will remember that there is art to medicine as well as science, and that warmth, sympathy, and understanding may outweigh the surgeon's knife or the chemist's drug.

I will not be ashamed to say "I know not," nor will I fail to call in my colleagues when the skills of another are needed for a patient's recovery.

I will respect the privacy of my patients, for their problems are not disclosed to me that the world may know. Most especially must I tread with care in matters of life and death. If it is given me to save a life, all thanks. But it may also be within my power to take a life; this awesome responsibility must be faced with great humbleness and awareness of my own frailty. Above all, I must not play at God.

I will remember that I do not treat a fever chart, a cancerous growth, but a sick human being, whose illness may affect the person's family and economic stability. My responsibility includes these related problems, if I am to care adequately for the sick.

I will prevent disease whenever I can, for prevention is preferable to cure.

I will remember that I remain a member of society, with special obligations to all my fellow human beings, those sound of mind and body as well as the infirm.

If I do not violate this oath, may I enjoy life and art, respected while I live and remembered with affection thereafter. May I always act so as to preserve the finest traditions of my calling and may I long experience the joy of healing those who seek my help.

This modern version of the oath emphasizes doctors' responsibilities to stress prevention over cure, not to be ashamed to ask for help when needed, and to keep in mind the psychological aspects of disease (Wright 2003).

The professional ethics of medicine in the United States developed with full awareness of this history and depended on the concepts from Hippocrates to Gregory and Percival. The first items of discussion at the organizational meeting of the AMA in 1847 were the establishment of a code of ethics and the creation of minimal requirements for medical education. The AMA's initial *Principles of Medical Ethics* (1958) were based on the Hippocratic tradition and Percival's Code and have remained relatively unchanged until recent years. These early principles strongly emphasized the physician as the purveyor of ethical standards relating to medicine and directed the physician to care for his individual patient to the best of his ability at all times and to act in a professional manner in all relationships with patients and colleagues. These principles helped the physician to understand his relationship with his patients and with the larger community and also helped the patients and the culture to understand and depend on this relationship.

Thus the popular image of the caring but highly paternalistic physician developed. Even though minor changes to the AMA's *Principles* were made along the way, the mutual understanding that they fostered worked well for most physicians and their patients. Paternalism was seen not as a problem but as a covenant requiring the physician to act as a benevolent parent with greater knowledge, and the patient in return to not question the advice of the physician and follow the physician's recommendations.

The 1957 revision of AMA's *Principles of Medical Ethics* stated, "A physician should . . . not dispose of his services under terms or conditions which tend to interfere with or impair the free and complete exercise of his medical judgment and skill or tend to cause a deterioration of the quality of medical care." In other words, the physician was in charge. By the 2001 revision, however, this section was completely deleted, and new principles—including an admonition to obey the law, a strong support of patient rights, and support of access to medical care for all people—had been added. Why this occurred is explained later in this chapter. The current version is as follows (AMA 2001).

American Medical Association *Principles of Medical Ethics*

Preamble

The medical profession has long subscribed to a body of ethical statements developed primarily for the benefit of the patient. As a member of this profession, a physician must recognize responsibility to patients first and foremost, as well as to society, to other health professionals and to self. The following Principles adopted by the American Medical Association are not laws, but standards of conduct which define the essentials of honorable behavior for the physician.

Principles of Medical Ethics

I. A physician shall be dedicated to providing competent medical care, with compassion and respect for human dignity and rights.

II. A physician shall uphold the standards of professionalism, be honest in all professional interactions, and strive to report physicians deficient in character or competence, or engaging in fraud or deceptions, to appropriate entities.

III. A physician shall respect the law and also recognize a responsibility to seek changes in those requirements which are contrary to the best interests of the patient.

IV. A physician shall respect the rights of patients, colleagues, and other health professionals, and shall safeguard patient confidences and privacy within the constraints of the law.

V. A physician shall continue to study, apply, and advance scientific knowledge, maintain a commitment to medical education, make relevant information available to patients, colleagues, and the public, obtain consultation, and use the talents of other health professionals when indicated.

VI. A physician shall, in the provision of appropriate patient care, except in emergencies, be free to choose whom to serve, with whom to associate, and the environment in which to provide medical care.

VII. A physician shall recognize a responsibility to participate in activities contributing to the improvement of the community and the betterment of public health.

VIII. A physician shall, while caring for a patient, regard responsibility to the patient as paramount.

IX. A physician shall support access to medical care for all people.

Nursing Ethics

Nursing as a profession has had a shorter history but one that meshed with the history of medicine until very recently. The origin of professional **nursing ethics** began with Florence Nightingale and her concepts of necessary and responsible obedience to the physician as developed during the Crimean War (1854–1857). Nightingale had a significant influence during this war through her organizational work. She subsequently founded the Nightingale Nursing School in London in 1860, and her ideas of preventive medicine were advanced through a paper in 1893. In this paper and others, she emphasized the need to treat the sick person rather than the disease, that prevention is much better than cure, that hospitalization does not necessarily lead to health, and that nursing must hold to its ideals as represented by the **Florence Nightingale Pledge** (Gretter 1893), often made by gradating nurses (Bishop and Goldie 1962).

Nursing ethics
A subset of applied ethics concerned with the activities and decisions made in the field of nursing.

Florence Nightingale Pledge
The pledge often made by graduating nurses that emphasizes the duty of the nurse to obey the physician as part of the nurse's duty to care for the patient. It calls for responsible obedience, with the needs of the patient being the primary consideration.

Florence Nightingale Pledge

I solemnly pledge myself before God and in the presence of this assembly, to pass my life in purity and to practice my profession faithfully. I will abstain from whatever is deleterious and mischievous, and will not take or knowingly administer any harmful drug. I will do all in my power to maintain and elevate the standard of my profession, and will hold in confidence all personal matters committed to my keeping and all family affairs coming to my knowledge in the practice of my calling. With loyalty will I endeavor to aid the physician in his work, and devote myself to the welfare of those committed to my care.

Nightingale emphasized the duty of the nurse to obey the physician as a part of her duty to care for the patient. She called for responsible— not blind—obedience, with the needs of the patient being the primary consideration.

Nightingale's influence on the profession of nursing continued unabated until a number of changes in the last half of the twentieth century. The American Nurses Association (ANA) changed the Nightingale ideals of caring for the patient by supporting physicians and others in these endeavors to a position of "client advocacy." This change was instituted to enable the nurse to practice on her own based on an usually unwritten contract with the "client" (Husted and Husted 1991). This basic change in ethics from a caring, patient-centered ideal with an emphasis on beneficence toward the patient to one of a contract with the client was controversial, so much so that ANA's most recent Code of Ethics for Nurses (2001) has reverted to the more traditional stance of "caring for the patient" while noting that "the patient" may be "an individual, family, group, or community."

American Nurses Association: Code of Ethics for Nurses

1. The nurse, in all professional relationships, practices with compassion and respect for the inherent dignity, worth and uniqueness of every individual, unrestricted by considerations of social or economic status, personal attributes, or the nature of health problems.

2. The nurse's primary commitment is to the patient, whether an individual, family, group, or community.

3. The nurse promotes, advocates for and strives to protect the health, safety and rights of the patient.

4. The nurse is responsible and accountable for individual nursing practice and determines the appropriate delegation of tasks consistent with the nurse's obligation to provide optimum patient care.

5. The nurse owes the same duties to self as others, including the responsibility to preserve integrity and safety, to maintain competence and to continue personal and professional growth.

6. The nurse participates in establishing, maintaining and improving health care environments and conditions of employment conducive to the provision of quality health care and consistent with the values of the profession through individual and collective action.

7. The nurse participates in the advancement of the profession through contributions to practice, education, administration and knowledge development.

8. The nurse collaborates with other health professionals and the public in promoting community, national, and international efforts to meet health needs.

9. The profession of nursing, as represented by associations and their members, is responsible for articulating values, for maintaining the integrity of the profession and its practice and for shaping social policy.

Until the second half of the twentieth century, physicians and nurses were the recognized purveyors of the ethics of patient care and were looked on to provide answers to ethical issues and problems. This responsibility fell mainly to the physicians, but nurses were also sought out for ethical advice and, in partnership with physicians, helped maintain the traditional tenets of professional ethics in medicine. Nurses at times had conflicts of interest because they were expected to adhere to their primary ethical mandate of putting the patient's well-being first while acting as an employee of a hospital or other healthcare organization (HCO) that had the responsibility to oversee the patient's care. Physicians were not placed in these conflict situations until recently, but with the growth of physicians also being employees of the HCO, they too are now grappling with these conflict issues.

After World War II, numerous other groups demanded and were given professional status in fields related to healthcare. Chaplains, social workers, psychologists, and technicians of all types are now all considered healthcare professionals, each group with its own code and list of principles that fundamentally define the moral basis for their particular profession. The origin for most of these ethical statements can be traced to the aforementioned codes of ethics of physicians and nurses, but each group's perspective is specifically defined based on its areas of responsibility. Although a commitment to patients is at the center of all of these codes of ethics, the codes do differ, and differing areas of responsibility and accountability can cause

Case Study

A nurse with an excellent reputation maintained her clinical competence by reading not only nursing journals but also any publications related to her primary area of nursing. After being hired by a large hospital three years ago, she received frequent promotions to become head nurse for the obstetrics (OB) ward. One of the floor nurses came to her recently and asked to talk privately. This nurse told the head nurse that one of the prominent OB doctors was noted to "smell of alcohol" at three recent deliveries and asked what she should do. She stated that she did not want any trouble but was concerned about the issue, even though there had been no discernible difficulties related to patient care. The head nurse thanked the floor nurse for the information and told her she would take care of the matter. That evening the physician in question was making rounds and the head nurse asked to speak to him. The nurse told him of the rumor of his drinking, which caused him to become angry and demand to know who had started the rumor. The head nurse refused to name the source of her information and told the physician that she had to report this incident to the hospital administration. The physician informed her that he was a member of the hospital's board of directors, and he would see to it that the head nurse was fired if this rumor resulted in any further fallout. He also expected that the person who reported him would be punished in some manner. He then left. How should this issue be resolved?

conflict among professionals who strive to deliver appropriate care to patients.

Healthcare Executive Ethics

ACHE is an organization representing healthcare executives and administrators. The college's first president, Charles A. Wordell, recognized that professionalization of the field was critical to healthcare management and could not be accomplished without standards (ACHE 2008).

Like the AMA and ANA, ACHE educates its members in all areas of the profession, formulates recommendations and guidelines, and disseminates information. Each organization produces a widely esteemed journal—the *Journal of the American Medical Association*, the *Online Journal of Issues in Nursing*, and the *Journal of Healthcare Management*. Moreover, all three organizations are concerned about what *professionalism* means in their respective professions, their members' commitment to professionalism, and their professional behavior.

ACHE's first code of ethics was published in 1941, and the code has been evolving ever since in response to changing circumstances. For instance, in 2007 the college introduced a standard to provide guidance to executives concerning their relationships with vendors and revised the standard in 2011 (ACHE 2011b). But since 1941, the code has emphasized the healthcare executive's or administrator's commitment to those she serves, especially patients and their families. Today, the code focuses on how healthcare executives and administrators are expected to behave and on the responsibilities healthcare executives and administrators have to the hospital's stakeholders (ACHE 2011a).

American College of Healthcare Executives Code of Ethics

Preamble

The purpose of the *Code of Ethics* of the American College of Healthcare Executives is to serve as a standard of conduct for members. It contains standards of ethical behavior for healthcare executives in their professional relationships. These relationships include colleagues, patients or others served; members of the healthcare executive's organization and other organizations; the community; and society as a whole.

The *Code of Ethics* also incorporates standards of ethical behavior governing individual behavior, particularly when that conduct directly relates to the role and identity of the healthcare executive.

The fundamental objectives of the healthcare management profession are to maintain or enhance the overall quality of life, dignity and well-being of every individual needing healthcare service and to create a more equitable, accessible, effective and efficient healthcare system.

Healthcare executives have an obligation to act in ways that will merit the trust, confidence, and respect of healthcare professionals and the general public. Therefore, healthcare executives should lead lives that embody an exemplary system of values and ethics.

In fulfilling their commitments and obligations to patients or others served, healthcare executives function as moral advocates and models. Since every management decision affects the health and well-being of both individuals and communities, healthcare executives must carefully evaluate the possible outcomes of their decisions. In organizations that deliver healthcare services, they must work to safeguard and foster the rights, interests and prerogatives of patients or others served.

The role of moral advocate requires that healthcare executives take actions necessary to promote such rights, interests and prerogatives.

Being a model means that decisions and actions will reflect personal integrity and ethical leadership that others will seek to emulate.

I. The Healthcare Executive's Responsibilities to the Profession of Healthcare Management

The healthcare executive shall:

A. Uphold the *Code of Ethics* and mission of the American College of Healthcare Executives;

B. Conduct professional activities with honesty, integrity, respect, fairness and good faith in a manner that will reflect well upon the profession;

C. Comply with all laws and regulations pertaining to healthcare management in the jurisdictions in which the healthcare executive is located or conducts professional activities;

D. Maintain competence and proficiency in healthcare management by implementing a personal program of assessment and continuing professional education;

E. Avoid the improper exploitation of professional relationships for personal gain;

F. Disclose financial and other conflicts of interest;

G. Use this *Code* to further the interests of the profession and not for selfish reasons;

H. Respect professional confidences;

I. Enhance the dignity and image of the healthcare management profession through positive public information programs; and

J. Refrain from participating in any activity that demeans the credibility and dignity of the healthcare management profession.

II.   The Healthcare Executive's Responsibilities to Patients or Others Served

The healthcare executive shall, within the scope of his or her authority:

A. Work to ensure the existence of a process to evaluate the quality of care or service rendered;

B. Avoid practicing or facilitating discrimination and institute safeguards to prevent discriminatory organizational practices;

C. Work to ensure the existence of a process that will advise patients or others served of the rights, opportunities, responsibilities and risks regarding available healthcare services;

D. Work to ensure that there is a process in place to facilitate the resolution of conflicts that may arise when values of patients and their families differ from those of employees and physicians;

E. Demonstrate zero tolerance for any abuse of power that compromises patients or others served;

F. Work to provide a process that ensures the autonomy and self-determination of patients or others served;

G. Work to ensure the existence of procedures that will safeguard the confidentiality and privacy of patients or others served; and

H. Work to ensure the existence of an ongoing process and procedures to review, develop and consistently implement evidence-based clinical practices throughout the organization.

III.   The Healthcare Executive's Responsibilities to the Organization

The healthcare executive shall, within the scope of his or her authority:

A. Provide healthcare services consistent with available resources, and when there are limited resources, work to ensure the existence of a resource allocation process that considers ethical ramifications;

B. Conduct both competitive and cooperative activities in ways that improve community healthcare services;

C. Lead the organization in the use and improvement of standards of management and sound business practices;

D. Respect the customs and practices of patients or others served, consistent with the organization's philosophy;

E. Be truthful in all forms of professional and organizational communication, and avoid disseminating information that is false, misleading or deceptive;

F. Report negative financial and other information promptly and accurately, and initiate appropriate action;

G. Prevent fraud and abuse and aggressive accounting practices that may result in disputable financial reports;

H. Create an organizational environment in which both clinical and management mistakes are minimized and, when they do occur, are disclosed and addressed effectively;

I. Implement an organizational code of ethics and monitor compliance; and

J. Provide ethics resources and mechanisms for staff to address ethical organizational and clinical issues.

IV. The Healthcare Executive's Responsibilities to Employees

Healthcare executives have ethical and professional obligations to the employees they manage that encompass but are not limited to:

A. Creating a work environment that promotes ethical conduct;

B. Providing a work environment that encourages a free expression of ethical concerns and provides mechanisms for discussing and addressing such concerns;

C. Promoting a healthy work environment which includes freedom from harassment, sexual and other, and coercion of any kind, especially to perform illegal or unethical acts;

D. Promoting a culture of inclusivity that seeks to prevent discrimination on the basis of race, ethnicity, religion, gender, sexual orientation, age or disability;

E. Providing a work environment that promotes the proper use of employees' knowledge and skills; and

F. Providing a safe and healthy work environment.

V. The Healthcare Executive's Responsibilities to Community and Society

The healthcare executive shall:

A. Work to identify and meet the healthcare needs of the community;

B. Work to support access to healthcare services for all people;

C. Encourage and participate in public dialogue on healthcare policy issues, and advocate solutions that will improve health status and promote quality healthcare;

D. Apply short- and long-term assessments to management decisions affecting both community and society; and

E. Provide prospective patients and others with adequate and accurate information, enabling them to make enlightened decisions regarding services.

VI.   The Healthcare Executive's Responsibility to Report Violations of the Code

A member of ACHE who has reasonable grounds to believe that another member has violated this *Code* has a duty to communicate such facts to the Ethics Committee.

Societal Influences on Codes of Ethics and Professional Principles

Note that professional organizations, in whatever field, change their codes of ethics in response to a number of variables, including technological change, a growing societal consensus on a belief or value, or a cultural shift in society. For example, note the widespread discontent with the original Hippocratic Oath and the adaption of a more modern version by nearly all medical schools for their graduating students (Lasagna 1964). Recent years have also seen a much greater attention to influences in society, such as "rights movements," the development of specific ethical standards for medical research, the involvement of courts in healthcare decisions, the rise of secular bioethics, the influence of academic institutions, the acceptance of gender-based equality, and so on. But perhaps most important in recent years, "patient rights" have become a prominent value within the American culture.

Tuskegee Experiment
A US Public Health Service clinical study (1932–1972) that tracked the progression of untreated syphilis in black men even after effective treatments had been developed.

The patient rights movement was stimulated by a number of ethical scandals related to patient care and research. Examples include the **Tuskegee Experiment** (sponsored by the US Public Health Service from 1932 to 1972), a study of the natural progression of syphilis using black men as the only subjects and which continued long after good treatment for the disease had been developed, and the **Willowbrook hepatitis study** (1965), which tested a vaccine for hepatitis B without adequate consent on children housed in an institution for the mentally disabled (Fletcher, Miller, and Spencer 1997). At the same time numerous patient care problems related to "right to die" issues—in which a patient was kept physiologically alive by newly developed technology (e.g., respirators, highly effective antibiotics) over the objection of the patient or his appropriate surrogate—received much press attention. The resulting debate called into question who had the authority to refuse medical interventions and whether physicians and HCO administrations could override a request by a patient or surrogate to stop life-sustaining interventions (Fletcher and Davis 2005).

Willowbrook hepatitis study
A clinical study in which a hepatitis B vaccine was tested without proper consent in children housed in an institution for the mentally disabled.

Soon it became obvious that physicians, who often had little knowledge of a specific patient's values, were making value decisions for the patient—decisions on which life and death and appropriate treatment depended. No longer could each physician be depended on to know or understand what the patient's moral stance in a particular situation would be.

But even though professional bodies strove to keep pace with and mirror societal changes, major disagreements among professionals within these organizations occurred and no doubt will continue to occur in the future as society either forms new, or discards older, beliefs or values. The accompanying case illustrates.

In spite of long-standing traditional values, codes of ethics have changed as a consensus has formed around the importance of patient rights. But what was to take the place of the caring physician in ethically problematic situations? And what of HCO rules that contradicted the patient's desires? How could such issues be considered while still maintaining the idea of the beneficence of the physician and the social mandate of the HCO that had prevailed throughout history?

In this instance, the federal and state governments and accrediting bodies became involved, acting as protectors of patients as subjects in human research experiments, followed soon by ways to protect a patient's rights to make an informed decision, even when these decisions could hasten death. Would patients and their families be required to accept the recommendations of healthcare professionals? Who should patients and their families turn to if recommendations were questioned, particularly in life-and-death situations? Who or what entity was to have the ultimate

Case Study

In 1988 the AMA's Council on Ethical and Judicial Affairs (CEJA) (the body within the AMA that has the responsibility to recommend changes in the AMA *Principles of Medical Ethics* to the AMA House of Delegates) was asked to study the ethical issues associated with using organs from anencephalic infants before the infants met the criteria for death. Infants with this disorder are born without a forebrain (the front part of the brain) and a cerebrum (the thinking and coordinating part of the brain). The remaining brain tissue is often exposed—not covered by bone or skin. A baby born with anencephaly is usually blind, deaf, unconscious, and unable to feel pain. Although some individuals with anencephaly may be born with a rudimentary brain stem, the lack of a functioning cerebrum permanently rules out the possibility of ever gaining consciousness. Reflex actions such as breathing and responses to sound or touch may occur (NINDS 2010).

Some members of the AMA shared the sentiment to make a special case and allow the harvesting of organs for transplantation from this class of patients because of the great need for organs from infants. The CEJA studied the matter and made a recommendation in 1988 based on the fact that the anencephalic infant was obviously human and alive, that these infants, even though destined to die within a short period of time, should be given the same consideration as other human infants who did not have the dire prognosis. The matter was brought up again in 1994, and the opinion was radically revised. The CEJA (1994) report stated: "It is ethically permissible to consider the anencephalic infant as a potential organ donor, although alive still under the present definition of death."

This single opinion reversed a primary obligation of physicians (to protect the patient). Predictably significant disagreement with this action occurred in the AMA House of Delegates and elsewhere. At its next meeting, the House of Delegates voted against this change, and the CEJA reverted to the 1988 opinion that requires determination of death prior to using the organs from an anencephalic infant for transplantation.

authority to decide the treatment of the patient? Courts, commissions, and legislatures have all weighed in on these issues, increasing the patient's authority to make healthcare decisions and in some cases leaving the physician and the HCO as advisers and not, as in the past, decision makers themselves.

The confusion that surrounded the patient rights issue led to the development of ethics committees in almost all HCOs. These groups were formed to help with patient care decisions, and they had varying degrees of authority. One or more physicians were often members of these committees, but nurses, chaplains, social workers, administrators, and hospital and outside lawyers were also members. Also, one or more community representatives who had no attachments with the HCO were often made members of the ethics committee. These community members were there to speak for the community's values during the committee's deliberations. (See Chapter 6 for further discussion of ethics committees and ethics consultation services.)

Many physicians who adhered to a traditional Hippocratic view were dismayed by what appeared to them to be interference in the doctor–patient relationship by nonclinical personnel and a wavering of the commitment to the traditional professional values that previously defined the professional obligations and the ethics of the practice of medicine. Patients and their families, too, were often confused and were not always willing to make difficult treatment decisions.

And what of the administrative staff of the HCO? What is the appropriate role for those charged by their ethical codes to enhance the ability of the HCO and clinicians in caring for the patient? What should happen when disagreements occur? What mechanisms for dispute resolution should be available in each HCO, and where does the final authority reside for these issues—with the physician, with the entire clinical staff, or with the HCO via its administration or through a committee structure? And most important, who prevails if a dispute arises about the appropriate ethical response to a patient care ethical dilemma—the clinical professionals or the healthcare administration and executives?

Though The Joint Commission is attempting to provide clarity to some of these questions through mandating the HCO's attention to clinical ethics issues (see Chapter 6) and mandating leadership's attention to the culture and climate of the HCO (see Chapter 14), confusion still exists. And this confusion will surely intensify as society continues to evolve, along with new forms of healthcare delivery.

Development of the Healthcare System in the United States

The US healthcare system throughout its development owes much of its form and function to its history in the United States and the economic, social, and political conditions under which it operates. Society has always paid attention to the healthcare system and those who direct the system and function within it. Changes throughout the history of the United States have had profound influence on healthcare delivery. However, in spite of changing modes of healthcare delivery, healthcare ethics changed little until the mid-twentieth century.

While professional organizations were wrestling with societal influences, such as the "rights" movements and how best to reflect these influences in their professional obligations, the healthcare system changed dramatically. It became bureaucratized; physicians and other healthcare professionals began to specialize and narrow their perspective to smaller areas of patient care; the number of malpractice lawsuits increased, with both physicians and HCOs being singled out; employment-based health insurance became the most frequent method of paying for healthcare; training at all levels became more common; and of course, competition among HCOs became fierce as employers increasingly favored managed care organizations. In addition, efforts were made to align provider incentives with payer incentives to control costs.

These changes added to the complexity of the work of the HCO, leading occasionally to a divergence of the cooperative roles of administrators and physicians. Roles and responsibilities enlarged or shrank depending on specifics, creating some confusion about professional duties and responsibilities. In some cases, the medical staff and the administrative staff viewed each other as enemies in their attempts to deliver healthcare to their mutual patients, forgetting that both had patient care as their priority and that cooperation was needed to ensure its achievement.

Professional Ethics in Today's Healthcare System

Doctors, nurses, healthcare executives and administrators, and other professionals in the HCO, in spite of their differing roles and responsibilities, are bound together through their codes of ethics and in their commitment to the welfare of their patients. But as noted previously, this is a time of dramatic change in healthcare. And we can expect dramatic changes in the near future as cost control measures must be imposed on the system.

All professionals who are a part of the system, as well as those involved in the payment for healthcare (governments at all levels, insurance companies, charities, other payers, and some individuals), are aware that each of these groups can and often does affect how patients are treated. Changes in one part of the system may have unforeseen and unintended consequences affecting the system as a whole or specific areas within the system. Answers to important questions are sometimes difficult to come by or are not ideal. So

Case Study

A well-respected oncologist admitted a patient with a rapidly progressive breast cancer for treatment with an expensive cancer drug that, although still controversial, had shown good results (prolonging expected survival time many months and sometimes years). Previously, the cost of the drug had been borne by the manufacturer and a private charity, but these funders announced that they could no longer defray the expense of treatment for any new patients because of financial constraints. The oncologist was aware that payment for the treatment of her new patient would have to be borne by the hospital. Shortly after the patient's admission, the oncologist received a call from the hospital administrator informing her that the hospital could not pay for the drug for her patient and that arrangements for payment would have to be made before the drug regimen was begun because the budget for compassionate care had been completely depleted for this fiscal year. The physician angrily told the administrator that she had supported the hospital in many ways, including financial donations to the building fund, and she expected the hospital to reciprocate and respond to her patient's need for the expensive drug. The administrator replied that the board would not approve, so he could not agree to that request. Who is right? What should be done?

the larger question becomes, how is the ethics of patient access and care to be handled within an environment of scarce resources? Should each patient receive the treatment recommended and desired to the extent possible while the appropriate resources are available? Is some method of "ethical rationing" to be developed? Who decides and under what rules? Do these changes leave room for any nonchanging ethical values for physicians, nurses and other clinicians, healthcare administrators, health insurance executives, politicians, and society as a whole?

The healthcare system has been consolidating for more than two decades. Greater consolidation means more regulations for HCOs, both internal—to standardize in the interest of quality, safety, and efficiency—and external—to control the quality, safety, and costs of large sources of expense. Moreover, in response to the Patient Protection and Affordable Care Act (ACA) (see Chapter 13), more consolidation is expected. Larger entities tend to be more complex. They are not as flexible as smaller entities because of the additional layers of the organization. Moreover, without clearly stated rules and regulations, people within the organization, regulators, and payers would waste precious time and resources tracking down appropriate functions and the answers they need. In addition, as payer resources become increasingly scarce, politicians and others will seek more ways to control costs. So providers, both individual and institutional, can expect more regulation and oversight from state and federal governments and other payer organizations.

As we continue down the road of greater consolidation, clinical decisions may become more constrained by rules and regulations. Physicians may believe that their position as a healer—based on the ideal of beneficence for the individual patient—is threatened. Nurses and other clinicians may increasingly become purveyors of HCO policy rather than advocates for their individual patients, and HCO executives and administrators may be pressured to look on their institutions as businesses measured not only by patient care outcomes but as the conservers of the resources allocated for medical care by increasing government mandates and regulations. All of these possibilities threaten the core professional and ethical commitment healthcare professionals have to their patients as well as the HCO's commitment to the goal of providing excellent care at a reasonable price.

Practical Advice

Healthcare administrators and clinical professionals beginning their career in today's healthcare system often question specifically how a particular ethical dilemma should be handled. Codes of ethics for their particular profession offer clear advice on how to approach a particular type of ethical problem but cannot be expected to have ready answers to a specific problematic case with unique features. For the young healthcare executive, referring to the ACHE Code of Ethics may cause confusion because it may be too general or too specific to apply to a unique case. Moreover, in covering the accepted ethical obligations to several groups of stakeholders, the code may add to confusion because of inherent conflicts in determining which obligations take precedence.

The young healthcare administrator may refer patient care–based ethical dilemmas to the hospital's ethics committee, if one is available, but advice from this body may be open to interpretation; seldom does an ethics committee give specific answers unless it has been given decision-making authority. The HCO's attorney may help with legal issues but, although legal questions usually accompany ethical issues, the law does not often give a complete or satisfactory answer to the problem. The mission and values of the HCO should be considered, but they might be contradictory and confusing. Finally, after all possible areas of help are considered, the knowledge and character of the healthcare executive will determine the direction of the response. Therefore, before making a decision, the junior healthcare executive must understand the ethical dilemma and its implications and must gather all pertinent information and understand the parameters (e.g., mission and values, legal boundaries, hospital bylaws and guidelines, community standards) within which a decision must fall. In addition, she must understand the consequences of her decision. Furthermore, she must be able to withstand pressure from stakeholders who would decide differently on the issue at hand. And she needs to understand the level of support from the board and senior executives and have a plan to follow through after the decision is made. The entire decision-making process should be transparent from beginning to end.

Ultimately, the responsibility of the young administrator is to foster an environment in which difficult decisions can be made openly and transparently within the appropriate parameters. To foster such an environment, the young administrator should consider supporting one or more ethics committees or subcommittees—one with patient care responsibility and one with organizational responsibility. Moreover, the young administrator should support mechanisms to ensure the two committees or subcommittees have ongoing collaboration and communication. An ethics committee with organizational responsibility could

- put in place ongoing education concerning ethical issues and how they affect the overall operation of the HCO,
- install a process for addressing controversial ethical issues that affect the overall operation of the HCO,
- offer a moral space to discuss the perspectives of differing stakeholders, and
- recognize and support the professionalism of the HCO's employees—no matter what their role—thereby fostering respect and cooperation among the professional groups that staff the HCO.

Indeed, such a committee could develop a realistic code for all professionals associated with the HCO, ensuring that the organization has ethics embedded in its entire decision-making process. A comprehensive ethics program for the entire HCO and all its stakeholders, with individual decisions concerning ethical issues being dependent on this process and the individual character and virtues of the individual administrators, should ensure such an environment.

Conclusion

Historically we have seen the development of revered sets of ethical principles overseeing the ethics of all organizations and professionals involved in healthcare. The public wants the healthcare of the community to be an important aspect of life for the community in general and the individuals that it comprises. And the public wants to trust its professionals and HCOs.

During the rapid changes in the healthcare system over the past 25 years there has been a greater consolidation of patient care in HCOs, and more physicians are becoming an integral part of the HCO beyond the traditional role as members of the medical staff. This development can be expected to accelerate as provisions of the ACA are implemented. As physicians become administrators and employees, their obligations increasingly align with the HCO rather than with individual patients. Thus, power in the HCO shifts away from clinicians to executives and administrators.

This shift means that an HCO's mission and values become important in the development and maintenance of the ethical principles of professional groups who practice within the HCO. As such, healthcare executives, administrators, and healthcare professional groups devoted to the ethics of medical practice need to look closely at what this means. Physicians practicing under the auspices of an HCO need to develop a revised code based on tradition and modern reality: a code that still emphasizes the character and virtues expected of healthcare professionals throughout history while recognizing the changes in the healthcare system and what these changes mean to the ethical stance of the healthcare professionals. This model accepts that the HCO will become the purveyor of the ethical principles that guide its healthcare professionals. It also implies that HCO executives and administrators must take seriously their responsibility for providing an environment that encourages the ethical and moral commitment of its professionals to their core obligations to patients.

Patients in particular and the population in general agree that the practice of medicine and the overall delivery of healthcare should be moral enterprises, and the work required to enforce this is as important as any other work of the HCO. Physicians and other clinicians *and* healthcare executives and administrators must work together toward this goal. Without a common ethical framework underlying the activities and values of the HCO, the ethical underpinning of the present healthcare delivery system is left as an entity without a conscience that will be doomed to satisfy few and gradually lose its bearings.

Ed Pellegrino (1998), a physician and bioethicist, stated: "No human being can escape the reality of being sick and being cared for. All must seriously contemplate what a divided profession without a common set of moral commitments would mean. Most important we are obligated to ask how patients might fare in the hands of a profession in tatters."

We cannot go back to the days when the doctor was expected to always act in the individual patient's best interest without consideration of others in the society, and the patient was obliged to follow the physician's advice or change physicians. Nor should we want to. But we should be able to expect that a healthcare professional will be truthful about the influences that guide her as an adviser. We should also expect that healthcare administrators will adhere to stated mission and values and will work with the professional staff to develop a more modern code of ethics for each clinical group, a code that will always maintain a strong ethical basis for their clinical practices.

Points to Remember

- The healthcare leader should be knowledgeable about the content of the codes and principles of ethics for physicians, nurses, and healthcare administrators.
- Codes and principles change over time in response to changes in the environment, in healthcare experience, in societal expectations, in ethical concepts and reasoning, and in healthcare science and technology.
- These changes in codes and principles are often difficult and contentious and take time to develop and be accepted.
- Differences in the codes and principles among different professions may lead to ethical uncertainty and conflicts within a healthcare organization.

References

American College of Healthcare Executives (ACHE). 2011a. *ACHE Code of Ethics.* Accessed March 25, 2013. www.ache.org/ABT_ACHE/code.cfm.

———. 2011b. "Considerations for Healthcare Executive–Supplier Interactions." Accessed March 26, 2013. www.ache.org/policy/execsuppliers.cfm.

———. 2008. "Remembering ACHE's 75th Anniversary." Accessed March 26, 2013. www.ache.org/ABT_ACHE/ACHE_75th.cfm.

American Medical Association (AMA). 2006. *Code of Medical Ethics of the American Medical Association.* Chicago: American Medical Association.

———. 2001. *Code of Medical Ethics of the American Medical Association.* Chicago: American Medical Association.

———. 1958. *Principles of Medical Ethics.* Chicago: American Medical Association.

American Medical Association Council on Ethical and Judicial Affairs (CEJA). 1994. "CEJA Report 5 – I-94: The Use of Anencephalic Neonates as Organ Donors." Accessed March 26, 2013. www.ama-assn.org/resources/doc/ethics/ceja_5i94.pdf.

———. 1988. "CEJA Report C – I-88: Anencephalic Infants as Organ Donors." Accessed March 26, 2013. www.ama-assn.org/resources/doc/ethics/ceja_ci88.pdf.

American Nurses Association. 2001. *Code of Ethics for Nurses.* Silver Spring, MD: American Nurses Association.

Areen, J., S. Goldberg, L. Gostin, P. Jacobson, and P. King. 1984. *Law, Science and Medicine.* Mineola, NY: Foundation Press.

Barber, B. 1988. "Professions and Emerging Professions." In *Ethical Issues in Professional Life,* edited by J. Callahan, 35–38. New York: Oxford University Press.

Bishop, N., and S. Goldie. 1962. *A Bio-bibliography of Florence Nightingale*. London: Dawsons of Pall Mall for the International Council of Nurses.

Burns, C. R. (ed.). 1977. *Legacies in Ethics and Medicine*. New York: Science History Publications.

Fletcher, J., and W. Davis. 2005. *Fletcher's Introduction to Clinical Ethics*, 3rd ed. Frederick, MD: University Publishing Group.

Fletcher, J. C., F. G. Miller, and E. M. Spencer. 1997. *Introduction to Clinical Ethics*, 2nd ed. Frederick, MD: University Publishing Group.

Gretter, L. E. 1893. "Florence Nightingale Pledge." *American Nurses Association*. Accessed March 25, 2013. http://nursingworld.org/FunctionalMenuCategories /AboutANA/WhereWeComeFrom/FlorenceNightingalePledge.aspx.

Hammurabi. 1772 BCE. *Code of Hammurabi*. Accessed March 25, 2013. www .innovateus.net/content/medicine-code-hammurabi.

Hippocrates. n.d. "The Hippocratic Oath." Translated by Michael North. www.nlm .nih.gov/hmd/greek/greek_oath.html.

Husted, G. L., and J. H. Husted. 1991. *Ethical Decision Making in Nursing*. St. Louis, MO: Mosby Year Book.

Joint Commission. 2013. "Standard LD 04.02.03, Elements of Performance 1–7." *Hospital Accreditation Standards*. Oakbrook Terrace, IL: The Joint Commission.

Jonsen, A. 1990. *The New Medicine and the Old Ethics*. Cambridge, MA: Harvard University Press.

Lasagna, L. 1964. "The Hippocratic Oath: Modern Version." Nova. Accessed March 25, 2013. www.pbs.org/wgbh/nova/body/hippocratic-oath-today.html.

Leake, C. (ed.). 1927. *Percival's Medical Ethics*. Baltimore, MD: Williams and Wilkins.

McCullough, L. 1998. *John Gregory and the Invention of Professional Medical Ethics and the Profession of Medicine*. Dordrecht, The Netherlands: Kluwer Academic Publishers.

National Institute of Neurological Disorders and Stroke (NINDS). 2010. "NINDS Anencephaly Information Page." Accessed March 26, 2013. www.ninds.nih .gov/disorders/anencephaly/anencephaly.htm.

Orr, R. D., N. Pang, E. D. Pellegrino, and M. Siegler. 1997. "Use of the Hippocratic Oath: A Review of Twentieth-Century Practice and a Content Analysis of Oaths Administered in Medical Schools in the U.S. and Canada in 1993." *The Journal of Clinical Ethics* 8 (Winter): 377–88.

Pellegrino, E. 1998. "Rethinking the Hippocratic Oath." In *Last Rights? Assisted Suicide and Euthanasia Debated*, edited by M. M. Uhlmann, 256–61. Washington, DC: Ethics and Public Policy Center.

Spencer, E., A. Mills, M. Rorty, and P. Werhane. 2000. *Organization Ethics in Health Care*. New York: Oxford University Press.

Wright, P. 2003. "Louis Lasagna." *Lancet* 362 (9393): 25.

6

ORGANIZATIONAL ADMINISTRATION AND THE CLINICAL ETHICS MECHANISM: A QUESTION OF RESPECT

Mark H. Waymack

This chapter is relevant to the following competencies identified in the ACHE Competencies Assessment Tool (see p. xxv):

Leadership
- Potential impacts and consequences of decision making in situations both internal and external

Professionalism
- Ethics committee's roles, structure, and functions
- Consequences of unethical actions
- Cultural and spiritual diversity for patients and staff as they relate to healthcare needs
- Professional standards and codes of ethical behavior
- Serve as the ethical guide for the organization

Knowledge of the Healthcare Environment
- The patient's perspective (e.g., cultural differences and expectations)

Learning Objectives

After completing this chapter, the reader will understand

- the general distinction between clinical and organizational ethics,
- the importance of organizational leadership supporting the work of clinical ethics in the healthcare organization, and
- how senior administration can effectively support clinical ethics work.

Introduction

Clinical ethics
Focuses on ethical issues associated with the delivery of patient care.

Organizational ethics
Focuses on the structure and conduct of the organization that makes the delivery of patient care possible.

Clinical ethics mechanism
An individual or group that grapples with ethical issues confronted by the care of particular patients, with a view toward resolving specific care issues. Sometimes called a clinical ethics service or committee.

Broadly speaking, this chapter examines the relationship between the administrators of a healthcare organization and that organization's **clinical ethics** activities and structures. Abstractly, what is the relationship between **organizational ethics** and clinical ethics? More concretely, what responsibilities or even authority should a senior administrator exercise over **clinical ethics mechanisms** and activities?

Some features of the relationship between organizational ethics and clinical ethics render it remarkably complex. The ethics of the relationship between organizational administration and practicing professionals is complex to begin with. Practicing professionals, such as physicians, enjoy some measure of professional autonomy in their practice decisions; consequently, prudent administrators tend to stay out of the physician–patient relationship and the physician's decisions about a patient's care. However, physicians do not receive complete carte blanche from the organization: They are expected to adhere to generally recognized practice parameters and abide by the rules and expectations of the institution. For example, a physician would not have the leeway to perform an elective tubal ligation in a Catholic hospital that has polices against such practices, nor would a hospital permit electroconvulsive therapy to be performed for a diagnosis of "shyness." Still, when it comes to professional practice, administrators tend to respect the professional judgment of the certified and licensed professional. After all, patients go to the oncologist or the neurosurgeon precisely because of her confirmed expertise. Most patients would not profess to know much about the standards or details of neurosurgery or oncology. But US society has long held a much more democratic notion of ethics expertise. After all, most people think of themselves as reasonably decent, ethically speaking. And if people are reasonably ethically good, then they must (seemingly) be reasonably well versed in their knowledge of ethics. If knowledge of ethics, or moral right and wrong, is widely spread in such a democratic fashion, then why all this fuss about clinical ethics in the first place? What could clinical ethics be about and why would it be needed in healthcare organizations?

How does clinical ethics differ from organizational ethics? This issue is not simple. Inevitably some overlap exists. In the end, the distinction might have more to do with emphasis or focus than any bright conceptual difference. One might think of the difference in these terms: physicians and nurses (for example) deliver patient care in a way that hospitals and skilled nursing facilities do not. Hospitals and nursing facilities, on the other hand, provide a special environment in which that patient care can be delivered. Clinical ethics, then, concerns the actual delivery of patient care. Organizational ethics, on the other hand, is about the place and the conduct of the structure, the organization, that makes the delivery of that care possible. Clinical ethics pays little or no heed to the organization's relations to its vendors, to the organization's debt ratio, or to whether certain staff employees are unionized or not. (And these, of course, are only a few of many possible examples.) Similarly, an organizational ethics committee would not typically have any direct interest or involvement into whether in the case of an elderly man with early-to-moderate dementia the medical team should go with the care options chosen by his adult offspring, or with what he himself says, or whether there might be compelling reasons to seek a court-appointed guardianship for healthcare decision-making. Nevertheless, instances may occur where the outcome of a clinical ethics deliberation concerning an individual patient may well adversely affect the organization or challenge its stated mission or some of its policies; or analogously, organizational deliberations may directly affect particular clinical ethics decision making with an individual patient. This situation is especially evident when one thinks of mission and policy formation or even budget issues. The practical outcome of this distinction is either that organizational ethics are addressed through a single, overarching mechanism or, more frequently, through separate institutional mechanisms for clinical and organizational ethics. When the mechanisms are separate, good communication must happen between them, both on a regular basis and with respect to individual cases whose resolution may have organizational impact or vice versa.

A crucial feature of a healthy relationship between administration and clinical ethics is based on senior administration's responsibility for effective leadership of the organization as a whole. Effective leadership includes moral leadership; hence, senior administrators cannot stand entirely apart from clinical ethics. However, articulating precisely what the relationship of administration to clinical ethics should be is not easy. The relationship between senior administration in the organization and the clinical ethics mechanisms and activities should include four major features:

1. respect on the part of administration for the work of the clinical ethics mechanism;
2. oversight of the clinical ethics work, especially in regard to its policies and procedures;
3. ongoing quality improvement; and
4. support for the clinical ethics mechanism and activities.

The first point is about attitude. The appropriate attitude arises from an appreciation of what the clinical ethics service does, and it is then expressed in terms of actions. Points 2 and 3 are both kinds of oversight, ensuring that the clinical ethics mechanism does what it is supposed to do and is working to do it well. Point 4 is about senior administration making it possible for the clinical ethics mechanism to succeed in its tasks and challenges.

What Is Clinical Ethics?

To be clear on what clinical ethics, particularly a clinical ethics mechanism or service, is, framing this section in terms of its history may be helpful.

Clinical ethics, in one sense, has been a part of the healing profession since time immemorial. In the Western tradition, one of the early documents concerning clinical ethics is the Hippocratic Oath, expressing the professional commitments of the Hippocratic school of healing (which was one of several healing traditions in the ancient world). Since then, while the particular moral principles might have varied by time and place, ethics has been an accepted part of the medical profession.

However, for the more than two millennia between Hippocrates and the 1970s, clinical ethics was not seen as a discipline, nor was it a central or controversial part of physician training. Rather, ethics was generally regarded as "common knowledge" within the profession and was rarely discussed outside of the profession itself.

The period immediately following World War II, particularly in the United States, saw enormous increases and advances in the technology of medicine. This period witnessed the introduction of such interventions as antibiotics, a proliferation of vaccines, ever-increasing sophistication in imaging (CT scans and MRIs), the invention of the intensive care unit and the trauma center, the ventilator/respirator, the medicalization of the feeding tube, and the introduction of chemotherapy and radiation therapies, to name but a few. The rate of medical innovation during this period was staggering. Although medicine seemed to be operating under a "technological imperative"—if you have technology you must use it—patients, families, and even many health professionals were increasingly worried that the outcomes of the use of such technologies were not always desirable. For example, keeping a loved one alive on a ventilator might sound good until one realizes that the loved one will never regain consciousness.

Things came to a head with the infamous case of Karen Ann Quinlan, a permanently comatose young woman who was kept alive on a respirator (and feeding tube). Her parents asked the physicians to turn off the respirator, a request the physicians adamantly refused, arguing that that would be tantamount to killing their patient, something that physicians are sworn never to do. The parents persisted, and the case finally wound up in the New Jersey State Supreme Court. The court concluded that as long as all the members of a "prognosis committee" agreed on the irreversible nature of Quinlan's condition, and if the parents remained firm in their resolve, then removing the respirator would be legally appropriate. (In an interesting twist, when the respirator was turned off and removed, to her parents' surprise, Quinlan breathed on her own. She lived another ten years, without ever regaining any consciousness, before dying of a respiratory infection.)

In the wake of the Quinlan case, two aspects of clinical ethics came together. First, a bioethics debate, including discussion of medical ethics that had been simmering in professional circles, burst onto the public scene. Both medical professionals and the public at large looked for assistance in deliberating clinical ethics problems. And from the ranks of principally philosophers and theologians emerged a new breed called "ethicists." Second, the Quinlan court decision had directed that a committee of experts be formed to carefully consider the case and either confirm or deny the proposed course of action.

In the 1980s, clinical ethics became increasingly complex and contentious. In vitro fertilization, surrogate motherhood, abortion, embryonic stem cell harvesting and research, genetic therapy and genetic enhancement, cosmetic surgery and cosmetic neurology, and extensive use of life support technology are all complex clinical ethics issues driven by new technology posing previously unasked and unanswered questions. The parallel rise of patient rights and respect for patient autonomy have also posed ethical questions. These include such issues as patient informed consent, a "right" to participate in biomedical research trials, and a revisiting of the questions of euthanasia and assisted suicide. Additionally, immigration into the United States has created a more culturally diverse population in the past 30 years. Cultural differences can include different moral attitudes toward healthcare and technology as well as differing understandings of the basic ethics of the provider–patient relationship. Finally, changes in financing and reimbursement policies have altered and challenged the traditional ethics of the physician–patient relationship.

The rapid rate of change in medical technology, social customs and laws, and even financial policies all come together to ensure that the fuzzy edges of clinical ethics will persist, and thus the activity of clinical ethics will not disappear any time soon in the United States. (For a fuller version of this history, see Levine 2007.)

The Emergence of the Clinical Ethics Mechanism

Buried in the Karen Ann Quinlan court decision was the direction to form a "prognosis committee" to review Quinlan's status. Though this was not, strictly speaking, an ethics committee, the decision did put forward the idea of a committee as a desirable resolution mechanism. Not only does such a committee provide safety in numbers, but some wisdom can emerge in interpersonal deliberation about these weighty ethical issues.

By the late 1980s, perplexed by myriad new medical ethics problems and confronted by discontented and questioning patients and family members, hospitals and medical staff borrowed the precedent of the Quinlan prognosis committee and radically transformed it into a recognizable clinical ethics service, thus creating and formalizing clinical ethics services in their institutions. (I use the term clinical ethics *service* loosely here. I do not mean to imply that clinical ethics is, or should be, a service in the formal sense in which many hospitals use the term.) External pressure, such as in the form of the Nursing Home Reform Act of 1987 and the Patient Self-Determination Act of 1990, sparked even more widespread interest in the development of such clinical ethics services. Recognizing a trend and judging it to be valuable, The Joint Commission began to consider the presence and availability of clinical ethics mechanisms as one measure in the accreditation process. Ethics language was explicitly incorporated in The Joint Commission's requirements in 1991, and has been periodically revised since then.

In the 1990s, the vagaries of the prognosis committee had begun to coalesce into the more recognizable form that is today's clinical ethics mechanism. First, two dominant styles of clinical ethics mechanisms emerged: a committee model and a **consult** service model. The committee model appealed to those who cherished a more democratic conception of ethics expertise and thought what the ethics work needed was a committee of professionals of good, moral, professional sense. The earliest committees tended to be composed almost exclusively of physician members, with perhaps some room made for a PhD in philosophy or theology. But gradually, the advantages to a committee of diverse membership (particularly nursing and social work in addition to medicine, and in terms of racial, ethnic, and educational diversity) came to be seen. Still, as committees grew in size, it became clear that doing clinical ethics with a committee of a dozen or more is an intrusive and unwieldy process. Many of these large committees created a smaller subcommittee that was tasked with taking all clinical ethics calls.

Clinical ethics consult
A model in which the clinical ethics mechanism is provided by an individual or a small group of experts as a consulting service.

The second model was a clinical ethics consulting service. Here the need for a committee was minimized, and the ethics service would be provided by one or a couple of ethics experts in a consultation model. The smaller mechanisms presumably benefitted by the expertise of the ethics consultants as well as their avoidance of a bureaucratic committee process. On the other hand, such consulting services did place what ethics power there might be in very few hands, concentrated under the rubric of "ethical expertise," an idea that has remained vague and problematic. Accordingly, in such models the consulting team commonly reports on a regular basis to an overall committee—thus combining an ethics committee with an ethics consulting service.

Both of these clinical ethics service models persist today, with different institutions having their own preferences. Accreditation bodies have not expressed any clear preference for one model over another.

Trying to discuss the forms of clinical ethics mechanisms without also considering the functions that have coalesced under these services is awkward. And once again, the services or functions now commonly attached to the clinical ethics service have historical roots. By the early 1990s, a triad of duties had become firmly placed: clinical consultation, policy, and education (Hall 2000; Ross et al. 1993).

Consultation

The first and most commonly recognized function is clinical ethics consultation. When ethically contentious, difficult, awkward cases arise, the clinical ethics service is there to assist. What should be done in the case of conflict between physician and patient or family? Is what the physician, the patient, or the family wishes ethically (professionally and institutionally) permissible? Although pointing to some common reasons that cases arise as pointedly ethics cases may be possible, enumerating all the possible reasons that might spark a request for ethics consultation is impossible. Furthermore, what triggers these concerns is deeply influenced by the context of care. Acute care settings tend to give rise to different questions than long-term care or rehabilitation care, for example.

Policy

Second, clinical ethics mechanisms became tasked with formulating clinical ethics policies. Awkward cases, particularly those driven by differences of opinion and conviction, may point out the need for applicable policies. Indeed, well-articulated and promulgated policies can not only help decide some of these cases, they can effectively keep the cases from becoming contentious in the first place. The need for policy was also motivated by (indeed, forced by) such federal legislation as the Nursing Home Reform Act of 1987, the Patient Self Determination Act of 1990, and the "Baby Doe" regulations imposed during the Reagan presidency (Levine 2007). Institutions were required to have standing policies on the withholding or withdrawal of life-support care, such as feeding tubes or respirators, and on advising all admitted patients of their rights to execute an advance directive or other treatment plan. Although various constraints existed, a "one size fits all" solution was not expected. End-of-life care policies for a Catholic or Orthodox Jewish skilled nursing facility might well differ from those policies guiding decision making in a public acute care hospital. What had become important was that the institution clarify its ethics policies and inform all those involved of these policies.

Education

Given this mandate to inform, the third member of the troika of clinical ethics duties emerged: education. In the minds of many, education emerged as perhaps the most important of the three duties (Hall 2000; Spencer et al. 2000). First, many problems or situations that came before the clinical ethics committee or consultants as cases could well have been avoided altogether if those involved had fully understood the institutional ethics policies to begin with. (This is by no means true of all problematic cases.) Second, even if the institution had exceptionally wonderful clinical ethics policies, those policies would remain impotent unless everyone providing care was aware of and understood them. And third, the twin tasks of articulating policy and educating staff (professional and otherwise) in the spirit and content of those policies serve as a mechanism to compel the organization to think clearly and articulately about what its central clinical ethics commitments ought to, and shall, be.

Administrative Engagement

First and foremost, senior administration should have respect for the work that an effective clinical ethics mechanism performs for patients, families, professionals, staff, and the organization itself. Additionally, the healthcare administrator should actively engage with the clinical ethics mechanism in three ways: oversight of policy, quality improvement, and institutional support.

Oversight of Policy

The delivery of healthcare is inescapably a team project, especially for care delivered within the setting of healthcare institutions. Individual professionals are the ones who provide hands-on care, but that care is provided within the context and infrastructure of the hospital, the long-term care institution, or other organization. What both of these parties—professionals and organizations—contribute to healthcare delivery is laden with values, including moral values. Serious effort should be taken, therefore, to ensure that in the delivery of that care, individual professional and organizational moral commitments should overlap.

Healthcare organizations are not all—just by virtue of being healthcare organizations—morally identical. Catholic hospitals have differing moral commitments than entirely secular, public hospitals. An Orthodox Jewish nursing home will have different moral strictures than a secular, for-profit nursing home. Even an academic teaching hospital may well have different moral commitments than nonacademic organizations. As noted previously, professional moral commitments are also part of this equation. And the background moral commitments of the society in which both the profession and the organization exist have a place. US society, for example, in terms of both moral and legal values, places a great deal of weight on individual patient autonomy. These moral values are reflected in organizational policies that cover such ground as expectations of informed consent, what is acceptable or unacceptable in end-of-life care, or what is acceptable or unacceptable in the creation of life, such as with fertility interventions. Ideally, such policies give the organization a chance to echo the moral and professional values articulated elsewhere in its mission and values statements as a healthcare organization.

An administrator's oversight of the clinical ethics service's contribution to policy formation may include

1. ensuring that those tasked to draft such policies provide adequate representation of these various points of view and commitments,
2. ensuring that any compromises among conflicting values represented in the policy drafts are compromises that the organization is comfortable with,
3. ensuring that the draft policies both fulfill and conform to legal expectations in the United States, and
4. ensuring that draft policies are periodically reviewed and affirmed by the appropriate bodies within the organization (for example, perhaps both the professional staff representation and the governing board of the organization).

Quality Improvement

The best organizations are keen not just to function but to function well. Quality review thus becomes a standard and persistent feature of good management. Therefore, healthcare organizations measure post-op infections from surgery, infections attributed to iatrogenic causes, complications in particular heart surgeries, falls on each floor of a nursing home, and other numbers. Biostatisticians and bioinformaticists may be employed to keep tabs on outcomes and trends so that quick and appropriate responses can be made to any unexpected or abnormal adverse outcomes. Accrediting bodies—and payers—may themselves be interested in just such data.

The thoughtful and committed administrator will want to consider not just that a clinical ethics mechanism exists but that it performs—preferably that it performs well. However, the administrator faces a perplexing difficulty: Clinical ethics committees may have membership, they may have meetings, they may take phone calls. But what do they actually do? In evaluating them or pondering their improvement, what kind of information should the administrator be looking for? What would constitute good outcomes versus unexpectedly adverse outcomes? And how could that information, whatever it is, be adequately captured in some kind of database? In short, knowing whether the clinical ethics mechanism is doing its job well, that it is functioning adequately or excellently, requires knowledge—and precision—about what constitutes a good outcome for a clinical ethics intervention. But this is where rubrics tend to fail. Is it a good outcome if the patient is happy? Not necessarily. Sometimes, no matter what medicine has available, a patient will die and a family may be upset, even angry. This may be no fault of medicine and no fault of an ethics consultation, but the patient's family may still be unhappy. Does that mean that the ethics consultation was not of good quality? Such an inference would seem to be unwarranted.

Right answer model
The idea that a good clinical ethics consultation outcome would be the identification and implementation of the right answer.

Three distinct ways of understanding the desired goals of clinical ethics consultation exist: the **right answer model**, the **mediation model**, and the **facilitation model**.

The right answer model presumes that such a thing as a right answer exists (and correlatively that professional expertise qualifies someone to identify or voice that right answer). In a right answer model a good clinical ethics consultation outcome would be the identification and implementation of that right answer. This model may make some sense in small, tightly knit communities that have a pervasive common sense of moral values and widespread recognition of who the relevant moral experts might be. Such a top-down model is not unheard of in certain communities, but it remains controversial in a society as culturally, ethnically, and morally diverse as the United States. On the other hand, buying completely into some kind of radical moral relativism or moral subjectivism would be foolish. Even a diverse society has broad areas of moral agreement, though sometimes that agreement is not noticed precisely because no articulated disagreement exists. US society does share a deep commitment to such values as the right of individual self-determination, and hence the legal requirement of informed consent. So although the right answer model may have some kernel of truth in it, this model should be approached with a large measure of caution, even skepticism.

Mediation model
Aims for an answer that comes out of discussion between the involved parties, acknowledges various points of view and concerns, and is acceptable to the parties involved, even if it might not be the first-choice outcome.

Facilitation model
The goal of the consultation is to help those involved articulate the ethical issues in conflict and explore how best to resolve those issues.

The mediation model, quite to the contrary, does not presume that there is any one right answer. What the ethics consultation aims for in this model is an answer that comes out of discussion between the various involved parties, that has paid heed to the various points of view and concerns, and that is acceptable to the various parties involved, even if it might not be the first choice outcome for anyone in particular. In this model, the answer is only right because it is the product of a certain kind of mediation process.

Expertise in this model would consist more of mediation skills than any content knowledge of moral truths.

Further, in the mediation model, the good outcome, the quality product, so to speak, is the one that comes out of this process and most conforms to an evolving consensus among the participants. If wide discussion involving all the relevant parties has occurred, and if the resolution is something that each party is happy (or at least okay) with, then that in itself counts as a quality outcome for the ethics intervention.

The facilitation model is perhaps the model most favored by the professional bioethics community, though this is by no means unanimous. At the core of the facilitation model is the conviction that moral values—particularly in the intense circumstances of healthcare, where life and death are often on the line—are not necessarily easy to discern clearly or to articulate. The goal of the consultation, then, is to deftly tease into the open what the various ethical conflicts might be and then through discussion and deliberation to sort through how best to navigate the troubled waters. To do this well requires a lot of moral knowledge, such as that gained through academic training, a good deal of practical experience, and excellent interpersonal skills.

Although many bioethicists seem to favor this model, identifying or measuring good outcomes with it has proven perplexing. The moral wisdom of including a variety of moral perspectives and exercising a variety of moral and interpersonal skills makes the criteria for success in consultation complex and vague. Fundamental moral principles and relevant legal considerations are certainly part of the knowledge base and are expected to be incorporated in the outcome. And commitment to central healthcare ethics concepts—such as patient autonomy, effective informed consent, and professional integrity—and adherence to organizational values and commitments are all part of any desired outcome.

This does not make quality review or outcomes assessment impossible, just complex. One can imagine an ethics mechanism coming up with key steps that should be taken (and documented) in any clinical ethics consultation. Were the relevant parties consulted? Were ethically appropriate decision makers identified? Were communication questions addressed? Did appropriate discussion occur of exactly what the perceived ethical issues are? Were a variety of strategies or options considered? Was all of this done in a timely fashion? In post-consultation reflection, were any lessons considered for future cases? And were there appropriate and adequate follow through and follow up? Yes, these questions are complex and not amenable to quantification, but they are still capable of some meaningful documentation and assessment.

A similar concern is evident when it comes to the question of expertise in clinical ethics. One supposed strength of the specialist consulting model was that it made use of clinical ethicists' professional expertise. On the other hand, the large committee model purports to respect a more democratic notion of ethics expertise. But whichever view one takes, what constitutes expertise in clinical ethics is still painfully unclear. What qualifies a particular individual to be a member of a clinical ethics committee or as a leader in ethics consultation? If the hospital is looking for a leading clinician to head up the cardiovascular team, candidates can be gauged by generally accepted criteria. Statistically, how have their patients fared in the past? Are the physicians board certified? What does their revenue stream look like? How many articles have they published? No such board certification exists for clinical ethicists. Simply having a higher educational degree, such as a PhD, is not in itself an adequate indicator or evidence of excellence in clinical ethics consulting. Writing a dissertation is quite a different task than conducting an ethics consultation, and the skill set required for each is substantially different.

American Society for Bioethics and Humanities The leading national organization for professionals in bioethics.

The **American Society for Bioethics and Humanities** (ASBH), the leading national organization for professionals in bioethics, has attempted to answer the skills and qualifications questions. After much deliberation, drafting, open discussion, and further deliberation and editing, the ASBH published a document sketching out a general consensus (though not necessarily unanimous) of the kind of training, knowledge base, and skills set that should be found in a clinical ethicist (ASBH 2010).

A second aspect of quality review, therefore, could be a knowledge and skills inventory of the ethics service members. For although appropriately skilled persons are not guaranteed to succeed, they are far more likely to succeed than those who conspicuously lack the relevant knowledge and skills.

Finally, any serious effort at quality review should include deliberate thought into both short-term and long-term ideas of how the clinical ethics mechanism can be improved, including a strategic plan for making that improvement a reality. Doing a decent job is simply not enough: continuous improvement is preferred. Senior administration might be especially helpful in this regard. Those individuals who gravitate toward clinical ethics work are not necessarily well equipped with the management and administration skills of such long-term strategic planning. This area is, therefore, excellent for collaborative effort between the clinical ethics leadership and senior administration, constructively combining different skills sets.

Support

The clinical ethics service thus provides services to patients, families, professionals, and the organization that may be difficult to quantify but are in keeping with the values of the professions and the values of the healthcare organization. The same is true of MRI scans, cardiac catheterization, barium scans, and appendectomies. But scans, catheterizations, and surgeries all typically produce a lucrative revenue stream in a well-run facility. Clinical ethics, like pastoral care, is a service that generates no real revenue. Quite the contrary, it serves as an upfront drain on the budget. Its ethics personnel could be employed doing something more "constructive" (i.e., generating revenue), and the office space it inhabits might have been used by some service that did generate direct revenue. Even the time of the personnel involved could have been used for some far more profitable endeavor.

We should, however, at least consider the possibility that a well-functioning ethics mechanism can have a positive impact on the financial bottom line. Good communication and problem solving by the ethics mechanism may help avoid unnecessary and undesired treatments. More important, good communication may also defuse the kinds of misunderstandings, anger, and resentment that can drive lawsuits as well as "defensive medicine." Though these things might be true, the purpose or the goal of the ethics mechanism is not just saving money for the institution.

So let us assume, for the sake of argument, that clinical ethics work is one of those items that will never be a revenue generator, much less a profit center. Nevertheless, the services it provides are central to the endeavor of healthcare as an intensely human, personal, and professional value-laden activity. Indeed, without a flourishing clinical ethics mechanism, a healthcare organization performing in an excellent manner is highly unlikely. A vibrant clinical ethics mechanism, therefore, it not a luxury item for the organization.

For a clinical ethics service to survive, and to flourish, it needs the meaningful support of the organization. So what does that support look like? It takes several different forms:

Financial

Clearly, the clinical ethics service needs financial support from the organization to do its work. The service will need some office and support staff hours, some professional salaried time, and possibly some contractual fees for outside ethical expertise on a retainer basis. An accessible and functional office space is also needed. With a large clinical ethics committee (some institutions have committees with membership of two dozen or more), various clinical departments must be willing to commit professional time to this non-revenue-generating activity. Furthermore, some ethics services activities will incur further expenses, such as educational endeavors both within the organization itself as well as educational outreach to the community, not to mention educational training for the ethics mechanism members themselves. How should an organization think of this money? Thinking in terms of necessary overhead is probably more constructive than thinking in terms of case-based costs. Thinking of it as overhead weaves the service into the fabric of the organization, whereas thinking of it as cost for services rendered raises further fraught issues of reimbursements and unauthorized cost shifting.

Institutional Support

"Institutional support" means more than just money. Does the administration behave in ways that convey throughout the organization that leadership takes the ethics work seriously and values the efforts of those who are dedicated to it? Is the physical location of the clinical ethics office tucked away in a janitor's closet in a back hall somewhere? Or does it occupy a space that both those working in the organization and patients and families can readily find? In other words, does the organization take pride in its clinical ethics services, or does it show its lack of investment or even its disrespect by effectively hiding and ignoring it? Similarly, does the clinical ethics mechanism show up occasionally in internal media in the organization (e.g., newsletters, featured centers)? Is the service ever mentioned in the image the organization projects, such as for marketing purposes?

Does the organization not only allow but affirmatively set aside resources for and insist upon continuing education activities for all those who serve in the clinical ethics program, whether it be a committee or consultant model? Whether such efforts take the shape of in-service training seminars, an annual retreat for all committee members, earmarked funding for participation in bioethics conferences, or other options, such efforts can not only improve the ethics and facilitating skills of the clinical ethics program members, they can also improve the function of the program as a program and can help avoid burnout in those professionals who devote time to clinical ethics work. Think of these efforts as how one nurtures, sustains, and even improves a clinical ethics program.

Next, does the organization behave as an organization in ways that bolster the clinical ethics program or detract from it? For example, when annual reviews for professional and staff personnel come around, does the review process acknowledge and

---

Case Study

Elizabeth J. was airlifted from a rural hospital to an urban teaching hospital. She is 55 years old and apparently suffering from a newly acquired blood disorder: For some reason, she is no longer producing her own clotting factor. With significant internal bleeding and airway obstruction, she is rushed through the ED into the ICU. Once the initial dangers are stabilized, the team begins to administer a typical therapy for clotting disorders: porcine-produced clotting factor. But this treatment spurs an allergic reaction in Elizabeth J. After much intensive care, the medical team, in desperation, tries an experimental drug under a compassionate use dispensation. The experimental clotting factor works, though it, of course, does not cure Elizabeth J. of her clotting disorder. It simply saves her from bleeding to death.

Elizabeth J. is now stabilized, and the time has come to talk about discharge planning. But some clinicians are concerned: They have not cured Elizabeth J. And once she is sent home, she is liable to bump into something or somehow start another bleeding incident. Her current hospitalization has cost $1.7 million, in no small part because the only drug that worked was experimental. Medicaid has agreed to pay $42,000. The rest will have to be written off as uncollectable bad debt.

(continued)

appropriately reward efforts contributed to the clinical ethics activities, or are such individuals penalized (e.g., for not having as many revenue-generating hours in the clinic because of hours spent doing ethics work)?

Leadership

Perhaps most important is that the healthcare organization's senior administrators—its leaders—accept and perform their roles as moral leaders within the organization. Moral leadership is important for many facets of the organization's character and activities. But such leadership is crucial for the effectiveness of any clinical ethics program. Senior administrators need not be hands-on in the clinical ethics programs.

(continued from previous page)

Members of the clinical ethics committee are deeply divided in their discussion. Some argue that their clinical obligation is to do "whatever is best" for the individual patient. Clearly, if Elizabeth J. returns (as is likely), she will benefit from another course of the experimental drug. Other members of the committee worry that the financial stress imposed upon their medical unit, especially if Elizabeth J. returns, would undermine what they can offer future patients. They insist that the medical team should craft a discharge plan that strongly discourages Elizabeth J. from returning to your hospital, even though they acknowledge that her local community hospital will not be able to provide the life-saving care that your hospital has provided.

What should the clinical ethics committee advise for the discharge planning? To what degree does a medical professional's ethical obligation to advocate for the patient in her care at this moment trump an obligation to conserve scarce resources to potentially benefit unknown patients in the future? What is the organization's ethical obligation in this case?

However, the real attitude toward moral values that senior administrators display as leaders intimately affects the ethics of what happens at the clinical level. If an adverse message is broadcast—that the organization does not take moral commitments seriously—then the clinical ethics program has little chance of working effectively. It is far more likely to be idle, nonfunctioning "window dressing" for an organization that places little or no value on its work. On the other hand, if senior administrators demonstrate a commitment to ethical values as part of the nature and conduct of the healthcare organization, then the clinical ethics programs are far more likely to be respected, supported, appreciated, and used as part of the everyday life of the organization. This is something the ethical administrator and leader will certainly want to strive for.

Conclusion

The purpose of this chapter has not been to provide a how-to manual for a clinical ethics program. Rather, it has been intended to give administrators some insight into the nature and value of what a thriving clinical ethics program can provide for the healthcare organization. And once the nature of its value is understood, how administrators can facilitate the functioning and improvement of the clinical ethics program without having their own clinical ethics expertise becomes easier to see.

Points to Remember

- Although clinical ethics and organizational ethics may overlap, clinical ethics focuses on the delivery of patient care while organizational ethics focuses on the structure and the conduct of the organization that makes the delivery of that care possible. A decision in one realm often has ramifications for decisions and activities in another realm.
- The services or functions that are now commonly attached to the clinical ethics service or clinical ethics mechanisms are generally 1) consultation, 2) education, and 3) formulation of clinical ethics policies.
- Senior administration should have respect for the work that an effective clinical ethics mechanism performs for patients, families, professionals, staff, and the organization itself. Moreover, administrators should support and oversee this work.

References

American Society for Bioethics and Humanities (ASBH). 2010. *Core Competences for Health Care Ethics Consultation,* 2nd ed. Glenview, IL: American Society for Bioethics and Humanities.

Hall, R. T. 2000. *An Introduction to Healthcare Organizational Ethics.* New York: Oxford University Press.

Joint Commission. 2012. *Hospital Accreditation Standards.* Oakbrook Terrace, IL: The Joint Commission.

Levine, C. 2007. "Analyzing Pandora's Box: The History of Bioethics." In *The Ethics of Bioethics: Mapping the Moral Landscape*, edited by L. Eckenwiler and F. Cohn, 3–23. Baltimore, MD: Johns Hopkins University Press.

Ross, J. W., J. W. Glaser, J. D. Rasinski-Gregory, J. M. Gibson, and C. Bayler. 1993. *Health Care Ethics Committees: The Next Generation.* Chicago: American Hospital Publishing.

Spencer, E. M., A. E. Mills, M. V. Rorty, and P. H. Werhane. 2000. *Organization Ethics in Health Care.* New York: Oxford University Press.

MORAL DISTRESS AND THE HEALTHCARE ORGANIZATION

Ann B. Hamric, Elizabeth G. Epstein, and Kenneth R. White

This chapter is relevant to the following competencies identified in the ACHE Competencies Assessment Tool (see p. xxv):

Communication and Relationship Management
- Demonstrate effective interpersonal relations
- Facilitate conflict and alternative dispute resolution

Leadership
- Potential impacts and consequences of decision making in situations both internal and external
- Foster an environment of mutual trust

Professionalism
- Mentor, advise, and coach

Business Skills and Knowledge
- Organizational dynamics, political realities, and culture
- Principles and practices of management and organizational behavior

Learning Objectives

After completing this chapter, the reader will be able to

- define moral distress, moral residue, and the Crescendo Effect;
- discuss common sources of moral distress in the healthcare setting;
- discuss three implications of the Crescendo Effect for healthcare organizations;

- describe how unaddressed moral distress can damage healthcare providers, teams, administrators, and organizations; and
- develop three strategies for addressing moral distress at these organizational levels:
  - Patient level
  - Team/unit level
  - Organization/systems level

Introduction

The provision of healthcare to sick and vulnerable individuals represents a profoundly moral practice. Healthcare professionals are (or ought to be) socialized into being effective moral agents rather than simply skilled technicians. As such, supporting and safeguarding the moral integrity of providers is a key obligation of leaders in healthcare organizations. Ethical issues are commonplace in healthcare organizations—whether they are specific to a patient, health professional, caregiving team, or manager. Typically, ethical problems involve a particular patient or a particular event. The classic understanding of an ethical dilemma involves identifying the most ethically justifiable option among competing choices. Once the decision is reached and the event passed, the ethical dilemma may no longer exist. Ethical problems can also emanate from managerial decisions that could affect groups of employees, physicians, patients, or external stakeholders. Although challenging, ethical problems often generate productive debate on the pros and cons of available options. In this way, discourse can be a healthy sign that the appropriateness of various treatment options or managerial decisions is being considered and that members of the healthcare team are morally engaged and genuinely concerned about the decisions that govern the outcomes of care they provide.

Moral distress
Occurs when individuals perceive that they are constrained from taking an ethically appropriate action. As a result, they experience compromised moral agency.

Similarly, **moral distress** is a common experience in every healthcare setting, not only for healthcare providers and caregiving teams but for managers, executives, and leaders. Moral distress occurs when an individual knows or thinks he knows the ethically appropriate action to take but is constrained from taking the action (Jameton 1984). In contrast to classic ethical dilemmas that focus on identifying the ethically justifiable action in a particular situation, however, moral distress extends beyond the particular patient or event and reflects deeper problems related to unit or system practices and environments. For senior-level managers, moral distress may emanate from interactions and relationships with trustees, senior executives, physicians, and other key stakeholders. Although examples of moral distress exist in the healthcare management literature (ACHE 2011b; Boyle et al. 2001; Suhonen et al. 2011; Worthley 1997), they are described under the rubric of organizational or managerial ethics. Whether patient-related or a matter affecting employees, physicians, or community healthcare services, moral distress often is not recognized in ethical deliberations at the individual patient, unit, ethics committee, or senior management and governance levels. This situation is a problem because the experience of moral distress is neither productive nor healthy. Rather, moral distress can damage individuals, teams, units, and even institutions. Administrators at every level of a healthcare institution must understand moral distress as it relates to demonstrated competencies and ethical practices (ACHE 2011a, 2011b; Healthcare Leadership Alliance 2010) and the dangers it poses to individuals within healthcare organizations and to organizations themselves. In this understanding, moral distress can be a critically important warning sign for administrators that something is not right and more investigation is necessary. Further, early attention to experiences of moral distress and explicit strategies to manage moral distress in the workplace can contribute to healthier work environments, more satisfied stakeholders, and a transformational organizational culture.

Moral distress has been present among caregiving professionals in healthcare organizations for many years; it was identified and named in the nursing literature almost 30 years ago (Jameton 1984). But the phenomenon has only recently garnered sustained attention leading to systematic research, particularly in disciplines such as medicine and respiratory therapy (Hamric and Blackhall 2007; Schwenzer and Wang 2006; Wiggleton et al. 2010). Although a fundamental competency for healthcare executives is promoting a positive ethical climate in healthcare organizations (see Chapter 14), a paucity of research exists articulating the healthcare leader's role in addressing moral distress (Bell and Breslin 2008; Suhonen et al. 2011). This chapter addresses moral distress, its root causes, and its manifestations at individual patient/family, workgroup/team, and organizational/systems levels. Our goal is for administrators to understand moral distress—and its potentially damaging consequences for themselves and for individual providers—and to make the connection to managerial, professional, and organizational ethics to develop shared values that sustain healthy work environments and cultures in which caregiving occurs. Strategies to address moral distress and minimize its occurrence are presented.

Understanding Moral Distress

Moral distress was initially defined as occurring when a person cannot carry out what she believes to be an ethically appropriate action because of institutional constraints (Jameton 1984). We now understand that moral distress

Compassion fatigue
The inability to continue to provide help and care in crisis situations because of repeated exposure to these situations.

Burnout
Emotional or physical exhaustion caused by prolonged stress or frustration.

Psychological distress
The physical and emotional symptoms that arise in stressful or emotional circumstances.

emanates from a variety of root causes, including factors internal to the individual, clinical situations, and external constraints (i.e., hierarchies, fear of legal action, restrictive policies) (Hamric 2012). The combination of the presence of a moral obligation or core value and constraint from acting on that obligation or value is what makes moral distress unique from other concepts, such as compassion fatigue, burnout, or psychological distress (Epstein and Hamric 2009). **Compassion fatigue** in the healthcare setting is the inability to continue to provide help and care in crisis situations because of repeated exposure to these situations (Figley 1995). **Burnout** is described as emotional or physical exhaustion caused by prolonged stress or frustration. **Psychological distress** describes the physical and emotional symptoms that arise in stressful or emotional circumstances. While all contain similar elements, only moral distress involves the compromise of a moral obligation or core value. This distinction is important because this moral component so profoundly affects one's experience of her moral integrity and view of her profession. This perceived compromise to one's moral integrity may be linked to an increased risk of burnout among healthcare providers (Meltzer and Huckabay 2004) and to administrators as well, as can be seen in the following case:

I have been a healthcare administrator for more than 30 years. For the first 24 years in less senior administrative positions and with various CEOs at the helm, I was always able to advocate for our patients and employees. However, in the past six years in the position of chief operating officer, I have gone through two CEOs and repeatedly had to survive moral distress created by a lack of corrective action regarding inappropriate physician behavior, specifically lack of responsiveness to patient care concerns.

I receive regular complaints about one particular doctor who will not return pages, is not responsive in timely rounding, and is disrespectful to staff. Problem reports are regularly filed. Patient outcomes are not the best. The chief medical officer (CMO) is a former medical practice colleague of the offending physician. When problems with this physician arise, the CMO says he will follow up, but nothing is done. The CEO's response is that the physician is a top admitter and has a busy practice. I believe that we are placing our patients in danger, and it keeps me up at night. On most issues I have the support of the newest CEO, however, physicians with high volumes seem to be untouchable when it comes to disciplinary action.

As a seasoned administrator I know the importance of juggling financial concerns with quality of care and competing stakeholder interests. However, I feel like my hands are tied when it comes to protecting and advocating for better patient care. I am at the end of my rope and ready to leave the profession because

I believe too many decisions are made for financial reasons at the expense of patient care quality. The mission and values of this organization are a sham.

Levels at Which Moral Distress Is Experienced

Moral distress is complex because it can manifest at one or more of three levels:

1. patient/family,
2. unit/team, and
3. organization/system.

Most often, moral distress is initiated by a particular patient situation, and most literature on moral distress emphasizes this level (Epstein and Delgado 2010; Hamric 2010; Ulrich, Hamric, and Grady 2010). However, moral distress is rarely if ever *only* about that particular case. On digging more deeply, team, unit, and even system problems that underlie these individual patient situations become clear—poor communication routines between providers, lack of unit-to-unit interaction, lack of policy to guide appropriate action, inadequate staffing, inappropriate use of resources, and hierarchical hospital structures that limit providers' abilities to be assertive.

These different levels of involvement become apparent when clinicians, for example, would call to discuss a particular patient problem and within five minutes had related similar stories involving numerous other patients. A sense of repeated encounters revealed that the root problems were within the team or unit or with the larger system. An example illustrates this point:

An ethics consultant was approached by a nurse manager to lead a team discussion of a patient who had received inadequate pain management upon admission. As the discussion proceeded, nurses began recounting other situations, and the real problem was quickly identified as the structure of the medical team managing this group of patients with gastrointestinal (GI) disorders and complex pain management needs. The GI team signed off to a resident on an internal medicine service on Friday afternoon and did not have any contact with their patients until Monday morning. Nurses were unable to obtain adequate pain management orders from these medicine residents when patients were admitted on the weekend. The nurses were distressed in feeling "in the middle" between patients who were clearly in pain and requesting or demanding stronger pain medicine and house officers who would not order such medication because of their unfamiliarity with the complexities of the patients' problems.

As the nurses discussed the situation, they understood the reluctance of the internal medicine residents to prescribe sufficient pain medications because the patients were unstable and complex to manage. Further, they recognized that the root cause was really the structure of the GI medical team and its system of weekend coverage; this identification allowed for different strategies focused on team communications and processes to ensure GI team coverage and pain management protocols that staff could employ on weekends.

To extend the example to the organization and system level, consider what may be discovered on further investigation:

Near the first of July every year when the newly minted house staff arrive on the scene, the administrator-on-call is regularly called by the house supervisor on weekends because house staff are unable to locate the GI attending physician to obtain pain control orders. The administrator's hands are tied because he has been warned in the past not to get involved in the medical management of a patient and that the "chief resident or fellow will sort it out."

In this example, the moral distress is elevated to the organization level, the root cause is ignored, and the problem is perpetuated. The policy or accepted practice produces an outcome again and again that causes moral distress.

Crescendo Effect
A model describing the interaction over time between increasing moral distress in repeated situations and increasing moral residue that lingers in the aftermath of recurring moral distress.

The Crescendo Effect

The recurrence of morally distressing problems in similar clinical situations can give rise to the **Crescendo Effect** (Exhibit 7.1). Short-term moral distress occurs as a clinical situation or organizational event develops. As the situation unfolds, the levels of moral distress among providers and managers and administrators may increase or crescendo. When the situation resolves, the level of moral distress drops significantly. Moral distress levels, however, do not necessarily return to zero once a situation is ended. Rather, after experiences where moral distress is not acknowledged or addressed, a residual amount of distress remains. This long-term component of moral distress is more commonly called **moral residue** (Webster and Bayliss 2000). Many providers vividly remember morally distressing situations as if they occurred just the day before. The frustration, anger, and hurt are quickly recalled. Repeated exposure to moral distress may lead to ever-increasing levels of moral residue. This moral residue crescendo is thought to be at least partly responsible for negative outcomes, such as moral numbness, burnout, and leaving a healthcare profession (Epstein and Hamric 2009). This model was derived from studies of nurses and physicians; while to our knowledge no study of moral distress and related outcomes among administrators has yet been undertaken, the model may apply to administrators as well.

Moral residue
Feelings that linger after a morally distressing situation that caused an individual to be seriously compromised.

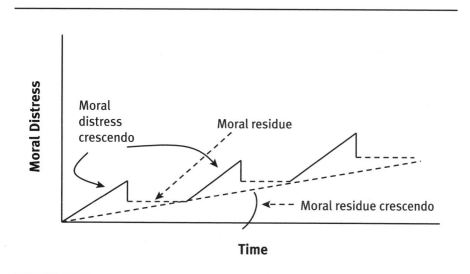

EXHIBIT 7.1
Moral Distress and Moral Residue Crescendos

Source: Epstein and Hamric (2009).

Moral distress and moral residue are often described together using the broader sense of the term *moral distress*. However, clinicians, unit managers, and healthcare administrators must understand the differences in terms, as these two elements of the Crescendo Effect have different consequences, require different skill sets for management, and need different intervention plans.

In the healthcare organization, the Crescendo Effect may arise from top-down decisions (governance to executive management, executive to middle management, middle management to frontline unit management); from bottom-up situations (patient to provider or caregiving team); or between team members (nurse to doctor, between nurses or caregiving team members). This chapter concentrates on the caregiving team's moral distress at the individual provider level, administrator or leader moral distress at the organizational level, and the connections between them.

Moral Distress and the Individual

Emotional strain is unavoidable in the high-intensity milieu of the modern healthcare organization. Situations can occur daily that evoke strong emotions, such as anger, sadness, relief, frustration, and anxiety. Individuals who are morally distressed can exhibit any of these emotions. In fact, moral distress is *always* emotionally distressing. Added to these, however are emotions that reveal compromises to one's moral integrity—decreased self-worth, powerlessness, guilt, and self-blame (Elpern, Covert, and Kleinpell 2005; Gordon and Hamric 2006; Wilkinson 1988). For providers, the sadness, the suffering, or even patient deaths are not problematic. Rather, the moments of being unheard, of feeling required to inflict pain on individuals who will not reap benefit, of being unable to advocate for the vulnerable, are most dangerous and most likely to affect them for months, years, and decades. These moments can take an enormous toll on providers. For administrators, moral distress caused by situations such as being unable to convince a governing board to make a difficult decision or being unable to advocate for staff in the face of severe cost pressure may also exact a toll on the administrator's moral agency. Consider the following case:

MA was a 62-year-old man who, during a complex surgical procedure, suffered serious complications including cardiac arrest. CPR was successful and MA was admitted to the medical intensive care unit for recovery. Over the next few days, it became apparent that neurological damage had occurred. MA was unable to move his left side and could not speak. Because he tracked movement of people in the room and was able to nod and shake his head, the initial belief was that MA would recover some neurological function in time, and that he would need long-term rehabilitation for maximal progress. After two weeks in the hospital, he was transferred to a transitional care facility, approximately two miles from the hospital. This new facility provides medical care and rehabilitation and is designed to be used for patients who are likely to be able to return home within three to five months.

MA continued to live at the transitional care facility for more than a year. During that time he did not regain motor or speech function and suffered repeated strokes. With each stroke, he was taken by ambulance to the acute care hospital. Each time, he recovered and was returned to the transitional care facility. However, after each transfer, MA was in worse neurological condition. After his fourth stroke, his kidneys failed and he required dialysis. He also suffered calciphylaxis, an extremely painful condition of vascular calcification and tissue necrosis due to poor kidney function. MA's worsening condition, and his need for more intensive nursing, physical therapy, and respiratory therapy support, dismayed the transitional care team because they lacked staffing to provide the level of care he required. They questioned the appropriateness of his repeated admissions to their facility, given the reality that he would not be able to return home. They increasingly expressed their moral distress over providing care that they did not believe was of benefit to MA. However, his family was adamant that MA continue to receive aggressive treatment and remain in the transitional care facility, despite his deteriorating condition.

The transitional care administrator felt trapped in the middle. While she understood and respected the staff's objections, the unit was new and trying to establish its place in the community—an angry family was the last thing they needed in terms of publicity. In addition, building positive referral patterns was necessary to keep the unit's census high enough to ensure financial viability. The acute care hospital exerted strong financial pressure to have MA returned to the transitional care unit each time his clinical situation stabilized—the hospital had its own problems with length of stay that compromised reimbursement, and one of its solutions was to discharge patients such as MA as soon as possible. The administrator struggled with the facility's need to serve as a necessary bridge for patients in their transition from the acute care hospital to home and the concerns of her staff that MA was not the type of patient they had "signed on for." Two nurses and a respiratory therapist resigned as a result of this case.

Note the elements of staff powerlessness, of being unheard and unable to act on their core obligations of effective rehabilitation and provision of quality care. But also note the administrator's moral uncertainty over this situation. The administrator also may be experiencing moral distress if she believes that her chief obligations are to advocate for her staff and to ensure appropriate admissions to the transitional care facility.

Epstein and Hamric (2009) described three potential outcomes of moral distress: becoming "routinized" to the moral dimensions of problematic cases (Chambliss 1996), **conscientious objection** (Catlin et al. 2008), or burnout and leaving the profession (Corley 1995; Meltzer and Huckabay 2004). In a recent study (Hamric, Borchers, and Epstein 2012), moral distress levels were significantly higher in providers who were considering leaving their positions because of moral distress, with 11 percent of ICU physician participants and 20 percent of the nurse participants reporting that they were considering leaving their positions because of moral distress.

> **Conscientious objection**
> Refusal to perform a specific legal role, responsibility, or other activity because of moral or other personal beliefs.

Moral Distress and Organizational Leadership

Moral distress is described but not named in the management literature. Leaders and researchers call it *ethical challenges in practice* (Bosa 2010; Nelson et al. 2009), *conscientious objection* (Morton and Kirkwood 2009), *organizational ethics* (Suhonen et al. 2011), *clash of personal and organizational values* (Badaracco 1998), *promise making, keeping, and rescinding* (ACHE 2011b), and *conflicts in priority setting and resource allocation* (Mitton et al. 2011). Mitton, Peacock, and Storch (2010) identified two examples of moral distress among healthcare managers:

1. Managers having to "sell" a direction or decision that they themselves do not believe in
2. Managers breaking their obligations to staff or colleagues

Other examples of moral distress arise from the way resources are allocated, decisions about powerful people who may be acting unethically, and a conflict of personal and organizational values. One board member described an example of moral distress:

As chairperson of the compensation committee of the board of trustees, I am responsible for conducting an annual performance review of the CEO. Understanding the true picture of a CEO's performance is sometimes difficult because the board relies on the CEO to submit agenda items, summary reports, and to keep the board informed. Before the board chairperson and I met to discuss the CEO's performance, the CEO approached the chairperson to request a $100,000 increase in compensation to be comparable with some national salary study. I believe the CEO is doing a good job, but a salary increase of that magnitude is unwarranted. This creates moral distress because I am confident we could find another CEO for far less money and we could use that money to hire more nurses.

Sarbanes-Oxley Act of 2002
A federal law requiring organizations to place a greater emphasis on corporate responsibility, regulatory compliance, and ethics at all levels of management and governance.

The implementation of the **Sarbanes-Oxley Act of 2002** required a greater emphasis on corporate responsibility and regulatory compliance with more focus on issues of ethics at all levels of management and governance. Although the law applies to publicly owned entities, many healthcare organizations responded by implementing similar policies about ethical issues such as divulging conflict of interest and anonymous reporting of suspected violations. An increasing emphasis on healthy work environments is intended to reduce horizontal violence (bullying), harassment, and fear related to speaking up about potentially unethical, illegal, or procedural issues that may violate the organization's policies.

With increased emphasis on transformational leadership and evidence-based management as pathways to high-performing healthcare organizations (White and Griffith 2010), identifying and dealing with moral distress represents an important commitment to shared values, transparency in decision making, and improving an organization's ethical climate (Bell and Breslin 2008). In exploratory work in Canada, Mitton, Peacock, and Storch (2010) found the most often reported consequence of moral distress among healthcare managers to be serious personal health problems without taking sick time off. Other reported consequences included decreased productivity, impaired workplace relationships, diminished staff morale, and impaired family and interpersonal relationships caused by not being able to leave work behind.

Strategies to Address Moral Distress

A major concern about moral distress and moral residue in the workplace is that repeated situations of moral distress will lead those with valuable skills and knowledge to feel disempowered and leave their position or even their profession. In the current healthcare climate, where patient care is clinically and ethically complex, healthcare professionals who are engaged and skilled in the clinical and moral aspects of their work and administrators with skill in managing complex organizations are critical to any organization's success. To maintain this highly skilled and sophisticated workforce, attention to moral distress and moral residue is a necessary role of the organizational leader. Building an organizational culture committed to minimizing the Crescendo Effect will take time and sustained effort at all levels of an organization's leadership. Efforts at individual team levels that are not supported by the larger institution are unlikely to result in a meaningful change; likewise, top-level administrative dictates will not necessarily lead to unit-level changes without clinicians seeing the need and having the skills to address moral distress.

Patient and Unit-Level Strategies

In spite of recent attention to the problems of moral distress, few reports of evidence-based interventions exist, and those that do have focused on nurses and providing education. This section surveys interventions that have been proposed but have yet to be studied systematically.

While the previous discussion clearly shows that strategies for addressing moral distress and preventing the buildup of moral residue must go beyond the presenting case, the case may present a place to start. Individual clinicians must be encouraged to recognize and speak up about their moral distress (Gordon and Hamric 2006; Hamric 2000; Hamric, Davis, and Childress 2006). Ulrich, Hamric, and Grady (2010) recommend open dialogue that includes patients, providers, and administrative personnel. Expressions of concern by any clinician should be seen as an opportunity for dialogue, not ignored or minimized. Promoting proactive, preventive-oriented discussions of moral distress among teams is most critical, because moral distress is often experienced by different team members in different ways (Hamric, Davis, and Childress 2006). Some team members may not experience moral distress at all, even though their colleagues do. Recognizing moral distress and the subjective nature of the experience is the first step. Educational programs to define and discuss moral distress can take the form of continuing education, time for ethics conversations on interdisciplinary bedside rounds, or scheduled grand rounds—the particular strategy selected needs to be woven into the educational approaches already in place and supported by clinicians and administrators. An informal unit-based ethics conversation program for nurses is well described by Helft and colleagues (2009). Interdisciplinary conversations that include at best all caregiving team members but at least nurses and physicians are important to highlight the various perspectives of different disciplines. While educational strategies are an important initial approach to highlight the problem of moral distress and they can validate the experiences of providers, education by itself is probably insufficient to result in meaningful change in institutional cultures.

Team discussions need to focus first on open and respectful communication that seeks to identify the root causes of moral distress. Ground rules may need to be established to create a safe space where every person is respected, heard, and does not fear reprisal. Recognizing that conversations about moral distress are challenging, even for well-functioning teams, is important. Experiences of moral distress threaten one's core values and sense of obligation; individuals may feel vulnerable sharing such deep-seated sources of their moral integrity, especially when their views are threatened or in conflict with others. Facilitators familiar with moral distress who can keep the discussion focused and respectful may be helpful in these conversations (Helft et al. 2009); leaders must tangibly support taking time from busy clinician schedules for such dialogues.

Patient situations leading to moral distress are often characterized by poor communication and lack of clear-cut patient treatment goals. The importance of early and ongoing conversations among team members, patients, and their families about the goals of treatment needs to be emphasized by organizational and clinical leaders. Hamric and Blackhall (2007) noted that most successful interventions to improve decision making at the end of life involved two characteristics: they improved communication within the team, and they brought nursing and physician perspectives together with the perspectives of patients and their caregivers. Ulrich, Hamric, and Grady (2010) further recommended interdisciplinary education and collegial practice as two strategies to decrease moral distress. Administrators have a crucial role to play in developing and supporting strategies at both unit and team levels of their organizations.

A nurse manager, reflecting on the toll moral distress was taking in nursing staff turnover, offered a number of strategies for unit-level leaders. While these strategies focus on nursing, they are useful for anyone in a leadership position. Her "sensible solutions" included (Coles 2010)

- know your staff,
- educate your staff,
- challenge the culture,
- use your resources, and
- match staffing to the requirements of the patients' conditions using objective data.

System-Level Strategies

Because of each institution's unique culture, no single strategy to address moral distress is universally applicable. The strategies presented in this section are intended to serve not as "cookbooks" but as launching points for discussion and development of tailored, workable approaches that meet a particular organization's needs and capabilities.

Organizational leaders are advocates for the institution's mission and values. An important aspect of this advocacy role is to apply the organization's mission and values to all levels of the organization, from high-level administration to individual units (Iltis 2005). Thus, mission and value statements can and should be used to guide intervention development and implementation. For example, suppose that the respiratory therapy staff on a medical ICU at Hospital A have reported moral distress when patients undergo multiple intubation attempts by interns before a more skilled professional intubates the patient. They feel that, in some but not all cases, patient care is compromised. If the mission of Hospital A includes a statement about teaching as a primary focus, the strategy to address the staff's moral distress might be very different than if the mission statement clearly states that efficient, highly skilled patient care is the primary focus. In either case, strategies may include adjustments in practice routines, improved communication between attending physicians and respiratory therapy, or changes in patient monitoring. In the teaching-intensive situation, changes in practice routines might include increased recovery time between attempts or increased respiratory therapy involvement. In the patient-care-focused situation, agreement on limits for intubation attempts may be more appropriate. In both cases, moral distress is addressed, but the solutions differ based on institutional mission. Tailored interventions, therefore, will likely be more successful in creating a culture that responds purposefully to moral distress.

Ethics consultation services (ECS) deserve special mention. (See Chapter 6 for a description of an ethics consultation service.) Having an ethics committee is not enough. Consultation services need to be available at all times, and staff need to know how to access them and be supported in doing so (Gordon and Hamric 2006); consultation needs to be effective, and ongoing evaluation is necessary. However, even with these features, ethics consultants who only focus on the case may not be effective in helping staff recognize and decrease their moral distress. Because moral distress goes beyond the case, clinicians who only think to call the ECS for a problematic case and facilitators who don't look beyond the case may miss the unit/team and organizational/system issues that are causing recurrent problems and a buildup of moral residue.

Two national organizations have addressed the issue of moral distress. The **American Association of Critical-Care Nurses** (AACN) developed a position statement on moral distress and proposed prescriptive strategies for employers to use to decrease moral distress and create a healthy work environment (AACN 2008). These and other strategies described in the literature are listed in Exhibit 7.2.

American Association of Critical-Care Nurses
A professional association focused on providing its members the knowledge, skills, and abilities they need to provide optimal care to critically ill patients.

EXHIBIT 7.2 Strategies to Mitigate the Harmful Effects of Moral Distress	Implement interdisciplinary strategies to recognize and name the experience of moral distress.
	Establish mechanisms to monitor the clinical and organizational climate to identify recurring situations that result in moral distress.
	Develop systematic processes for • reviewing and analyzing the system issues enabling situations that cause moral distress to occur and • taking corrective action.
	Consider unit-based ethics conversations facilitated by a clinical ethicist (Wocial et al. 2010).
	Develop a moral distress consultation service (Epstein and Hamric 2009).
	Create support systems that include the following: • Employee assistance programs • Protocols for advance care planning (end-of-life care) • Ethics committees • Critical stress debriefings, counseling, and spiritual services after difficult and traumatic occurrences • Grief counseling • The services of an ethicist
	Extend the purpose of ethics committees (beyond bioethics) to include consideration of managerial and organizational ethics policies, issues, and problem-solving mechanisms.
	Be familiar with professional codes of ethics and ethical policy statements (e.g., American College of Healthcare Executives, American Nurses' Association's *Code of Ethics for Nurses*).
	Create healthy workplace policies and initiatives.
	Create interdisciplinary forums to discuss patient goals of care and divergent opinions in an open, respectful environment.
	Develop policies that support unobstructed access to resources such as the ethics committees.
	Ensure nurses and other clinical staff are represented on institutional ethics committees with full participation in all decision making.
	Provide education and tools to manage and decrease moral distress in the work environment.

The US Department of Veterans Affairs (VA 2013) has developed a set of materials as part of its **IntegratedEthics Initiative**. Based on quality improvement principles and strategies for organizational change, the

IntegratedEthics initiative is a comprehensive, systemwide program with three components: ethics consultation, preventive ethics, and ethical leadership. The latter two components of the initiative have utility for any healthcare organization dealing with moral distress. Preventive ethics describes a quality improvement system that focuses on recurrent ethical problems at unit or systems levels and addresses moral distress explicitly. Ethical leadership focuses on helping leaders create responsive ethical environments. While a full description of this initiative is beyond the scope of this chapter, the reader is encouraged to examine the detailed materials that have been developed by the VA's National Center for Ethics in Health Care.

In summary, the strategies for addressing moral distress emanate from a commitment to ethics and ethical decision making that is consistent with the organization's mission, vision, and values. A number of the strategies listed here are not explicitly aimed at managing moral distress. Rather, leaders and managers who develop a culture anchored in sound ethical decision making and procedures to use when ethical issues arise should find it easier to manage moral distress. Strategies that have been adopted by nurses and the clinical professions are a first step but may be inadequate to address what appears to be a pervasive phenomenon from a systems perspective. The American College of Healthcare Executives has led in promoting ethics policy statements, improving ethics education, and raising awareness of leadership's role in establishing an ethical organizational climate. More could be done by including moral distress and explicitly naming ways to manage it.

> **IntegratedEthics Initiative**
> A comprehensive, systemwide ethics program based on quality improvement principles and strategies for organizational change; developed by the US Department of Veterans Affairs. The initiative has three components: ethics consultation, preventive ethics, and ethical leadership.

Conclusion

Moral distress and moral residue are real phenomena that can compromise the moral integrity of healthcare providers and staff at all levels of an organization. Dealing with these damaging phenomena is a challenge for administrators and clinicians alike. The management literature is only beginning to discuss moral distress and to identify specific strategies to address it. Institutional leaders must first acknowledge that moral distress may be a real and serious issue in their organization. They need to identify the Crescendo Effect as it occurs in recurrent patient, unit, or management situations. Strategies for minimizing moral distress will need to be developed at patient/family, unit/team, and organizational/systems levels for moral distress to be mitigated throughout an organization. Knowledge and skill in managing moral distress must be evident at all levels of an organization, from the night staff personnel to the top level administrators to the governing board.

Points to Remember

- *Moral distress* occurs in situations where an individual knows or thinks she knows the ethically appropriate action but is constrained from taking that action. *Moral residue* describes the feelings that remain after situations of moral distress, when an individual feels that her moral integrity has been compromised. The *Crescendo Effect* hypothesizes that these two phenomena gradually increase in situations of repeated, unaddressed moral distress.
- Moral distress arises at individual/patient, unit/team, and organizational/system levels.
- Experiences of moral distress are not limited to any one profession. Any healthcare provider, manager, or administrator can experience moral distress and moral residue.
- The management literature is beginning to address moral distress, but more studies of administrators are needed. In addition, more strategies for minimizing moral distress need to be developed and studied.
- A focus on ethics is necessary but not sufficient to deal with the Crescendo Effect.

Cases and Questions

1. Consider the following case:

   Lisa was an experienced nurse who had left an orthopedic unit for a 40-bed inpatient surgical ICU six months ago. She made the change to critical care because of the ability to focus on one or two patients; as Lisa stated, "I loved caring for and really getting to know my patients." The culture on this unit was to rotate nurses to care for different patients every two to three days, even if the patient the nurse had cared for and come to know well was still in the unit. Lisa met with her unit manager and requested to be assigned the same patient each shift she worked; the manager agreed. Lisa's second long-term patient was Mr. George.

   Mr. George was a 67-year-old Caucasian man who was admitted to the ICU following bilateral carotid endarterectomies for severe carotid stenosis. He had a long history of smoking, mild COPD, and peripheral arterial disease. Mr. George was married and had no children. He lived at home with his wife of many years. He was retired from his work as a salesman and the couple had relocated to the area four months before his surgery.

Mrs. George was a thin, quiet, unassuming woman. She would come to the hospital early each morning and sit at his bedside holding his hand during every visiting period. She confided in Lisa that she was intimidated by the setting and the surgeon and just wanted to take him home. She also expressed the difficulty she was facing personally with her husband hospitalized as she tried to get situated in their new home and learn her way around a new city. She did not know many people in the area as they had just relocated when Mr. George became increasingly ill and hospitalized. As she said, "He is the people person. I don't know anyone here."

Lisa cared for Mr. George nearly every shift she worked for five weeks. Immediately post op Mr. George was alert and responsive and, although he was intubated, he was able to follow commands and communicate using hand signals and a whiteboard. He had a wonderful sense of humor and took the ups and downs in stride. However, Mr. George's condition progressively deteriorated, with his post-op course complicated by pleural effusions, a deep vein thrombosis in the right leg, and a pneumothorax requiring a chest tube. He remained ventilator-dependent and failed several attempts to wean from the ventilator. He eventually received a tracheotomy.

Mr. George was taken back to surgery six times for different procedures and with each event he grew worse. No one was talking to Mrs. George about her husband's prognosis. She would sign consents for procedures or surgeries asking very few questions of the physician. Her questions would come later, and finding a surgeon or resident available to speak with her was difficult.

On several occasions Lisa's charge nurse encouraged her to take a different assignment, and during two shifts she was told that her assignment would be to care for patients other than Mr. George. The management team was worried that she was getting too involved and becoming too close to the patient and his wife. However, Lisa continued to request to care for Mr. George. She had grown close to his wife and realized that she was a main source of support for this frightened woman who had few contacts in this new city. Even though Mrs. George did receive social work and pastoral care consultations during her husband's hospitalization, she always sought out Lisa to talk with.

After a long weekend off, Lisa arrived at work on Monday morning and was told that Mr. George had had a very bad night. He had coded twice and survived. His wife had been called and was on the way in. The resident was coming up to see her to speak to her about withdrawing support. Lisa went in to see Mr. George. He was puffy, swollen, unresponsive, and hardly resembled the man who had arrived on the unit five weeks earlier. The physicians met with Mrs. George, and the decision was made to withdraw the ventilator and the vasopressors. Mrs. George was to be allowed to sit at her husband's bedside as much as she wanted. By 10:00 a.m., the ventilator had been turned off and the drugs had been weaned down. Mr. George did not die. By three o'clock in the afternoon Mr. George had been extubated and his breathing became agonal but still Mr. George did not die.

Around 4:00 p.m., the ICU received a call from the emergency department that they needed a bed for a patient who had suffered a drug overdose. The charge nurse approached Lisa and told her that they were going to move Mr. George downstairs to the medical unit and that she would be getting the new admission. The charge nurse said that he was the only patient who was stable enough to move. Lisa requested to be allowed to accompany them to the new unit but was told no and a transport team arrived to move Mr. George downstairs. Lisa again spoke to the charge nurse and told her that she believed it was wrong for Mr. and Mrs. George to be transferred off the unit when he could die at any moment. The charge nurse was sympathetic but said that she had no choice because "We need the bed." Lisa asked a third time if someone else could care for the new patient so that she could at least accompany the George's to his new room but was again told no; instead, she was instructed to prepare Mr. George's room for the new admission.

As Lisa tells the story, she comments, "I did as I was told. I cleaned the room and received report from the ED. I admitted a 27-year-old patient who had attempted suicide by taking an overdose of Tylenol. She had been given activated charcoal and was vomiting and had severe diarrhea. She was loud and angry and difficult. I was feeling overwhelmed and could not stop thinking about Mr. and Mrs. George. One of my colleagues helped me get my new patient settled in and at 6:45 p.m. I was able to give report to the oncoming shift. By 7:30 p.m. I had completed all of the admission paperwork and could finally leave the unit. I ran down three flights of stairs and down the hall to Mr. George's new room. Mr. George had died and Mrs. George was gone." (The authors thank Lisa Manthey, RN, for writing and sharing this case.) Identify the sources of moral distress in this case. What were the root causes of Lisa's moral distress? Could she have explored other options? What steps could you take as an administrator to prevent or minimize what happened to Lisa?

2. Take one of the cases described in the chapter. Identify potential root causes for each level: patient/family, unit/team, and organization/ system. What strategies could you as an administrator employ to

help staff deal with their moral distress in this situation? What needs to change at an institutional level to prevent this situation from recurring?

3. Moral distress often has its origin in poor communication and lack of collaboration among healthcare team members. If you were to join an organization where this was an issue for a particular team, what strategies could you develop to work with teams to improve their communication and collaboration?

4. Because moral distress occurs at multiple levels, addressing this phenomenon is not a simple matter of developing institution-wide procedures or writing a mission statement about supporting ethical practice. Develop an approach for an institution-wide effort to acknowledge and address moral distress within an organization.

Note: The authors appreciate the distinctions between the terms *moral* and *ethical* as used in this text. However, these distinctions are not drawn in the moral distress literature; as a consequence, this chapter treats the terms interchangeably.

References

American Association of Critical-Care Nurses (AACN). 2008. "Position Statement on Moral Distress." Accessed March 8, 2013. www.aacn.org/WD/practice /Docs/Moral_Distress.pdf.

American College of Healthcare Executives (ACHE). 2011a. "Code of Ethics." Accessed March 8, 2013. www.ache.org/ABT_ACHE/code.cfm.

———. 2011b. "Ethical Policy Statements." Accessed March 8, 2013. www.ache .org/policy/index_ethics.cfm.

Badaracco, J. L. 1998. "The Discipline of Building Character." *Harvard Business Review* March–April: 104–13.

Bell, J., and J. M. Breslin. 2008. "Moral Distress as a Leadership Challenge." *JONA's Healthcare Law, Ethics, and Regulation* 10 (4): 94–97.

Bosa, I. M. 2010. "Ethical Budgets: A Critical Success Factor in Implementing New Public Management Accountability in Health Care." *Health Services Management Research* 23 (2): 76–83.

Boyle, P. J., E. R. DuBose, S. J. Ellingson, D. E. Guinn, and D. B. McCurdy. 2001. *Organizational Ethics in Health Care: Principles, Cases, and Practical Solutions.* San Francisco: Jossey-Bass.

Catlin, A., C. Armigo, D. Volat, E. Vale, M. A. Hadley, W. Gong, R. Bassir, and K. Anderson. 2008. "Conscientious Objection: A Potential Neonatal Nursing

Response to Care Orders That Cause Suffering at the End of Life? Study of a Concept." *Neonatal Network* 27 (2): 101–108.

Chambliss, D. 1996. *Beyond Caring: Hospitals, Nurses, and the Social Organization of Ethics.* Chicago: University of Chicago Press.

Coles, D. 2010. "Because We Can . . . Leadership Responsibility and the Moral Distress Dilemma." *Nursing Management* 41 (3): 26–30.

Corley, M. C. 1995. "Moral Distress of Critical Care Nurses." *American Journal of Critical Care* 4 (4): 280–85.

Elpern, E. H., B. Covert, and R. Kleinpell. 2005. "Moral Distress of Staff Nurses in a Medical Intensive Care Unit." *American Journal of Critical Care* 14 (6): 523–30.

Epstein, E. G., and A. B. Hamric. 2009. "Moral Distress, Moral Residue, and the Crescendo Effect." *Journal of Clinical Ethics* 20 (4): 330–42.

Epstein, E. G., and S. Delgado. 2010. "Understanding and Addressing Moral Distress." *Online Journal of Issues in Nursing* 15 (3): Manuscript 1.

Figley, C. R. 1995. *Compassion Fatigue: Coping with Secondary Traumatic Stress Disorder in Those Who Treated the Traumatized.* Bristol, PA: Brunner/Mazel.

Gordon, E. J., and A. B. Hamric. 2006. "The Courage to Stand Up: The Cultural Politics of Nurses' Access to Ethics Consultation." *Journal of Clinical Ethics* 17 (3): 231–54.

Hamric, A. B. 2012. "Empirical Research on Moral Distress: Issues, Challenges, and Opportunities." *HEC Forum* 24 (1): 39–49.

———. 2010. "Moral Distress and Nurse-Physician Relationships." *Virtual Mentor* 12 (1): 6–11. Accessed March 8, 2013. http://virtualmentor.ama-assn .org/2010/01/ccas1-1001.html.

———. 2000. "Moral Distress in Everyday Ethics." *Nursing Outlook* 48: 199–201.

Hamric, A. B., and L. J. Blackhall. 2007. "Nurse-Physician Perspectives on the Care of Dying Patients in Intensive Care Units: Collaboration, Moral Distress, and Ethical Climate." *Critical Care Medicine* 35 (2): 422–29.

Hamric, A. B., C. T. Borchers, and E. G. Epstein. 2012. "Development and Testing of an Instrument to Measure Moral Distress in Healthcare Professionals." *AJOB Primary Research* 3 (2): 1–9.

Hamric, A. B., W. S. Davis, and M. D. Childress. 2006. "Moral Distress in Health Care Professionals: What Is It and What Can We Do About It?" *Pharos of Alpha Omega Alpha Honor Society* 69 (1): 16–23.

Healthcare Leadership Alliance. 2010. "Competency Directory." Accessed February 13. www.healthcareleadershipalliance.org/directory.htm.

Helft, P. R., P. D. Bledsoe, M. Hancock, and L. D. Wocial. 2009. "Facilitated Ethics Conversations: A Novel Program for Managing Moral Distress in Bedside Nursing Staff." *JONA's Healthcare Law, Ethics, and Regulation* 11 (1): 27–33.

Iltis, A. S. 2005. "Values-Based Decision Making: Organizational Mission and Integrity." *HEC Forum* 17 (1): 6–17.

Jameton, A. 1984. *Nursing Practice: The Ethical Issues.* Englewood Cliffs, NJ: Prentice-Hall.

Meltzer, L. S., and L. M. Huckabay. 2004. "Critical Care Nurses' Perceptions of Futile Care and Its Effect on Burnout." *American Journal of Critical Care* 13 (3): 202–208.

Mitton, C., S. Peacock, and J. Storch. 2010. "Moral Distress Among Healthcare Managers: Conditions, Consequences, and Potential Responses." *Healthcare Policy* 6 (2): 99–112.

Mitton, C., S. Peacock, J. Storch, N. Smith, and E. Cornelissen. 2011. "Moral Distress Among Health Systems Managers: Exploratory Research in Two British Columbia Health Authorities." *Health Care Analysis* 19 (2): 107–21.

Morton, N. T., and K. W. Kirkwood. 2009. "Conscience and Conscientious Objection of Healthcare Professionals: Refocusing the Issue." *HEC Forum* 21 (4): 351–64.

Nelson, W., M. C. Rosenberg, J. Weiss, and M. Goodrich. 2009. "New Hampshire Critical Access Hospitals: CEOs' Report on Ethical Challenges." *Journal of Healthcare Management* 54 (4): 273–83.

Schwenzer, K. J., and L. Wang. 2006. "Assessing Moral Distress in Respiratory Care Practitioners." *Critical Care Medicine* 34 (12): 2967–73.

Suhonen, R., M. Stolt, H. Virtanen, and H. Leino-Kilpi. 2011. "Organizational Ethics: A Literature Review." *Nursing Ethics* 18 (3): 285–303.

Ulrich, C. M., A. B. Hamric, and C. Grady. 2010. "Moral Distress: A Growing Problem in the Health Professions?" *Hastings Center Report* 40 (1): 20–22.

US Department of Veterans Affairs. 2013. "IntegratedEthics: Improving Ethics Quality in Health Care." Accessed April 2. www.ethics.va.gov/integratedethics/index.asp.

Webster, G., and F. Bayliss. 2000. "Moral Residue." In *Margin of Error: The Ethics of Mistakes in the Practice of Medicine*, edited by S. Rubin and L. Zoloth. Hagerstown, MD: University Publishing Group.

White, K. R., and J. R. Griffith. 2010. *The Well-Managed Healthcare Organization.* 7th ed. Chicago: Health Administration Press.

Wiggleton, C., E. Petrusa, K. Loomis, J. Tarpley, M. Tarpley, M. L. O'Gorman, and B. Miller. 2010. "Medical Students' Experiences of Moral Distress: Development of a Web-Based Survey." *Academic Medicine* 85 (1): 111–17.

Wilkinson, J. M. 1988. "Moral Distress in Nursing Practice: Experience and Effect." *Nursing Forum* 23 (1): 16–29.

Wocial, L. D., M. Hancock, P. D. Bledsoe, A. Chamness, and P. R. Helft. 2010. "An Evaluation of Unit Based Ethics Conversations." *JONA's Healthcare Law, Ethics and Regulation* 12 (2): 48–54.

Worthley, J. A. 1997. *The Ethics of the Ordinary in Healthcare: Concepts and Cases.* Chicago: Health Administration Press.

ETHICS IN HEALTHCARE QUALITY IMPROVEMENT

Paul M. Schyve

This chapter is relevant to the following competencies identified in the ACHE Competencies Assessment Tool (see p. xxv):

Communication and Relationship Management
- Identify stakeholder needs/expectations
- Communicate organizational mission, vision, objectives, and priorities

Leadership
- Potential impacts and consequences of decision making in situations both internal and external
- Foster an environment of mutual trust
- Encourage a high level of commitment to the purpose and values of the organization
- Hold self and others accountable for organizational goal attainment
- Promote continuous organizational learning/improvement

Professionalism
- Serve as the ethical guide for the organization

Business Skills and Knowledge
- Build trust and cooperation between/among stakeholders

Learning Objectives

After completing this chapter, the reader will

- understand the role of quality improvement in healthcare,

- understand the basis for a moral obligation to engage in quality improvement in healthcare,
- recognize the ethical uncertainties and conflicts that arise within quality improvement activities in healthcare, and
- be able to apply quality improvement approaches to address ethical conflicts and uncertainties in healthcare.

Introduction

Quality improvement
An approach to managing quality that continuously improves the quality and performance of an organization's internal processes as well as its outputs.

Quality improvement (QI) is a phrase that has taken on a special meaning in industry and, more recently, in healthcare (Batalden and Davidoff 2007). It connotes more than just improving the quality of a specific product or service. It refers to an approach to managing quality that continuously improves the quality and performance of an organization's internal processes as well as its outputs. For this reason, it is often called "continuous quality improvement" or "performance improvement." QI can refer to any or all of three levels of organizational functioning:

1. the management of the entire organization—best exemplified in the performance criteria of the Malcolm Baldrige National Quality Award (National Institute of Standards and Technology 2013),
2. an approach to the management and improvement of quality within the organization, and
3. the use of specific tools to manage and improve quality.

This chapter focuses on QI in the latter two functions: an approach to managing and improving the quality of healthcare provided by the healthcare organization and the tools used within this approach.

Characteristics of QI

What characterizes a QI approach to improving quality (McEachern 1995)?

1. A QI approach thinks in terms of systems: the system creates (or destroys) quality. The system includes the processes that people work within; the people who are part of the system (e.g., practitioners, administrators, and other staff in healthcare); the resources that are consumed in the processes (e.g., technology, medications, and sutures in healthcare); and the information that flows through the people and processes (e.g., in the handovers among practitioners during transitions in the care of patients). QI has an axiom that every system is perfectly designed to produce the result it gets—whether good or bad;

therefore, if a different result is desired, the system must be changed. This focus on system change results in the use of tools that can describe and analyze the processes within the system and can identify how to redesign them.

2. A QI approach focuses on understanding the needs, perceptions, and satisfaction of the "customers" of any process—whether these customers are the recipients and users of internal processes within the organization (e.g., the physicians, nurses, and pharmacists in healthcare) or the external recipients and users of the organization's products and services (e.g., patients, patients' families, and communities). In the language of QI, *customer* does not always refer to the party that pays for a product or service—in this way, QI customers share characteristics with the stakeholders in an ethical conflict (see Chapter 4 on the role of stakeholders in addressing ethical conflicts). This understanding of customers' and other stakeholders' needs, perceptions, and satisfaction helps to determine the goals for changing the system.

3. A QI approach is data driven. That is, organizations rely on measurements of current performance of processes and their outputs and of the changed performance of processes and their outputs to understand the need for change, to develop proposed changes in processes, and to evaluate the results of the changes. This emphasis on data as an evidence base is accompanied by the use of statistical tools to understand the significance—and meaning—of the measurement data.

4. A QI approach includes a real-world trial of a proposed change to determine whether the change as designed produces the sought-after improvements in quality. If it does not, a cycle of design, trial, and measurement is repeated. QI is, therefore, experiential learning.

5. A QI approach is intended to bring about immediate improvements in quality for the participants in, and recipients of, the QI activities. In healthcare, for example, a QI project may be intended to benefit patients by increasing the reliability with which they receive the correct care, rather than intended to determine whether or not a specific care is the best (i.e., research).

Role of QI in Healthcare

QI is neither easy nor cheap. Its underlying systems approach is often at odds with the acculturation of many healthcare practitioners—especially physicians—who have been taught that they themselves, as individual professionals, are primarily responsible for the quality of the care their patients receive.

This acculturation begins during their professional training and is reinforced by the nature of the US medical liability system. Leaders and managers of a healthcare organization may experience this clinical professionalism as resistance to QI as it is described. So, one might wonder, why put out the effort?

The Need for Improvement in Healthcare

An investment in QI is a necessary response to the evidence that has accumulated over the past decade that the challenges facing healthcare are immense (Corrigan, Donaldson, and Kohn 2001a; Kohn, Corrigan, and Donaldson 2000). First, many widespread practices in healthcare today lack a good evidence base. And, even when an evidence base is established for a practice, the knowledge about the evidence base is often not effectively disseminated; the evidence-based practice is often not translated into implementable processes; and, when implementable processes are created, they are often not widely adopted in the real world of clinical practice. Second, today's practices—at both the individual and the organizational level—are resource intensive, with resulting unsustainable costs, as well as evidence of significant waste. Third, evidence exists of significant preventable harm to patients within the current healthcare system. Remember the axiom: Every system is perfectly designed to produce the result it gets—whether good or bad; therefore, if a different result is desired, the system must be changed. So, if society wants a sustainable healthcare system that uses evidence-based practices, which are provided without waste, and that avoid preventable harm, the system must change. That is the role of QI (Berwick 1989; Chassin and Loeb 2011).

Crossing the Quality Chasm: A New Health System for the 21st Century
A 2001 report from the Institute of Medicine detailing quality gaps in healthcare and proposing solutions for improvement.

In 2001, the Institute of Medicine (IOM) published *Crossing the Quality Chasm: A New Health System for the 21st Century*. Under the auspices of the IOM, a committee of national experts representing many stakeholder groups proposed and vetted six aims for the future healthcare system: The system should provide healthcare that is *safe, effective, patient-centered, timely, efficient*, and *equitable* (Corrigan, Donaldson, and Kohn 2001b). For each aim, the committee identified the gap between current performance and desired performance, and concluded that only sustained quality improvement at all levels of the healthcare system can close these gaps.

These six aims express something fundamental—safety, effectiveness, patient-centeredness, timeliness, efficiency, and equity. They are not *science*-based; rather, they are *values*-based. While it will take science to identify and develop evidence-based practices needed to achieve each aim, the aims themselves are values. As such, achieving them often generates ethical conversations about **moral conflicts** and uncertainties. Engaging in QI designed to "cross the quality chasm" will necessitate engaging in ethical deliberations.

Moral conflict
A disagreement or uncertainty about what actions to take when values conflict with each other.

A Moral Obligation to Engage in QI

Whether a healthcare leader or manager has a moral obligation to engage in QI depends on

1. whether society has a moral obligation to provide healthcare to its members,

2. whether a healthcare organization has a moral obligation to attempt to achieve the six value-based aims for this healthcare, and

3. whether the healthcare professionals working within the organization have a profession-based moral obligation to engage the organization in QI. That is, engaging in QI for the sake of engaging in QI is not a strong motivation. However, engaging in QI as a moral imperative would be a strong motivation.

Society's Moral Obligation

In a survey by the Pew Forum on Religion and Public Life (2003), 72 percent of Americans expressed the belief that society should provide for healthcare for all; this belief

Case Study

A 150-bed not-for-profit rural hospital serves two nearby towns, both of which help support the hospital through tax-based subsidies. The hospital is recognized by the community as providing high-quality care, and this judgment is corroborated by data in the Hospital Compare online database published by the US Centers for Medicare & Medicaid Services. One of the towns has had an influx of immigrants from Southeast Asian countries who speak very limited English. Hospital clinical staff have complained to the hospital's CEO that they are unable to provide high-quality care because of the language barrier, and they are afraid that soon a language-based serious adverse event will result in a patient's death. The CEO is sympathetic to staff's concerns and proposes to the hospital's board of trustees that the hospital's language interpretation services include hiring a full-time interpreter who speaks the most common of the languages used by the recent immigrants. The CEO points out that this proposal will help achieve equity in the quality and safety of care for the now diverse population served by the hospital. The board includes members representing each town served by the hospital. The board members from the town with the new immigrants support the proposal. The members from the other town do not; they believe that creating "equity" for the other town's immigrants will divert resources from the high-quality care their town's citizens currently receive. The CEO puzzles over how to develop a proposal that will achieve equity and also preserve the quality of care, and he initiates a QI project to develop better services for patients with limited English proficiency that will not sacrifice the quality of care for all.

- Who are the relevant stakeholder groups? That is, who will be affected by the change?
- What are each group's most important values?
- What techniques could be used to enable the stakeholder groups to learn each other's values and concerns and to identify shared values and priorities?
- What role should the CEO play in helping the stakeholder groups reach a resolution that also respects the CEO's values and integrity?
- Who has the final decision-making authority?

was held by majorities of those who identified themselves as Democrats, as Republicans, or as Independents. Further, a majority of all Americans saw this obligation as a *moral*, as well as political, issue (Pew Forum on Religion and Public Life 2003). This belief that the provision of basic healthcare is a moral obligation of American society is based on three American values (Levine et al. 2007):

1. *Equality of opportunity*, which is necessary to enable every person to fulfill the American goals of life, liberty, and the pursuit of happiness. For example, the inability to obtain healthcare by a racial or ethnic group would compromise—through the effect of untreated illness— equality of opportunity for members of that group.
2. *Justice*, which requires a fair allocation of social resources toward vital needs. Justice is compromised when one vital need—such as healthcare—wastes resources that could go to meeting other vital needs—such as education and housing.
3. *Compassion*, especially for the least fortunate, including those who are ill.

Considerable debate surrounds whether healthcare is an individual's right; about how the societal obligation would be best met (e.g., through not-for-profit versus for-profit financing; through single-payer versus multiple-payer reimbursement systems; through public sector versus private sector delivery of services); and about the accountabilities of various parties (e.g., patients, practitioners, provider organizations, health systems, state and local governments, the federal government). However, despite these debates, strong consensus exists that society has a moral obligation to provide for healthcare for all its members.

In addition to the consensus that society has a moral obligation to provide for healthcare for each of its members, healthcare is also widely

Public good
Goods made available to everyone (regardless of how they are delivered or financed) so that they benefit individual recipients and, in the aggregate, benefit society as a whole.

viewed as a **public good**. Public goods are goods that are made available to everyone (regardless of how they are delivered or financed) so that they benefit the individual recipient(s) and, in the aggregate, benefit society as a whole. Traditional examples of public goods in the United States are public safety, education, public health, and healthcare, because a safe, educated, and healthy populace is deemed to be prerequisite to a successful democracy and an economically productive society. Public goods, because of their societal as well as individual benefits, are themselves value-laden within a society, and their provision is considered to be a moral obligation.

Healthcare Organizations' Moral Obligation

If society has a moral obligation both to provide for healthcare to its members and to provide healthcare as a public good, society will justly expect that those who engage in delivering this healthcare—practitioners, such as doctors, nurses, and pharmacists; healthcare organizations and their leaders and managers; and healthcare policy makers—do so with the public's values for healthcare in mind. The public's values for healthcare are best represented by the six value-based aims published by the IOM: safety, effectiveness, patient-centeredness, timeliness, efficiency, and equity. Since their publication in 2001, these aims have been widely endorsed by the public as well as by healthcare professionals and healthcare policy makers (Berwick, Nolan, and Whittington 2008; Honoré et al. 2011). Therefore, the public presumes that those engaged in delivering healthcare have a moral obligation to attempt to achieve the six value-based aims. In turn, a healthcare organization's obligation to engage in QI derives from its moral obligation to achieve the societal values for healthcare that are reflected in these six value-based aims. Fulfillment of this moral obligation by an organization is substantially dependent on the organization's leaders and managers.

Professional Ethics

All those engaged in healthcare, whether they are clinicians or administrators, have a moral obligation to engage in QI. As long as an individual is engaged in providing the public good of healthcare, she is morally obligated to try to improve its quality.

This moral obligation is based not only on the healthcare organization's obligation but also on the nature of professionalism. As described in Chapter 5, among the attributes of professionalism is "primary orientation to community interests, rather than to individual self-interest"; this attribute aligns with the previous discussion about societal expectations that healthcare providers achieve the six value-based aims for healthcare. The healthcare professions participate in a social contract in which society authorizes the members of the profession to undertake certain skilled activities if the members meet certain obligations, one of which is competence. With the accelerating advance of science in medicine, competence requires that one continually learn and change one's practice accordingly. Principle V of the American Medical Association (2012) Principles of Medical Ethics is, "Continue to study, apply, and advance scientific knowledge." This principle identifies QI as a personal moral obligation of the physician. Further, specialty certifying boards now require physicians to maintain their certification by demonstrating continuing competence in practice-based learning—essentially, personal QI. With the recognition that quality and safety are created by the system of care (i.e., the combination of people, processes, resources, and information), demonstrating continuing competence in systems-based practice is also required by the certifying boards (Wynia and Kurlander 2007). This combination of practicing in a system and learning from this practice establishes an obligation for the physician to participate in organizational QI; the same expectation would apply, by analogy, to other healthcare professionals.

For healthcare executives, the American College of Healthcare Executives (2011) Code of Ethics requires that the executive

- maintain competence and proficiency in healthcare management by implementing a personal program of assessment and continuing professional education,
- work to ensure the existence of a process to evaluate the quality of care or service rendered,
- lead the organization in the use and improvement of standards of management and sound business practices, and
- create an organizational environment in which both clinical and management mistakes are minimized and, when they do occur, are disclosed and addressed effectively.

Taken together, these ethical obligations of the healthcare leader or manager point to an obligation to engage both himself and the organization—through his leadership and management—in QI. For an individual to conduct this leadership or management without reference to the six value-based aims articulated in the IOM report would suggest that the individual does not share society's underlying values for healthcare. And, if the aims *are* shared by the individual, to fail to make efforts to achieve them would suggest that the person does not place much importance on these specific aims relative to other aims (e.g., money, fame).

In summary, the clinical practitioners, the healthcare leaders and managers, and the healthcare organization itself all have moral obligations to engage in QI. The healthcare leader or manager has a crucial role in meeting these obligations.

Role of the Healthcare Executive in QI

The major advances in quality have occurred when improvement efforts are focused on the system (the processes, people, resources, and information that work together to achieve a result), not just on the performance of the individuals within the system. Large systems (e.g., the organization) are composed of subsystems, which are composed of microsystems. In healthcare, the team that works together to provide care to the patient is the **microsystem**. A system, a subsystem, and a microsystem each have a culture. This culture consists of the customary values, attitudes, beliefs, and behaviors held by those working throughout the system, subsystem, or microsystem and by the

Microsystem
The team that works together to provide care to the patient.

way they uniformly do their work. An organization that expects to continuously improve quality must embed the specific expectation for QI within the culture of the organization.

Culture of QI

A QI culture includes those characteristics described in the chapter Introduction: systems thinking and a focus on processes, attention to the customers of a process, data-driven decision making, experiential learning, continuous improvement, and intended immediate real-world benefit. In healthcare, the culture specifically focuses these characteristics on the aims of safety, effectiveness, patient-centeredness, timeliness, efficiency, and equity in the provision of care.

Leaders Shape Culture

An organization's culture—the customary values, attitudes, beliefs, and behaviors of those within the organization—is established by, or enabled by, its administrative and clinical leaders and managers. Only the leaders and managers of an organization can shape a sustainable QI culture in the organization. They establish and maintain the culture through their communications, through their behavior, by providing education to staff on the values and ways of the culture, by providing the resources needed to conduct the activities called for by the culture, and by rewarding those who fulfill the cultural expectations. When the leaders and managers are most successful, the culture becomes organic to the

Case Study

A clinical department manager in a multisite hospital has led her department from a failing, highly criticized enterprise to one that is much more efficient. She has improved patient and family satisfaction, improved physician and nurse satisfaction, increased patient volume, and improved the bottom line. Her achievement is recognized in the hospital's C-suite, and she is promoted to administrator for a division at one of the other hospital sites. When she arrives, she quickly recognizes that the same changes that were made in her previous department could benefit her new division. However, when she gently suggests two of these process changes, the staff and physicians tell her that the processes have been working just fine and that their motto is "If it ain't broke, don't fix it." On the one hand, she recognizes that the division is composed of highly competent people whom she would not want to lose. On the other hand, she wants to create a culture of QI so that the motto will become "If it's working OK, let's make it even better." She is, however, not sure how to start this transformation.

- Who are the relevant stakeholder groups? That is, who will be affected by the change?
- What are each group's most important values?
- What techniques could be used to enable the stakeholder groups to learn each other's values and concerns and to identify shared values and priorities?
- How can the administrator identify and recruit others in the division who can influence their colleagues to create a culture of QI?
- What role should the division administrator play in helping the stakeholder groups reach a resolution that also respects her values and integrity?
- Who has the final decision-making authority?

organization and lives on even as leaders and managers change. To shape a QI culture, healthcare leaders and managers should be personally committed to and involved in the following (Reinertsen 2008):

- Embedding a QI culture in the mission, vision, values, and code of conduct of the organization
- Developing sensitivity in themselves and others to the value conflicts among stakeholders regarding the aims of healthcare (see the discussion of moral imagination in Chapter 14)
- Engaging relevant stakeholders in resolving these conflicts (see the discussion of stakeholders in Chapter 4)
- Engaging the clinical professionals in QI
- Engaging the ultimate customer—patients and their families—in QI
- Reducing moral distress among staff with regard to the goals of QI within the organization (see the discussion of moral distress in Chapter 7)

The same activities can be applied to the subsystems within a healthcare organization and to the microsystems in which the patients are participants.

Ethical Challenges That Arise in Healthcare QI

This chapter has so far explored why there is a moral obligation in healthcare to engage in QI, why that engagement is a personal obligation of a leader or manager in a healthcare organization, and what the leader or manager might do to meet that obligation. But QI itself generates ethical challenges.

Value Conflicts

First, as with many values discussed in other chapters of this book, values may conflict with each other. Or, perhaps more accurately, the actions that could be taken to better achieve one value may compromise maximum achievement of another value. For example, timeliness and efficiency may be valued by all stakeholders, but (at least some) actions to improve efficiency—as measured by resource use—may compromise the timeliness of an intervention. Likewise, all stakeholders may value both effectiveness (as measured by the use of evidenced-based practices) and patient-centeredness (as measured by following a patient's preferences); but following the patient's preferences may mean using less-effective interventions. Such ethical conflicts arise in making decisions about the focus for using QI resources (e.g., whether a QI project should be initiated to focus on timeliness or on efficiency), and within a QI project, in making decisions about how the values should be balanced in deciding on the goals of the project (e.g., how much patient-centeredness can be compromised in the interest of improving safety). Hearing clinicians complain that the leaders' and managers' QI projects focus too much on efficiency with too little regard for their impact on effectiveness or patient-centeredness is common, as is hearing leaders and managers complain that the clinicians' QI projects do not focus enough on efficiency.

The Aim of Efficiency

Second, QI projects take resources. No matter the ultimate benefit, the process of QI itself can be intensive, certainly with the use of staff time and often with the use of other resources. If waste of resources is to be avoided—an aim, or value, for the healthcare system—resources should not be wasted in QI, just as they should not be wasted in clinical care. Using resources wisely in QI requires using robust, evidence-based QI techniques in identifying problems, learning from customers, analyzing processes, designing changes, and testing changes (Chassin 1998). Although these robust techniques—such as Lean to improve process efficiency (Doerman and Caldwell 2010) and Six Sigma to improve process effectiveness (De Feo and Early 2010; Pyzdek 2003)—are often labor-intensive, they are more likely to result in effective, sustainable changes than are other, less robust techniques. But having developed the correct technical solution to a problem is not enough. The QI resources are wasted if the correct solution cannot be successfully implemented. Therefore, QI also requires effective change management, including understanding the stakeholders in the change and working with them to implement the change.

Research in QI Projects

Third, in many QI projects both staff and patients must change what they do or receive. If these changes are experimental, or designed to be research, the QI project may either be or contain elements of human subject research—and must be treated as such from both an ethical and a regulatory perspective (Lynn et al. 2007). Even if no element of human subject research is involved, if the proposed changes create a risk of potential harm to affected patients, a moral obligation exists to obtain their consent for participation in the QI project. Criteria that differentiate between QI and research, and the forms of independent review for QI that is not research but that may cause harm to patients, are both in flux. These ethical conflicts and uncertainties, when they arise, should be considered by a healthcare organization's Institutional Review Board, ethics committee, and legal counsel before the healthcare leader or manager determines a course of action.

Complex System Change

Fourth, QI projects often result in changes in complex adaptive systems; most healthcare organizations are complex adaptive systems. When changes are made in **complex adaptive systems**, unexpected, unintended consequences almost always occur; when the complex adaptive system is an open system (i.e., it interacts with other systems), the unexpected, unintended consequences may occur in a system other than the focus of change (Zimmerman, Lindberg, and Plsek 2001). Because these unexpected, unintended consequences may be harmful—sometimes catastrophically so—engaging in QI creates an obligation to be vigilant for these unpredicted changes and to intervene as quickly as possible to prevent, or at least to mitigate, harm. In short, the moral obligation to engage in QI generates a derivative moral obligation of vigilance.

Complex adaptive system
A system composed of many interconnected parts (e.g., people), each with the freedom to act in ways that are not fully predictable but will affect other parts in the system, resulting in those parts also changing—often in unpredictable ways. As the parts change, the system's functions and outputs adapt, often unpredictably.

The Aim of Safety

Fifth, the ethical challenges created by QI can relate to the aim of patient safety. The conflicts between the six value-based aims often involve the aim of safety, whether the conflicts are over what QI project to undertake or what goals to set for a project. For example, the changes that an organization can make to better achieve the aims of patient-centeredness, timeliness, or efficiency may compromise the achievement of the aim of safety, and the changes that the organization can make to better achieve the aim of safety may compromise the achievement of the aims of patient-centeredness, timeliness, or efficiency. That the IOM report placed *safety* first in the list of aims for the healthcare system is meaningful (Corrigan, Donaldson, and Kohn 2001a). From the time of Hippocrates, the moral obligation has been "First, do no harm." Although this is one of the moral obligations of physicians and nurses, all those who take a position in healthcare—whether or not they are clinicians—should adopt this obligation as their own; if they cannot or will not, they should not be in healthcare. Does this mean that patient safety must be paramount at all costs to the other aims? No; the other aims are all to be honored in addressing moral conflicts and uncertainties in how to proceed in QI. Rather, it means that patient safety should always be considered and should receive an extra emphasis in the ethical deliberations.

Addressing Ethical Challenges with QI

The nature of QI—both its approach to managing quality and the tools it employs—can contribute to the resolution of other ethical conflicts and uncertainties within a healthcare organization. A QI activity begins with identifying a target for improvement, which may be a problem, a need for change, or simply the desire to improve the current level of performance. One of the first steps is to determine the customers of the process that is to be changed. But others in the process are also identified: those who carry out the process, those who supply the process with inputs, and those who will be affected by the process or by its outputs. The customers and the others involved in or affected by the process are all stakeholders in the process.

For each stakeholder group, its members' goals for the process are determined. Based on the current performance of the process and the stakeholders' goals, the goals for the QI activity are set. All QI activities begin with the desire to fully achieve all the multiple stakeholders' goals. But often no change can be designed that will do so. Instead, balancing the stakeholder's various goals is necessary. This balance is designed to identify changes that will optimally achieve each of the stakeholders' goals rather than maximally achieve every goal. Relative priorities among goals must be set and changes designed that will best achieve

Case Study

The chief operating officer (COO) of a large and successful ambulatory surgery center in a major metropolitan area has been directed by the center's physician-ownership board and its CEO to reduce expenses to bolster a slipping bottom line. The COO assembles a team comprising a surgeon, a nurse, a technician, a receptionist, a billing clerk, a patient, the chief financial officer (CFO), and a mid-level administrator. The team interviews many other staff members for ideas, measures selected current processes, and develops a list of the five changes that would yield the greatest savings. Two of the changes are to processes in the operating suites, one revises the intake process, one revises the billing process, and one streamlines the credentialing process for the physicians. Before implementing any of the changes, possible failure modes or adverse effects are identified and either the proposed change is modified or a monitoring system is established to provide an early warning of an adverse effect to enable its prevention or mitigation. Two months after the changes are put into effect, an unexpected increase in surgical-site infections is identified. A root cause analysis of the increase uncovers that one of the changes in the operating suite processes created a previously unrecognized risk of infection.

- Who are the relevant stakeholder groups? That is, who will be affected by the change?
- What are each group's most important values?
- What techniques could be used to enable the stakeholder groups to learn each other's values and concerns and to identify shared values and priorities?
- What role should the COO play in helping the stakeholder groups reach a resolution that also respects the COO's values and integrity?
- Who has the final decision-making authority?
- Under what circumstances should patients and their families be informed of unpredictable, unexpected risks when changes are made in care processes?

the highest-priority goals while still respecting the goals whose achievement is likely to be compromised. The process analysis and data analysis of QI are designed to identify the change options that would best achieve the higher priority goals while minimizing the compromise of the lower-priority goals.

Applying QI to Resolve Moral Conflicts

Now read the preceding paragraph, substituting the word "value" for "goal." The QI process

1. identifies all the stakeholders for a moral conflict or uncertainty,
2. determines each stakeholder's values,
3. determines relative priorities among the values,
4. attempts to design a resolution (change) that achieves the higher-priority values while minimizing the compromise of the lower-priority values, and
5. assesses the effect of the resolution (change) on the achievement of each of the values.

Thus, the principles and tools of QI can be useful in managing and resolving ethical conflicts and uncertainties. These principles and tools can help identify all the stakeholders and their values and can help the stakeholders set priorities among these values (see Chapters 4 and 14 for a discussion of this process in healthcare ethics). And these principles and tools of QI—such as those used in an integrated Lean-Six Sigma approach to improving quality (George 2002)—can also be used to design an optimal resolution when the actions to achieve one value are likely to compromise achievement of another.

Successful QI not only uses rigorous tools for identifying solutions, it also incorporates change management techniques. These techniques include robust methods for determining stakeholder goals and values (George et al. 2005), for identifying barriers to developing, accepting, and implementing resolutions, and for addressing those barriers. These techniques can further facilitate the resolution of ethical conflicts when used within the context of the QI process. The use of change management techniques is in part designed to reduce the discomfort among stakeholders with the changes to be made and with the compromise of their goals and values. Reduction of this discomfort in the case of moral conflict can reduce the associated moral distress for clinicians, nonclinical staff, and the administrators and managers themselves.

In summary, the use of QI principles and tools and of change management techniques may contribute to the resolution of especially intractable moral conflicts that lead to moral distress.

Conclusion

Although widespread agreement exists on the value-based aims that American society has for healthcare, the current healthcare system is far from achieving these aims. Only sustained and effective efforts to improve healthcare are likely to close the gaps between desire and reality. The approaches and tools of QI have been demonstrated to be effective in creating improvement, and healthcare organizations that have applied them on a continuous basis have made the most progress in achieving society's aims.

The adoption and use of QI throughout an organization depends on the organization's leaders and managers. Both society's expectation that healthcare will be managed as a public good rather than for private benefit and the professional codes of ethics for clinicians and for healthcare executives place a moral obligation on healthcare organization leaders and managers to engage their organizations in QI in order to achieve society's value-based aims for healthcare.

Although there is a moral obligation to engage in QI, the QI activities themselves can create ethical conflicts and uncertainties. These conflicts and uncertainties often relate to the prioritization of the value-based aims that the activities are designed to achieve. Additional ethical issues may be raised in specific

QI projects related to the involvement of human subjects in research or the risk of potential harm to affected patients and other participants.

Case Study

At a professional conference, the owner of a 100-bed assisted living facility learns about new ways to create patient-centered programming within assisted living settings. Intent on making care delivery at his own facility a more patient-centered experience for its residents, he asks the assisted living administrator to implement changes. The administrator has seen the effectiveness of a Six Sigma approach to improvement in a hospital where he was formerly employed. With the help of a consultant, he begins a Six Sigma project to make the residence more patient-centered. They progress through the design-measure-analyze-improve-control (DMAIC) phases of Six Sigma. In obtaining "the voice of the customer" during the design phase, staff learn that different stakeholders have different values. The residents most value their freedom, the residents' families most value the residents' safety, and staff most value efficiency. During the analyze and improve phases, staff are able to identify solutions that create more patient-centered programming with only minimally increased risk to the residents and that uses fewer resources (e.g., providing interactive videos for patients that identify options and the relative benefits, risks, and costs of each option). The goals are that residents are pleased and their families agree that the improved quality of life for their loved ones is worth the minimally increased risk.

- Who are the relevant stakeholder groups? That is, who will be affected by the change?
- What are each group's most important values?
- What techniques could be used to enable the stakeholder groups to learn each other's values and concerns and to identify shared values and priorities?
- What role should the administrator play in helping the stakeholder groups reach a resolution that also respects his values and integrity?
- Who has the final decision-making authority?
- Some staff members believe the resolution is not consistent with their commitment to "first, do no harm" and are at risk of moral distress. What can the administrator do to reduce this risk?

Fortunately, the approach and tools of QI are designed to identify the aims and values of stakeholders in the project, set priorities among these aims and values, and devise changes that will better achieve the higher-priority aims without negating the lower-priority aims. So within QI itself are the tools to help resolve the ethical conflicts and uncertainties that engagement in QI generates or uncovers.

Healthcare—its science, its delivery structure, its financing—is constantly changing. Failure to change in response is the death knell for a healthcare organization—and its leaders and managers. Engaging in QI is not only the right thing to do ethically, it is in the interest of the healthcare organization and the organization's leaders and managers themselves.

Points to Remember

- American society considers the provision of healthcare to all its members to be society's moral obligation.
- Society's value-based aims for healthcare are that it be safe, effective, patient-centered, timely, efficient, and equitable.
- Both societal expectations and professional codes of ethics establish a moral obligation for healthcare organizations and their leaders and managers to take actions to achieve these aims.
- QI comprises an approach and tools that can effectively reduce the significant gaps in achieving these aims in today's healthcare system (e.g., failure to provide evidence-based effective care, inefficiency and waste, preventable harm).
- QI is characterized by systems thinking and a focus on processes; attention to the customers of a process; data-driven decision making; experiential learning; continuous improvement; and immediate real-world benefit.
- Although a moral obligation, QI activities themselves generate or uncover moral conflicts and uncertainties.
- The approach and tools of QI are also suited to resolving the moral conflicts and uncertainties that are generated or uncovered—such as identifying stakeholders and their goals and values; setting priorities among goals and values; designing proposed changes that best balance them; and measuring their achievement.

References

American College of Healthcare Executives (ACHE). 2011. *ACHE Code of Ethics.* Accessed March 25, 2013. www.ache.org/ABT_ACHE/code.cfm.

American Medical Association (AMA). 2012. *Code of Medical Ethics of the American Medical Association*. Chicago: American Medical Association.

Batalden, P. B., and F. Davidoff. 2007. "What Is 'Quality Improvement' and How Can It Transform Healthcare?" *Quality and Safety in Health Care* 16 (1): 2–3.

Berwick, D. M. 1989. "Continuous Improvement as an Ideal in Health Care." *New England Journal of Medicine* 320 (1): 53–56.

Berwick, D. M., T. W. Nolan, and J. Whittington. 2008. "The Triple Aim: Care, Health and Cost." *Health Affairs* 27 (3): 759–69.

Chassin, M. R. 1998. "Is Health Care Ready for Six Sigma Quality?" *Milbank Quarterly* 76 (4): 565–91.

Chassin, M. R., and J. M. Loeb. 2011. "The Ongoing Quality Improvement Journey: Next Stop, High Reliability." *Health Affairs* 30 (4): 559–68.

Corrigan, J. M., M. S. Donaldson, and L. T. Kohn. 2001a. "A New Health System for the 21st Century." In *Crossing the Quality Chasm: A New Health System for the 21st Century,* edited by J. M. Corrigan, M. S. Donaldson, and L. T. Kohn, 24–40. Washington, DC: National Academies Press.

———. 2001b. "Improving the 21st Century Health Care System." In *Crossing the Quality Chasm: A New Health System for the 21st Century,* edited by J. M. Corrigan, M. S. Donaldson, and L. T. Kohn, 41–64. Washington, DC: National Academies Press.

De Feo, J. A., and J. F. Early. 2010. "Six Sigma: Improving Process Effectiveness." In *Juran's Quality Handbook: The Complete Guide to Performance Excellence,* 6th ed., edited by J. M. Juran and J. A. De Feo, 355–85. New York: The McGraw-Hill Companies, Inc.

Doerman, S. M., and R. K. Caldwell. 2010. "Lean Techniques: Improving Process Efficiency." In *Juran's Quality Handbook: The Complete Guide to Performance Excellence*, 6th ed., edited by J. M. Juran and J. A. De Feo, 327–54. New York: The McGraw-Hill Companies, Inc.

George, M. L. 2002. *Lean Six Sigma: Combining Six Sigma Quality with Lean Speed.* New York: The McGraw-Hill Companies, Inc.

George, M. L., D. Rowlands, M. Price., and J. Maxey. 2005. "Voice of the Customer (VOC)." In *The Lean Six Sigma Pocket Toolbook,* 55–68. New York: The McGraw-Hill Companies, Inc.

Honoré, P. A., D. Wright, D. M. Berwick, C. M. Clancy, P. Lee, J. Nowinski, and H. K. Koh. 2011. "Creating a Framework for Getting Quality into the Public Health System." *Health Affairs* 30 (4): 737–45.

Kohn, L. T., J. M. Corrigan, and M. S. Donaldson, 2000. "Errors in Health Care: A Leading Cause of Death and Injury." In *To Err Is Human: Building a Safer Health System,* edited by L. T. Kohn, J. M. Corrigan, and M. S. Donaldson. Washington, DC: National Academies Press.

Levine, M. A., M. K. Wynia, P. M. Schyve, J. R. Teagarden, D. A. Fleming, S. K. Donohue, R. J. Anderson, J. Sabin, and E. J. Emanuel. 2007. "Improving

Access to Health Care: A Consensus Ethical Framework to Guide Proposals for Reform." *Hastings Center Report* 37 (5): 14–19.

Lynn, J., M. A. Baily, M. Bottrell, B. Jennings, R. J. Levine, F. Davidoff, D. Casarett, J. Corrigan, E. Fox, M. K. Wynia, G. J. Agich, M. O'Kane, T. Speroff, P. Schyve, P. Batalden, S. Tunis, N. Berlinger, L. Cronenwett, M. Fritzmaurice, N. N. Dubler, and B. James. 2007. "The Ethics of Using Quality Improvement Methods in Health Care." *Annals of Internal Medicine* 146 (9): 666–73.

McEachern, J. E. 1995. "Introduction." In *Clinical CQI: A Book of Readings* by D. Neuhauser, J. E. McEachern, and L. Headrick, 1–23. Oakbrook Terrace, IL: The Joint Commission.

National Institute of Standards and Technology Malcolm Baldrige National Quality Award. 2013. *2013–2014 Health Care Criteria for Performance Excellence.* Accessed June 27. www.nist.gov/baldrige/publications/hc_criteria.cfm.

Pew Forum on Religion and Public Life. 2003. "Religion and Politics: Contention and Consensus." Accessed February 14. www.pewforum.org/Politics-and-Elections/Religion-and-Politics-Contention-and-Consensus.aspx.

Pyzdek, T. 2003. *The Six Sigma Handbook, Revised and Expanded.* New York: The McGraw-Hill Companies, Inc.

Reinertsen, J. L. 2008. "Leadership for Quality." In *The Health Care Quality Book: Vision, Strategy, and Tools*, 2nd ed., edited by E. R. Ransom, M. S. Joshi, D. B. Nash, and S. B. Ransom, 311–29. Chicago: Health Administration Press.

Wynia, M. K., and J. E. Kurlander. 2007. "Physician Ethics and Participation in Quality Improvement: Renewing a Professional Obligation." In *Health Care Improvement: Ethical and Regulatory Issues* by B. Jennings, M. A. Baily, M. Bottrell, and J. Lynn, 7–27. Garrison, NY: The Hastings Center.

Zimmerman, B., C. Lindberg, and P. Plsek. 2001. *Edgeware: Insights from Complexity Science for Health Care Leaders.* Irving, TX: VHA.

THE HEALTHCARE ORGANIZATION AS EMPLOYER: THE DEMANDS OF FAIRNESS AND THE HEALTHCARE ORGANIZATION

Leonard J. Weber

This chapter is relevant to the following competencies identified in the ACHE Competencies Assessment Tool (see p. xxv):

Communication and Relationship Management
- Identify stakeholder needs/expectations
- Sensitivity to what is correct behavior when communicating with diverse cultures, internal and external
- Communicate organizational mission, vision, objectives, and priorities
- Facilitate conflict and alternative dispute resolution
- Labor relation strategies

Leadership
- Adhere to legal and regulatory standards

Professionalism
- Organizational business and personal ethics
- Adhere to ethical business principles

Knowledge of the Healthcare Environment
- Workforce issues

Business Skills and Knowledge
- Compensation and benefits practices
- Organizational policies and procedures and their functions
- Develop employee benefit and assistance plans
- Potential impacts and consequences of human resources

Learning Objectives

After completing this chapter, the reader will be able to

- explain an ethically significant difference between mandating influenza vaccination for the public and mandating influenza vaccination for healthcare workers,
- state a common ethical objection to a policy making nonsmoking a condition of employment in a healthcare organization,
- provide an explanation of the widespread sense that there is something "wrong" about the compensation level of healthcare executives, and
- explain why it can be ethically dangerous to identify a positive vote of employees for union representation as a failure on the part of management.

Introduction

How to be fair in employing and managing staff is one of the most challenging demands placed on healthcare administrators. While all agree that good ethics requires fairness or justice in the treatment of employees, determining what *fairness* means in specific settings is often difficult when faced with complex, emotion-laden, and controversial issues, such as downsizing, wages and salaries, employee health-related behavior, whistle-blowing, performance evaluations, and collective bargaining. Fairness requires that the needs, interests, and concerns of employees be considered in relationship to the needs, interests, and concerns of other relevant stakeholders. Careful and insightful stakeholder analysis is never simple.

Understanding the demands of fairness and identifying best ethical practices in employee-related issues and policies is difficult but not impossible. Best ethical practices are not primarily determined by a review of what other organizations are doing or by getting a legal opinion. Rather, they are determined by considering the perspectives and priorities that are highlighted when the issues are explored explicitly as issues of fairness and ethics. The ethical organization consistently includes careful ethical analysis in the process of making decisions on key or controversial issues. Executives have a responsibility to ensure that this occurs.

Maintaining good ethics is not easy. Many situations occur in which the right or best thing to do is not immediately clear, all relevant responsibilities considered. This chapter briefly discusses four employee-related ethical issues commonly found in healthcare organizations. They are examples of the effort to ground the search for organizational policies and practices in an explicit exploration of the meaning and demands of fairness.

While these reviews of the issues are too brief to be considered position papers on how to proceed, they do point toward some specific conclusions. Ethical analysis is, after all, not neutral, and a commitment to fairness necessarily includes advocacy of particular approaches. Taken together, these four issues identify many of the concepts and concerns that healthcare leaders need to consider as they work out the implications of a commitment to fairness to employees:

1. Policy mandating influenza vaccination of employees in a healthcare organization
2. Policy prohibiting tobacco use as a condition of employment
3. Just compensation, both for those who are the lowest paid in the organization and for executives
4. Response to an effort to select a collective bargaining agent

Mandatory Influenza Vaccinations

In recent years the number of healthcare provider organizations that have implemented mandatory annual vaccination of employees for seasonal influenza has increased significantly (Immunization Action Coalition 2013). Despite the intense concern in 2009 and 2010 about H1N1 influenza, these institutional policies mandate seasonal influenza vaccination and are being instituted as regular policy, not as a response to a new or unusually severe epidemic.

Mandating influenza vaccination is a significant change from past practices in many organizations, which had previously strongly encouraged vaccination. Mandatory vaccination of employees has encountered some resistance, and the questions that have been raised about the extent to which employers are justified in mandating employee health-related behavior need to be addressed.

Supporters of mandatory vaccination often make the following points:

- Vaccination of healthcare workers has been shown to lower patient mortality.
- After years of efforts of encouraging healthcare workers to get seasonal flu vaccinations, only about 40 percent of healthcare employees typically get the shots.
- Requiring flu vaccination is not a significant departure from previous healthcare standards. Requirements have already existed for mandatory

rubella, measles, mumps, hepatitis B, and varicella vaccinations and for annual TB screening for healthcare workers.

The argument in support of a mandatory vaccination program is often based on the need of healthcare workers to protect public health and the failure of a voluntary program to achieve the desired result. "Despite considerable evidence that the vaccination of health care workers benefits workers, their patients, their families, and their institutions, few health care professionals take advantage of vaccination programs unless these programs are actively promoted or required as a condition of employment. Even when programs are actively promoted, their increases in vaccination rates generally remain below levels required to achieve herd immunity and, therefore, are unlikely to secure the potential benefits from high rates of vaccination" (Anikeeva, Braunack-Mayer, and Rogers 2009).

Some employees and some supporters of employee rights might object to a requirement for an annual influenza shot for a variety of reasons. Three concerns are particularly worth noting:

1. Some have doubts about the effectiveness or safety of flu shots. They are not convinced that vaccination will protect employees themselves or others in their workplace. They may also question the strength of the evidence supporting the conclusion that a mandatory vaccination policy is more effective than voluntary vaccinations in protecting the health of patients and employees.

2. Some object that the informed-consent right to decline unwanted treatment is being violated by policies that deny or restrict the freedom of employees to say no.

3. Some see required vaccination as excessive involvement by employers in the private lives of employees. They argue, for example, that how employees take care of their own health is their own business and should not be controlled by the employer.

Informed consent
The right of individuals to decide whether (1) to accept recommended healthcare services, and (2) to receive the information needed to make the decision.

In the general population, many adults choose not to be vaccinated against seasonal influenza, even when they are part of a vulnerable group for whom vaccination is strongly recommended. In general, the standards of healthcare ethics support these individuals. The principle of **informed consent** means individuals have the right to decide whether to accept recommended vaccination, just as it means they have the right to decide whether to accept recommended surgery. All of us have the right, ordinarily, to decide for ourselves whether to be vaccinated.

The word *ordinarily* is a qualifier in that statement. The qualifier is necessary because our rights are limited by our responsibility to avoid placing others at unnecessary risk of significant harm. Rights are sometimes also limited by the specific responsibilities inherent in work-related roles.

The policies being discussed mandating vaccination are policies for healthcare workers, not the general public and not employees in other kinds of organizations. The argument in support of such policies is based on the fact that these workers are involved directly or indirectly in patient care, which is relevant in terms of what should be expected or required of them.

For the general public, restricting the freedom of individuals to decline healthcare has a sound ethical basis only when necessary to protect others from serious harm or to protect the common good. An extensive outbreak of a deadly infectious disease, for example, might justify quarantine or mandatory vaccination of the public. This general standard justifies mandatory healthcare only in public health emergencies.

The responsibilities of healthcare workers are different from those of the general public; the demands that can be placed on healthcare workers are also different. Although the nature of seasonal influenza clearly does not present the kind of emergency that would justify mandatory vaccination of the public, consider the specific circumstances of healthcare workers.

At the heart of professional healthcare ethics is the obligation to avoid harming those in one's care (see Chapter 5). At an organizational level, one of the implications of this responsibility is the need to limit as much as possible the infections patients acquire while in the staff's care.

Another aspect of healthcare professionalism is the subordination of one's own interests to the needs of those being cared for. This means that, at times, professionalism requires that healthcare workers stay on the job even when it means risking their own health. It also means making a daily commitment to doing what is needed for patient well-being rather than following their own preferences.

Good organizational policy recognizes both the general right of individuals to decide freely whether to accept healthcare interventions for themselves and the responsibility of healthcare workers to protect patients from harm. Although justifying an employer requirement designed to protect the employee's own health would be difficult, a requirement designed to protect against patient harm should be assessed differently.

Using this analysis, one can make a strong ethical case for a healthcare organization's mandate for annual seasonal influenza vaccination of employees when the following considerations apply:

- Substantial evidence exists that patients are put at significant risk—and suffer harm—when employees have seasonal influenza.
- Substantial evidence exists that the risks to patients will be reduced by increased vaccination of hospital staff.

- The organization has good reason to conclude that the level of staff vaccination necessary to protect patients will not be achieved by a voluntary program (even with incentives).
- The categories of employees included in a vaccination requirement are all those, and only those, necessary to achieve the patient safety goal. (Given the ways employees interact among themselves, this consideration may mean that all employees need to be included.)
- Covered employees for whom influenza vaccination is medically contraindicated are exempted from the requirement.
- Other exemptions for covered employees are limited to ensure the effectiveness of the program and fairness in its application.
- Consequences for nonexempted employees who refuse to comply with the requirement are no more severe than necessary to ensure the effectiveness of the program and fairness in its application.

These points are meant to reflect and implement the standard that healthcare-related mandates for employees are appropriate if necessary to protect patients from preventable harm, but they should be no more restrictive of individual freedom (to decide whether to accept healthcare interventions) than necessary to achieve that goal.

As the analysis of this issue illustrates, the demands of fairness require that executives pay careful attention to the ethical arguments on both sides of an issue and make a decision that can be explained in terms of key ethical responsibilities.

Nonsmoking as a Condition of Employment

Since the Cleveland Clinic stopped hiring smokers in 2007, the number of hospitals and health-related businesses instituting similar policies has gradually increased: "Hospitals in Florida, Georgia, Massachusetts, Missouri, Ohio, Pennsylvania, Tennessee and Texas, among others, stopped hiring smokers in the last year and more are openly considering the option" (Sulzberger 2011). These policies treat tobacco use as many employers have long treated illegal drugs. Job applicants are tested for nicotine in their bodies, and individuals testing positive are simply not eligible for employment.

That more healthcare organizations will be faced with the question of whether to institute policies of this sort is likely. Responding to this question is of significant organizational importance, not simply an HR issue. The decision made both contributes to and reflects the administration's understanding of employer ethics.

One can easily detect a variety of concerns in the different ways of approaching the issue. For some, the question is whether such a policy might promote healthier living and protect patients and staff from the smell that may accompany a smoker hours after the last cigarette. For some, a key concern is increasing worker productivity and reducing employer healthcare costs. For some, protecting employee off-the-job private behavior from control by employers is at the heart of the matter. Good ethical analysis requires recognizing all relevant concerns and responsibilities and identifying priorities among different responsibilities, goals, and consequences.

Sometimes a policy of not hiring smokers is seen as the next step in an effort to discourage smoking and to protect others from secondhand smoke. Banning smoking in the building and on the hospital property has not been successful in getting all employees to quit smoking, so why not simply refuse to hire smokers? The question, of course, is whether such a hiring policy is similar, in ethical significance, to a prohibition of smoking on campus or whether it is an entirely different kind of step.

Restricting certain employee personal behaviors on the job and at the worksite is reasonable and often necessary to provide for a safe working and service environment. Policies that ban tobacco use from healthcare campuses have widespread support. These onsite smoking restrictions have generally been considered ethically acceptable, even ethically required, because they contribute to a healthier environment for patients, coworkers, and visitors (without attempting to extend controls further than the worksite) (Roizen, Hasan, and Clive 2008; Williams et al. 2009).

Policies prohibiting workplace smoking benefit many and place minimal restrictions on the personal behavior of individual employees. They prevent smoking in the workplace, but do not attempt to control the employee's behavior away from work. When the employer prohibits a certain kind of employee behavior that applies to the employee offsite and outside of working hours, the connection between personal behavior and potential negative job impact is less clear and less direct, if it even exists.

Both the public and business ethicists have long recognized that hiring criteria, practices, and decisions need to be scrutinized carefully to avoid discrimination. Employment is of such fundamental importance that any practice that, intentionally or not, unfairly deprives some people of the opportunity for employment needs to identified and challenged. This concern—and the guidelines that have been developed over the years to address it—is relevant to the question of not hiring smokers.

The decades-long civil rights efforts to increase job opportunities for everyone regardless of ethnic, racial, or gender identity were gradually successful in leading to the recognition that some criteria or bases for hiring or not hiring individuals are irrelevant and unfair. While some forms of job discrimination are now widely recognized—and legally prohibited—a need for ongoing clarification of appropriate and inappropriate criteria for employment decisions remains. The groups legally protected from discrimination do not include all individuals who are sometimes rejected for unfair reasons.

In the study of business ethics in recent decades, the relationship between employers and employees emerged as one major area of focus, including the nature and limits of the right of employees to individual privacy and individual freedom. When is employer monitoring and mandating of employee behavior appropriate and when is it not? Emphasizing the distinction between behavior on the job and behavior off the job has become common in business ethics. The general standard is that employee off-the-job behavior should be respected as private (i.e., something employers should not inquire about) unless it is something that affects "the employee's work performance in a direct and serious manner" (Velasquez 2002).

The antidiscrimination movement and the attention paid to the nature of employee privacy have led to a common perspective on ethical hiring criteria: Hiring decisions based on any factors not directly related to the ability to do the job put individuals at risk of being deprived of employment opportunities unfairly. An ethical imperative exists to avoid making employment decisions on the basis of personal attributes, characteristics, or behaviors unless they can be shown to be directly related to job performance.

The key question, of course, is whether smoking offsite negatively affects work performance in a serious and direct manner. Making a convincing case that unless they engage in healthy behavior at all times, employees are failing to live up to their essential job responsibilities would be difficult. Smoking does have negative health consequences and can be expected to affect work performance at times. The same might be said, to a certain extent, of many other personal habits or behaviors—too much work, poor diet, heavy drinking, lack of exercise, too little rest, living in a stressful environment, a dangerous hobby.

That smoking is singled out is understandable. It is a behavior that has become less socially acceptable; it can be tested for in the lab and does not require personal assessments or self-reporting; and some argue that there is no "moderate" level of indulgence that is acceptable or healthy. Although singling out smoking is understandable, the differences may not mean that offsite smoking is not compatible with acceptable job performance while other offsite health-related behaviors are more compatible.

A requirement that all employees be nonsmokers may well save on the organization's healthcare costs. Of course, some nonsmokers' healthcare costs or health-related absenteeism can be expected to be higher than normal.

Consistency—treating similar cases similarly—is one aspect of fairness. If the key reason for a policy of hiring only nonsmokers is the smoker's likely future healthcare needs, should job applicants be tested for other conditions that suggest greater future healthcare needs?

As is evident in almost every discussion of presymptomatic genetic testing, widespread concern exists that an employer might use someone's predisposition to a genetic disease as a reason for deciding against that person's employment. And strong support exists for legislation prohibiting "genetic discrimination" in hiring and firing, such as the Genetic Information Nondiscrimination Act (2008).

The ethical standard of direct relationship to job performance is designed to ensure that hiring decisions will not be based on irrelevant—and therefore unfair—considerations. Expanding the concept of job performance to include potential future healthcare costs so that potential healthcare costs can be decisive in employment decisions appears to undermine the notion of fair employment opportunity that the concept is intended to protect.

If the state has not legislated differently (and about half of them have), the legal concept of "employment at will" permits employers to refuse to hire smokers. But the fact that the practice may be legal in a particular state does not by itself make it a sound ethical policy. Insisting that the private lives of employees are generally off-limits for employers is one of the most important protections against the misuse of hiring power by employers.

In the previous discussion of mandatory vaccinations, the distinctness of healthcare workers is described as a relevant and important consideration. Making demands of healthcare workers that are not appropriate to make of other kinds of employees or employees in other organizations can be appropriate at times. Those demands, however, are directly related to their work responsibilities and do not necessarily mean support for singling out healthcare employees for requirements or restrictions related to what they do outside of work.

Smoking is unhealthy behavior, unhealthy to oneself and others, and is voluntary in the sense that no one is forced to start and many are able to stop, given sufficient incentive, time, and effort. To provide a healthier environment, strong ethical support exists for banning smoking in the workplace. To promote health and to contain healthcare cost, providing smoking cessation programs and incentives for employees makes good sense. Making nonsmoking a condition of employment, however, seems to be a different kind of step, primarily because it allows employers to determine who gets employed based on behavior outside of the workplace.

Just Compensation

**Ethically accept-
able minimum
wage**
A "living wage"
that allows a full-
time employee to
be able to meet
the basic needs
of himself and a
small family. Not
the same as the
legal minimum
wage.

Historically, most of the attention paid to the meaning of just compensation in ethics has focused on wages on the lower end of the pay scale in healthcare organizations. The key concern was to identify the minimum level at which compensation can be considered just or fair. Recent years have seen as much concern focused on the high end of the pay scale—what is the point at which compensation of executives or others is too high to be fair?

An **ethically acceptable minimum wage**—not the same as the legal minimum—has long been understood to be a "living wage," one that allows a full-time employee to be able to meet the basic needs of himself and a small family. Anything less is exploitation, a violation of the employee's basic dignity and basic rights. This principle is commonly included in international documents of basic rights, such as the **United Nations Declaration of Human Rights,** ratified in 1948. A typical expression is found in the 1989 **Community Charter of the Fundamental Social Rights of Workers**: "Workers should be paid wages sufficient to support a decent standard of living for themselves and their family" (Commission of the European Community 1989).

Three points can be made to clarify the meaning of a living wage.

**United Nations
Declaration of
Human Rights**
Adopted in 1948
by the United
Nations General
Assembly to artic-
ulate the human
rights and funda-
mental freedoms
that are applicable
to every person,
everywhere. The
document is
meant to serve as
a bulwark against
oppression and
discrimination.

1. The minimum just or fair wage is not the same as the legal minimum wage. The legal minimum wage is created as legislation and therefore is the result of a variety of influences and compromises. It is not directly based on the actual cost of living—a quick review of the prices of housing, food, and transportation in the United States demonstrates that the federal minimum wage is not at all sufficient to meet the needs of an average-sized family.

2. The US federal poverty thresholds are based explicitly on a cost-of-living analysis (taking family size into account) and thus are much more helpful for those seeking to determine the amount of a just wage. These thresholds may also underestimate the real cost of living, however. The Census Bureau, which does the calculation, has since the 1960s used the cost of an economy food budget as the key measure. The cost of food is based on the US Department of Agriculture's food budget designed for families under economic stress. This figure is then multiplied by three to set the poverty thresholds (Hanson 2008). The actual cost of living for a family, according to other calculations, is typically considerably more than three times the purchase price of economy-level groceries (Economic Policy Institute 2008). Thus, a wage sufficient to put the worker right at the poverty level does not mean that one is earning a living wage.

**Community Char-
ter of Fundamental
Social Rights of
Workers**
A charter adopted
in 1989 by the
Commission of
the European
Community that
establishes the
major principles
on which the Euro-
pean labor law
model is based.

3. A just wage is not necessarily the same as the prevailing wage paid in the community for this kind of work. Given supply and demand, the possibility exists that the prevailing wage for some positions is not sufficient to meet the cost of living. The ethical standard of the living wage strongly asserts that "the market" is not the final criterion or standard to be used to determine fairness to employees.

In recent years, a number of healthcare organizations have made an explicit decision that no employee will be paid less than a living wage, a wage that is then usually defined in terms of a percentage (typically considerably over 100 percent) of the federal poverty level for a small family (Kushner and Gallagher 2007). Other methods can be used to calculate the amount of a living wage, such as the fair housing wage (the amount of money that a household would need to afford a rental unit at the fair market rent, using the federal affordability standard of paying no more than 30 percent of income for housing). For this discussion, the important point is that a standard of fairness exists that can be used for making these decisions and that the standard is based on the actual cost of living.

Until recently, most of the discussion and concern related to just compensation focused on the needs of those at or near the bottom of the wage scale. **Morale** in the organization suffers when people are underpaid. However, morale also suffers, perhaps as much, when employees perceive that someone at the top is overpaid. When executives have high compensation packages, many others in the organization may feel that they, by comparison, are not being treated fairly.

Morale
The state of an individual's or a group's feelings and willingness to accomplish assigned tasks.

As attention has turned to fairness in regard to those who are highly compensated, the point of reference has changed. The fairness question here is not whether such individuals are able to meet their basic needs but whether compensation is appropriate to the purpose and mission of the healthcare organization and whether an organization can justify paying some individuals so much more than others.

Finding published comments such as the following is increasingly common (Shinkman 2011): "There are hundreds of nonprofit hospital CEOs . . . compensated with millions of dollars while their institutions throw a few bread crumbs to the poor living in their service areas. Many of these institutions spend more on CEO pay than charity care. Alan Sager, a professor of health policy and management at Boston University, recently told *Crain's Chicago Business* what a lot of healthcare pay and governance experts dare not say: 'There's an enormous sense of self-entitlement among CEOs. It started in the for-profit corporate sector, but it has sloshed over into the non-profit hospital world.'"

When information about the (often seven-figure) total compensation of area healthcare CEOs is published in local newspapers, a strong negative reaction almost always follows, both from the public and from employees in the executive's own organization. Careful attention must always be given to the criteria used to determine the level of executive compensation in health services organizations; a critical review is an especially high priority at a time when many think that there is something wrong with the present level.

Boards and board committees often approach the question of executive compensation with a view to attracting and retaining talented managers. To be competitive in the search for good managers, conforming to market-driven compensation levels is normally considered necessary. Market analysis is an important tool, but just as with a living wage, analysis alone does not determine fair executive compensation.

- A market analysis requires a variety of decisions about the peer organizations to which the comparison is being made: Are the organizations in the region or national? What is the size of comparison organizations (and what determines size)? Do they have comparable missions? Are they in comparable communities? And at what level does the organization want its executive compensation to be compared with peers (in the top half, sixty-fifth percentile, or other level)?

- Is the market analysis conducted ethically and objectively? Who decides which organizations are appropriate peers (for example, how much of a role does the occupant of the position have in naming the peers)? The goal of fairness can be undermined by the way the process is managed.

- Market analysis does not address the question of how to design and monitor incentive compensation to ensure that the executive is rewarded only for extraordinary achievements in promoting the mission of the organization.

- Market analysis does not contribute much to understanding just compensation if, as is widely believed, executive compensation is excessive across the board. Using excessive pay elsewhere as the standard will result in excessive pay here—and contribute to continually raising the level.

- Even when well thought out and carefully done, market analysis does not provide the answer regarding what constitutes the just level of compensation for executives in a particular organization. It does not address the important question of internal equity.

Even when done well, market analysis examines only external equity or external comparison. The standards of internal equity are identified by specifying the limits to executive compensation compared to what others in the organization are receiving. In terms of fairness to all employees—and in terms of organizational morale and culture—internal equity is every bit as important as external equity in determining the level of executive compensation.

Identifying the ratio between the highest paid and the lowest paid employee or between the highest paid and the midlevel employee can be an enlightening experience for an organization—and then to engage in a reflective and fairness-driven conversation about what a most appropriate ratio might be, all relevant responsibilities considered. In helping to set compensation levels for executives in the organization, ethicists do not have a formula—such as cost of living for the lowest paid—to offer as a guiding standard. However, they recognize that using the marketplace as the only or the final arbiter of fairness in executive compensation is avoiding the hard work of ethical leadership and almost inevitably contributes to an upward spiraling process.

Union Organizing

Actions speak more loudly than words. No matter what administrators say about how much they value and respect employees, most employees assess the real nature of that respect based on the ways management addresses the kinds of issues discussed in this chapter. This assessment is certainly true in many organizations in regard to collective bargaining.

Many healthcare administrators are opposed to labor unions and see unions as interfering with the effective running of the organization. This opposition can be reinforced by a culture in which consulting firms regularly provide programs on how to prevent or defeat unionizing efforts. While managers are aware of the general *legal* protection of workers' right to unionize, they may not be as familiar with the *ethical foundation* for respecting workers' efforts to select a collective bargaining agent.

The right to form unions has long been recognized as a fundamental and essential human right (UN 1948). As a human right, this applies to all organizations that hire employees, whether for-profit or nonprofit. And, as a human right, the right of workers to bargain collectively makes binding claims on management and the public. To prevent workers from organizing is to deny them the opportunity to decide for themselves how to speak regarding decisions that affect them directly. Seeking to speak with a stronger and more unified voice by organizing is one way for workers to express themselves in an organization.

Hospital administrators understandably sometimes dislike organizing efforts and prefer that employees not select a particular union to represent them. In terms of good management–employee relationships and best ethical practices, however, the key questions are how to understand the meaning of unionizing efforts and what methods to use in responding to such efforts. Some responses demonstrate respect for employees and contribute to good relationships, while others can be quite destructive.

Taking seriously the human right of employees to organize for collective bargaining seems to suggest the following points:

- Describing the positive vote of employees for union representation as a failure on the part of management can be a trap. When people say that those organizations that get unions deserve them, they are saying that unions are an abnormal part of good management–employee relationships and that they occur only when management has failed to manage effectively. Besides being a questionable statement, this kind of thinking puts administration in the position of having to oppose union organizing efforts vigorously as a way of demonstrating that it has not failed.

- To observers, union organizing campaigns in healthcare organizations often seem to resemble the worst of hard-fought political campaigns— every tactic that one can legally get away with is used to win. Sometimes management employs "union prevention" consultants to conduct the most effective campaign. When the decision is made to fight vigorously to win the election, the great risk is that the fight will escalate and that both sides might use methods that contribute to a negative work environment in the future, whether employees select a bargaining agent or not.

- In any effort to encourage employees not to select a particular union to represent them, the case must be made in a way that is honest and nonintimidating. Distorting the potential negative implications of a pro-union vote undermines the goal of an informed decision on the part of employees. And practices such as mandatory one-on-one meetings with managers to discuss union representation can be intimidating to many employees. Every step being considered regarding communication with employees about the election should be scrutinized carefully in advance in terms of its long-term implications for management–employee relationships. Proposing it as a good strategy to win the election is not enough.

In healthcare organizations in the United States affiliated with the Roman Catholic Church, the ethics related to union organizing efforts have long been a topic of intense ethical interest. This interest has been sparked by the fact that two realities have existed side by side for some time. On the one hand, the social justice teaching of the Roman Catholic Church has, for well over a century, consistently emphasized the basic right of workers to form unions to secure what they consider fair working conditions. On the other hand, union organizing in Catholic healthcare institutions in recent decades has sometimes involved vigorous union-preventing efforts on the part of administration and attacks upon the organization's leadership by union organizers.

Although reasons and explanations that make the conjunction of these two realities more understandable may well exist, the question of "What is going on here?" has often been raised. In an effort to move beyond this contentious history, a group made up of Catholic bishops, Catholic health-care organizations, and labor unions met repeatedly over a two-year period to offer advice to both management and unionizing employees, resulting in the report *Respecting the Just Rights of Workers: Guidance and Options for Catholic Health Care and Unions* (USCCB 2009). The report merits careful consideration by both healthcare administrators and union organizers (and not only by those in Catholic organizations—the ethical principles identified and applied are not at all unique to the Catholic tradition).

The authors recognize that the key to maintaining high ethical standards at the time of union elections is to focus explicitly on a fair process. They emphasize the need for management and labor to reach mutual agreement on the means to be used to ensure free and fair choice in decisions about union representation. The document proposes that employers and unions create and sign "a written, enforceable Local Agreement" (USCCB 2009, 8) that outlines the rules that will be followed by each while the organizing effort is under way. A major portion of the document is devoted to identifying the principles that would protect a fair and just process and can be incorporated into such a document.

The Local Agreement is proposed as a way of ensuring a fair process by agreeing in advance on the rules that management and union organizers will abide by. Since a fair process requires accurate and truthful information, the standards that are proposed for guiding communication during an organizing campaign may be particularly worthy of attention.

Employers often see unions as unnecessary and as potentially disruptive of working relationships in an organization. They therefore want to prevent employees from selecting union representation. Good ethics is often more about the means used than about the end sought. And respectful long-term working relationships are established and protected more by adhering to the demands of fairness than by achieving a predetermined outcome.

Conclusion

Considerably more can be said about each of the issues discussed in this chapter. The purpose here is simply to demonstrate the kinds of perspectives and analysis that might be brought to the consideration of employee-related issues when the goal is to have organizational policies and practices based on a commitment to understand and implement the demands of fairness. Employees and prospective employees are, first of all, individuals who are owed the respect and protections owed all persons. As employees, they take on certain responsibilities and tasks, but they do not lose or give up the need to be treated with the kind of fairness that has been elaborated most clearly in the human rights and social ethics traditions.

Points to Remember

- In employee relationships, determining what *fairness* means is often difficult. Best practices are ensured by considering the perspectives and priorities that are highlighted when the issues are explored explicitly as issues of ethics, including fairness. Executives have a responsibility to include ethical analysis when making decisions on key or controversial issues. Consistency—treating similar cases similarly—is one aspect of fairness.

- Our rights are limited by our responsibility to avoid placing others, our employees and our patients, at unnecessary risk of significant harm. Rights are sometimes limited by work-related roles. Mandates for employees are appropriate if necessary to protect patients, but they should be no more restrictive of individual freedom than necessary to achieve that goal.

- Restricting certain employee behaviors on the job to provide a safe working environment is reasonable and often necessary. Making demands of healthcare workers can be appropriate, even if similar demands are not appropriate to make of other employees or employees in other organizations.

- Employment is of such fundamental importance that any practice that unfairly deprives some people of the opportunity for employment needs to be identified and challenged. The general standard is that employee off-the-job behavior should be respected as private unless it affects the employee's work performance in a direct and serious manner. An ethical imperative exists to avoid making employment decisions on the basis of personal attributes, characteristics, or behaviors unless they can be shown to be directly related to job performance.

- A just wage is not necessarily the same as the prevailing wage in the community for the same kind of work. The ethical standard of the living wage and the market is not the final criterion or standard to be used to determine fairness to employees. The standard of fairness is based on the actual cost of living.

- The question of fairness in high compensation is whether it is appropriate to the purpose and mission of the healthcare organization and justified for paying some individuals much more than others. The assumptions and the process in determining executive compensation must be scrutinized to clarify their objectivity and ethical implications, including internal equity. Internal equity is as important as external equity.
- The right to form unions is recognized as a fundamental and essential human right. Knowing the ethical foundation for respecting worker's efforts to select a collective bargaining agent is important. In terms of good management–employee relationships and best ethical practices, the key questions are how to understand the meaning of unionizing efforts and what methods to use to respond. The key to maintaining high ethical standards is to focus on a fair process.

References

Anikeeva, O., A. Braunack-Mayer, and W. Rogers. 2009. "Requiring Influenza Vaccination for Health Care Workers." *American Journal of Public Health* 99 (1): 24–29.

Commission of the European Community. 1989. "The Community Charter of the Fundamental Social Rights of Workers." Accessed April 8, 2013. http://europa.eu/legislation_summaries/glossary/social_charter_en.htm.

Economic Policy Institute. 2008. "Basic Family Budget Calculator." Accessed May 1, 2013. www.epi.org/resources/budget/.

Genetic Information Nondiscrimination Act of 2008. Pub. L. 110–233, 122 Stat. 881. www.eeoc.gov/laws/statutes/gina.cfm.

Hanson, K. 2008. "Mollie Orshansky's Strategy to Poverty Measurement as a Relationship Between Household Food Expenditures and Economy Food Plan." *Review of Agricultural Economics* 30 (3): 572–80.

Immunization Action Coalition. 2013. "Honor Roll for Patient Safety." Accessed May 1. www.immunize.org/honor-roll/influenza-mandates.asp.

Kushner, M., and J. Gallagher. 2007. "Calculating a Socially Just Wage." *Health Progress* 88 (5): 29–32.

Roizen, M. F., I. M. Hasan, and D. Clive. 2008. "Balancing Health Promotion and Healing." *Virtual Mentor* 10 (11): 700–707.

Shinkman, R. 2011. "The Problem of 8-Figure Hospital Paychecks and Near-Poor Patients." Published November 28. www.fiercehealthfinance.com/story/evaluating-eight-figure-paychecks-and-near-poor-patients/2011-11-28.

Sulzberger, A. G. 2011. "Hospitals Shift Smoking Bans to Smoker Bans." *New York Times* February 11.

United Nations (UN). 1948. "Article 23." *The Universal Declaration of Human Rights*. Accessed April 8, 2013. www.un.org/en/documents/udhr/index .shtml#a23.

United States Conference on Catholic Bishops (USCCB). 2009. *Respecting the Just Rights of Workers: Guidance and Options for Catholic Health Care and Unions*. Published June 22. http://old.usccb.org/sdwp/national/respecting_ the_just_rights_of_workers.pdf.

Velasquez, M. G. 2002. *Business Ethics: Concepts and Cases*, 5th ed. Upper Saddle River, NJ: Prentice Hall.

Williams, S. C., J. M. Hafner, D. J. Morton, A. L. Holm, S. M. Milberger, R. G. Koss, and J. M. Loeb. 2009. "The Adoption of Smoke-Free Hospital Campuses in the United States." *Tobacco Control* 18 (6): 451–58.

AN INTRODUCTION TO ENVIRONMENTAL AND SUSTAINABILITY ISSUES IN HEALTHCARE MANAGEMENT

Carrie R. Rich, J. Knox Singleton, and Seema S. Wadhwa

This chapter is relevant to the following competencies identified in the ACHE Competencies Assessment Tool (see p. xxv):

Communication and Relationship Management
- Identify stakeholder needs/expectations

Leadership
- Potential impacts and consequences of decision making in situations both internal and external
- Establish a compelling organizational vision and goals

Professionalism
- Serve as the ethical guide for the organization

Knowledge of the Healthcare Environment
- The interrelationships between access, quality, cost, resource allocation, accountability, and community
- The patient's perspective (e.g., cultural differences, expectations)

Business Skills and Knowledge
- Organizational mission, vision, objectives, and priorities

Learning Objectives

After completing this chapter, the reader will be able to

- explain what healthcare sustainability is,

- understand the relationship between sustainability ethics and clinical ethics,
- describe how sustainability relates to the mission of healthcare organizations, and
- explain why sustainability is an ethical imperative for healthcare organizations and their leaders.

What Is Sustainability?

Healthcare sustainability
Defined by "triple bottom line" practices that minimize environmental impact, fiscal waste, and negative effects on the community. Addressing sustainability issues is ethically consistent with providing safe, quality care.

Sustainability addresses a triple bottom line: people, planet, and profit, or social, environmental, and fiscal responsibility (Elkington 1998). **Healthcare sustainability** minimizes negative effects on the community, reduces the environmental impact of healthcare, and cuts fiscal waste. In many ways, the mission of healthcare mirrors the goals of sustainability. Sustainability can be an end goal or the framework for reaching an end goal. For the future of health, sustainability is a component of the healthcare leader's moral core. The cultural dynamic is shifting to a point where the conversation is no longer just about what impact we as a society are having on the environment but more so what impact the environment is having on human health (Boone 2012). Sustainability is aligned with a new paradigm of health, one focused on prevention and wellness. The concept of sustainability includes more than environmentalism and the threat to human health if we maintain the destructive environmental status quo (Dentzer 2011).

Sustainability includes maximizing the productive life cycle of investments in the healthcare system (Lüdeke-Freund 2009) and is a fundamental component of public health and well-being (WHO 2012). Core components of sustainable operations include energy management, water use reduction, environmentally preferable purchasing, health information technology, sustainable foods, green construction, and alternative transportation. These operational processes also create opportunities for cost savings.

Linking Environmental Ethics to Healthcare Ethics

Healthcare services have a direct stake in sustainability. Although sustainability is a shared value across a variety of human endeavors and industries, sustainability specifically aligns with the mission of healthcare organizations. All healthcare organizations share a mission to contribute to promoting and maintaining the health and well-being of the communities they serve. Being excellent at providing safe, quality care while ignoring the importance of environmental sustainability to healthcare would be ethically inconsistent. The goals of providing quality of care and environmental sustainability are interdependent; quality of care focused on improved patient and community health can be undone by the failure to operate the healthcare organization sustainably.

Sustainability is a strategy by which healthcare organizations can pursue the mission of healthcare. Often, the failures of sustainability efforts increase the burden of disease and the demand for health services within a community (CDC 2011). The effects of pollution on the public's health are clearly detrimental—in 1952, the deaths of 4,000 people in London were associated with widespread use of dirty fuels (World Resources Institute 1998). Currently, more than 455,000 premature deaths occur in the European Union's 27 member states each year because of air pollution from fine particles (Health and Environmental Alliance 2011). According to the United Nations Environment Programme (2012), the public health impacts of pollution range from respiratory abnormalities to skeletal muscular system impacts to central nervous system impacts.

The quality of the environment is affected by providing healthcare services (Rastogi 2010). The healthcare industry uses large amounts of increasingly scarce resources (Practice Greenhealth 2013). Generating waste is a necessary part of healthcare operations, but the creation of 7,000 tons of waste daily by the healthcare industry is considered by the American Hospital Association (2012) to be excessive and unsustainable. Much of the $10 billion that the healthcare industry spends annually on energy is wasted (Halvorson 2012). The opportunity exists to spend money more responsibly. With healthcare composing 17.3 percent of the gross domestic product (CMS 2012), fiscal responsibility is an ethical priority.

How healthcare organizations conduct business is as meaningful as their core mission of providing health services (Callender et al. 2003). Healthcare organizations have an ethical mandate to design their business practices and development strategies to achieve goals that are compatible with sustainability.

Wealth Versus Health

Wasting less intrinsically means saving more. Waste-reduction strategies often provide a starting point for healthcare organizations newly energized around sustainability because they can be highly visible (e.g., recycling) and a clear business case exists for sustainable waste management (Practice Greenhealth 2012). A combination of waste reduction and prevention strategies is saving millions of dollars annually in healthcare organizations across the United States (Brown 2012). Still, many healthcare organizations have yet to fully embrace sustainable practices.

Cost Implications: What Is the Ethical Bottom Line?

In some instances the implementation of a practice that supports sustainability conflicts with or competes with achieving the other values-based goals of a healthcare institution. This conflict usually involves allocation of limited resources. For example, in 2011, Inova faced a decision about purchasing environmentally preferable recycled content paper. The additional cost was $100,000 annually. Inova's leaders asked themselves what values and commitments should determine the decision to purchase environmentally preferable recycled paper content (Heath 2011). Their analysis included identifying and exploring all implications, including the true costs and opportunity costs of purchasing recycled paper. Factored into the decision was the impact that $100,000 could have if it was infused into other components of the organization's mission. Inova ultimately decided to purchase nonrecycled paper. In this instance, the decision was made by clarifying the relationship between the allocation of resources and the organization's values and priorities. Using the money saved by purchasing virgin paper to provide indigent care, at that moment, had a higher priority than did "going green." The values and issues related to implementing sustainable practices must be balanced and prioritized against other demands on the organization's resources. Those values and issues were made explicit in the decision-making and management processes, which reinforced the organization's ethics culture.

More broadly, ethical implications can challenge the fiscal responsibilities of a healthcare organization. For example, recycling alkaline batteries is not legally required. However, batteries contain many toxic materials. A healthcare organization's options include discarding batteries into a landfill or paying a premium to dispose of batteries through recycling. The ethical dilemma arises, when no regulatory requirement to behave in ethical manner exists, whether a healthcare organization should opt for the fiscally responsible but environmentally degrading option. Or should the healthcare organization opt for the environmentally responsible, more costly approach? Is this question more sensitive to healthcare organizations than to any other business because of their mission for health and wellness of the community?

How to Present Sustainability Without Degrading It

Significant cost savings are often associated with environmental sustainability efforts. These cost savings can be drivers to engage those within healthcare organizations who are not inherently engaged in sustainability. For instance, Hospital Corporation of America (HCA) saved more than $21 million in 2011 through single-use device reprocessing (Healthier Hospitals Initiative 2012a). Partners HealthCare had energy costs of $100 million. By developing a strategic management plan of energy conservation and efficiency mechanisms, they were able to reduce 9 percent of their total energy use in 18 months (Healthier Hospitals Initiative 2012c). Kaiser Permanente saved $4 million annually by purchasing environmentally responsible computers (Healthier Hospitals Initiative 2012b). These examples show not only cost savings but also a positive impact on the surrounding community, employees, and the environment.

The danger, however, is that sustainability is promoted solely as a cost-savings mechanism. This scenario risks emphasizing cost to the detriment of the social and environmental components of the triple bottom line. Two outcomes may result:

1. "Greenwashing," which means marketing items and processes as being environmentally responsible even when they do not meet such criteria (Hoffman and Hoffman 2009)
2. Supporting the longevity of a sustainability program only when there are associated cost savings

Sustainability is aligned not only with cost savings but also with community benefit, employee engagement strategy, brand promise, and the quality and safety imperative (Rich, Singleton, and Wadhwa 2012).

Defining Roles in Healthcare Sustainability

Each individual in healthcare has a unique responsibility when it comes to operationalizing ethics within environmental sustainability.

The Administrator's Role

Healthcare administrators have a professional and moral mandate to catalyze their organizations and their communities to address sustainability challenges. Many healthcare leaders do not recognize the relationship between sustainability and their obligation to improve the health and safety of patients, staff, and community; thus, they often do not recognize that sustainability should be part of their ethical decision-making framework.

The values inherent in sustainability are a dimension of the healthcare executive's professionalism; that is, a moral core commitment to work to enhance the well-being of the patients and the community that are served by the organization (see Chapter 5). The community appropriately looks to the executive leadership of healthcare organizations for competency in clarifying complex health-related issues and guidance in making decisions that impact quality of life. Communities expect healthcare leaders to be accountable for their business decisions, including the effects of their decisions on the environment (Thomas and Harris 2004). Healthcare leaders may be held to a higher standard of accountability than are the leaders of other industries because their professionalism embodies a commitment to the spirit of the Hippocratic Oath: "First, do no harm."

The promotion of sustainability is therefore a moral and ethical mandate for healthcare leaders. Because of their leadership skills, professional knowledge, and access to resources and status, healthcare executives can be expected to use their positions and the moral authority that accompanies these positions to raise the issue, bring community leadership together, and facilitate collaboration to make sustainability a reality. Few other people in the community have comparable platforms from which to inspire action.

The moral requisite is to make the goal of sustainability as explicit and as high a priority as is the goal of quality of care. Consider the use of chemicals in medical products and devices. At one point, intravenous (IV) fluids were packaged in glass vials. To reduce cost and improve functionality, IV bags are now made of plastic. One unintended consequence of switching to plastic bags has been the leaching of Bis(2-ethylhexyl) phthalate (DEHP) from plastic bags into humans. DEHP is known to cause gastrointestinal distress in humans (EPA 2000). To treat our most vulnerable population, babies in the neonatal intensive care unit (NICU), many hospitals have switched to non-DEHP IV bags. However, these bags cost more. Although many healthcare organizations made the change in the NICU, not all departments have made this switch. The ethical question remains: What is the line between clinical precaution and cost management? This question is a key consideration for the healthcare administrators aiming to define their role in sustainability.

The Clinician's Role

Clinicians play a vital role in leading sustainability initiatives within healthcare organizations because they are the face of healthcare to most patients. How clinicians carry themselves strongly represents the ethics of a healthcare organization. For instance, if a doctor is seen placing paper in a recycling bin as opposed the trash bin, the message conveyed is that the doctor cares about the environment in which her patients live.

Many organizational sustainability programs that exist today were created and driven by clinicians. For instance, sustainability programs at Inova, University of Maryland, Kaiser Permanente, and Gundersen Lutheran were originally inspired by clinicians who cared about the environments in which their patients are expected to heal (Cohen 2012).

The Patient's Role

Often, the responsibility of getting better is put on the patient's clinical team. This situation does not empower the most important stakeholder: the patient. In healthcare ethics, the opportunity exists to discuss the patient's responsibility, not only toward their individual health but also in fulfilling the health of the ecosystem in which he resides. Many of the illnesses that patients suffer from are linked with environmental factors (CDC 2011). Environmental sustainability is a responsibility that affects the individual's health and well-being as well as population health.

Individual Versus Public Health

The relationship between healthcare, environmentalism, and sustainability is unique. As Exhibit 10.1 shows, environmental conditions, such as socioeconomic and cultural conditions, are determinants of health for individuals, families, and communities.

Impact of Ethics Across the Supply Chain

How an organization spends its resources is a visible indicator of that organization's ethical values. Healthcare organizations have a unique opportunity to use purchasing power to align ethics with environmental sustainability.

EXHIBIT 10.1
Determinants
of Health

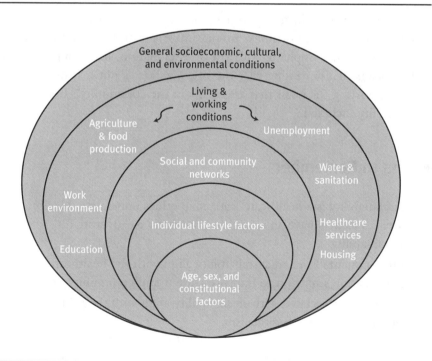

Adapted from "Measuring Deprivation" *Rural Health Good Practice Toolkit*. Available at www.ruralhealthgoodpractice.org.uk/index. php?page_name=section1_chapter4_measuring_deprivation.

What is the environment? In many senses, the environment can be defined as our outdoor surroundings. Others may consider the environment to be manufactured—the space in which we reside or work every day. For an ailing patient, the most important environment is the care environment. The care environment is where the patient goes to heal, is most vulnerable, and trusts the sanctity of the place. Kaiser Permanente understood this reality when building a cancer treatment center. Kaiser Permanente's goal was to build a cancer treatment center that was void of carcinogens. One would think that cancer centers would logically be carcinogen-free, but that is not the reality. In fact, when Kaiser Permanente embarked on its cancer treatment facility, no carpets free of volatile organic compounds (VOCs), a known carcinogen, existed. Kaiser Permanente leveraged its purchasing power to align with its organizational ethics and drove the market to create low-VOC carpet. This item is now available at major retailers for homeowners to make healthy decisions about their built environment. This example shows how the healthcare industry led ethical change by embracing a sustainability challenge (Healthier Hospitals Initiative 2012b).

Conclusion

The healthcare organization—with its influence, visibility, and resources—should take every opportunity to maximize positive community impact. While it starts by complying with law and regulation, leadership in sustainability means demonstrating that the organization is not just meeting code but is supporting the goals that are clearly in the community's best interests, sustainability included.

Points to Remember

- Sustainability is a healthcare leadership ethics imperative. Health services leaders have an ethical responsibility to advocate for sustainability.
- Environmentalism and sustainability align with the healthcare organization's mission to improve patient and community health.
- The values associated with sustainability align with the values associated with healthcare professionalism.

References

American Hospital Association (AHA). 2012. "Waste." Accessed April 1. www .sustainabilityroadmap.org/topics/waste.shtml.

Boone, T. 2012. "Creating a Culture of Sustainability: Leadership, Coordination and Performance Measurement Decisions in Healthcare." *Health Care Without Harm*. Published April 1. www.noharm.org/us_canada/reports/2012/apr/ rep2012-04-01.php.

Brown, J. 2012. "Benchmarking Sustainability in Health Care Awards Benchmark Report." *CleanMed*. Published April 1. www.cleanmed.org/2010/ downloads/presentations/C4/Brown.pdf.

Callender, A., D. Hastings, M. Hemsley, L. Morris, and M. Peregrine. 2003. "Corporate Responsibility and Healthcare Quality: A Resource for Health Care Boards of Directors." *The Office of Inspector General of the US Department of Health and Human Services and The American Health Lawyers Association*. Accessed July 27. http://oig.hhs.gov/fraud/docs/complianceguidance /CorporateResponsibilityFinal%209-4-07.pdf.

Centers for Disease Control and Prevention (CDC). 2011. "Environmental Hazards and Health Effects." National Center for Environmental Health. Published July 27. www.cdc.gov/nceh/ehhe/.

Centers for Medicare & Medicaid Services (CMS). 2012. "NHE Fact Sheet." Accessed January 3. www.cms.gov/Research-Statistics-Data-and-Systems/Statistics-Trends-and-Reports/NationalHealthExpendData/NHE-Fact-Sheet.html.

Cohen, G. 2012. "Introductory Remarks." CleanMed Annual Conference. Denver, Colorado, April 30.

Dentzer, S. 2011. "Embarking on a New Course: Environmental Health Coverage." *Health Affairs* 30 (5): 810.

Elkington, John. 1998. *Cannibals with Forks: The Triple Bottom Line of 21st Century Business*. Gabriela Island, BC, Canada: New Society Publishers.

Halvorson, G. 2012. "Sustainable Hospitals Can Help Bend the Cost Curve: Kaiser Permanente's Environmental Stewardship." *The Commonwealth Fund*. Published November 2. www.commonwealthfund.org/Blog/2012/Nov /Sustainable-Hospitals-Can-Help-Bend-the-Cost-Curve.aspx.

Health and Environmental Alliance. 2011. "Information Release: Research Quantifies Increased Life and Wealth from Cleaner Air." Accessed June 2, 2013. www .env-health.org/IMG/pdf/20110304_Aphekom_-_HEAL_Information_ Release.pdf.

Healthier Hospitals Initiative. 2012a. "Efficient Use of Resources: Reprocessing of Single Use Devices at HCA (Hospital Corporation of America)." Accessed January 2. http://healthierhospitals.org/get-inspired/case-studies /efficient-use-resources-reprocessing-single-use-devices-hca-hospital.

———. 2012b. "Kaiser Permanente | Electronic Products Environmental Assessment Tool (EPEAT) – Purchasing Environmentally Responsible Computers." Accessed January 2. http://healthierhospitals.org/get-inspired/case-studies /kaiser-permanente-electronic-products-environmental-assessment-tool-epeat-.

———. 2012c. "Partners Healthcare Strategic Energy Master Plan." Accessed January 2. http://healthierhospitals.org/get-inspired/case-studies/partners-healthcare-strategic-energy-master-plan.

Heath, S. 2011. Interview with author, March 10.

Hoffman, J., and M. Hoffman. 2009. "What Is Greenwashing?" *Scientific American*. Published April 1. www.scientificamerican.com/article .cfm?id=greenwashing-green-energy-hoffman.

Institute for Rural Health. "Measuring Deprivation." *Rural Health Good Practice Toolkit*. Available at www.nwpho.org.uk/reports/ruralhealth.pdf.

Lüdeke-Freund, F. 2009. "Business Model Concepts in Corporate Sustainability Contexts: From Rhetoric to a Generic Template for 'Business Models for Sustainability.'" Centre for Sustainability Management (CSM): Leuphana Universität Lüneburg. Accessed July 27. http://dx.doi.org/10.2139/ssrn.1544847.

Practice Greenhealth. 2013. "Energy, Water, & Climate." Accessed January 2. http://practicegreenhealth.org/topics/energy-water-climate.

———. 2012. "Inova Fairfax Hospital: Regulated Medical Waste Reduction and Minimization." Accessed July 27. http://practicegreenhealth.org/sites /default/files/uploadfiles/casestudy_inova_r6_web_1.pdf.

Rastogi, N. S. 2010. "Green Lantern: How Much Trash Does a Hospital Produce?" *Washington Post*. Published October 18. www.washingtonpost.com/wp-dyn /content/article/2010/10/18/AR2010101804465.html.

Rich, C., K. Singleton, and S. Wadhwa. 2012. *Sustainability for Healthcare Management: A Leadership Imperative*. Oxford, United Kingdom: Routledge.

Thomas, J., and J. Harris. 2004. "Environment: Value to the Investor." *Global Environmental Management Initiative*. Accessed July 27. www.gemi.org /resources/GEMI%20Clear%20Advantage.pdf.

United Nations Environment Programme (UNEP) Urban Environment Unit. 2012. "Environmental Pollution Impacts on Public Health: Implications of the Dandora Municipal Dumping Site in Nairobi, Kenya." Accessed July 27. www .unep.org/urban_environment/pdfs/dandorawastedump-reportsummary.pdf.

US Environmental Protection Agency (EPA). 2012. "What Is Sustainability? | What Is EPA Doing? | How Can I Help?" Accessed July 27. www.epa.gov /sustainability/basicinfo.htm.

———. 2000. "Bis(2-ethylhexyl) phthalate (DEHP)." Accessed January 6. www.epa .gov/ttnatw01/hlthef/eth-phth.html.

World Health Organization (WHO). 2012. "Putting Health at the Heart of Sustainable Development." Accessed July 27. www.who.int/hia/green_economy /health_sust_development/en/.

World Resources Institute. 1998. "Rising Energy Use: Health Effects of Air Pollution." Accessed July 27. www.wri.org/publication/content/8463.

EXTERNAL REQUIREMENTS FOR ETHICS IN HEALTHCARE ORGANIZATIONS

Ann E. Mills

This chapter is relevant to the following competencies identified in the ACHE Competencies Assessment Tool (see p. xxv):

Leadership
- Adhere to legal and regulatory standards

Professionalism
- Consequences of unethical actions
- Organizational business and personal ethics
- Uphold and act upon ethical and professional standards

Knowledge of the Healthcare Environment
- Corporate compliance laws and regulations
- Governmental, regulatory, professional, and accreditation agencies

Business Skills and Knowledge
- Organizational policies and procedures and their functions

Learning Objectives

After completing this chapter, the reader will be able to

- understand that the primary external sources of ethical expectations concerning a hospital are stakeholders,
- discuss the distinction between "law" and "ethics,"
- understand why the US Department of Health and Human Services (HHS) requires hospitals to develop "voluntary compliance programs,"

- know the requirements of HHS for developing ethics and compliance programs,
- know what The Joint Commission considers an appropriate culture for hospitals,
- identify the various orientations of ethics and compliance programs,
- reflect on the available evidence as to which orientation produces a more positive impact, and
- understand the power of organizations in affecting individual behavior.

Introduction

The primary sources of external ethical expectations concerning a hospital are its stakeholders. These include its patients, professionals, healthcare financing organizations, professional associations, the community in which the hospitals resides, and so on (see Chapter 4 for a more complete list of a hospital's stakeholders). Patients will expect, on entering a hospital, to be treated with courtesy and respect. Professionals will be guided by their professional associations as to their behavior when confronting an ethically problematic situation and will expect the hospital to acknowledge and support their professional codes of ethics. The community will expect the hospital to serve its needs.

This book shows that the hospital, as well as individuals affiliated or employed by the hospital, will often be confronted with a troublesome ethical situation or dilemma. Chapter 2 demonstrates how conflict can occur between the various missions and values of a hospital and how that conflict can translate into ethical conflict for the hospital as well as the individual. Some chapters discuss how certain types of ethical conflict can be resolved. For example, Chapter 5 discusses how ethical conflicts at the bedside might be resolved, and Chapter 2 offers a framework for thinking through ethical dilemmas that administrators might face.

This book stresses the importance of a healthcare organization having an appropriate culture, a culture that is legitimized by reflecting societal expectations and values so that it can meet the expectations of its stakeholders. (See Chapter 2 for a definition of culture and its important component, the ethical climate.)

But developing an appropriate organizational culture in hospitals is also required by judicial and accreditation authorities. The two primary judicial authorities creating laws and guidance aimed at creating an appropriate organization culture in hospitals are the United States Sentencing Commission (USSC) and the Office of Inspector General (OIG) in the Department of Health and Human Services (HHS).

The laws associated with the USSC concerning the creation and maintenance of an appropriate organizational culture are found in Chapter 8 of the Federal Sentencing Guidelines (FSG) (USSC 2010). In regard to organizational culture, the guidance offered to hospitals by the OIG is found in two documents that are discussed in more detail later in the chapter.

Even though the laws associated with the FSG and the guidance offered by OIG overlap, in hospitals, they are generally handled by two different functions. Legal counsel oversees requirements associated with the FSG, and a chief compliance officer oversees requirements associated with the OIG.

Because future administrators will probably be more concerned with how compliance issues impact the culture of a hospital, the chapter does not discuss the FSG. The interested student can find a discussion about the FSG in the Appendix.

This chapter begins with a brief discussion of the relationship between law and ethics. It looks more closely at the guidance offered by the OIG on what kind of culture it requires hospitals to develop and how to go about developing it. The chapter looks at the hurdles involved in using **compliance programs** as a tool in developing a hospital's organizational culture.

Compliance programs Guidelines designed to promote a culture that pays attention to ethics and encourages compliance with the law. Required by the Federal Sentencing Guidelines and the Office of Inspector General.

To be eligible to receive payment from Medicare, hospitals must meet certain conditions, and they must be certified to have met these conditions. Hospitals may gain certification by choosing to be reviewed by a state certification agency under contract to the Centers for Medicare & Medicaid Services (CMS) or be accredited by either The Joint Commission or the American Osteopathic Association. Because a large majority of hospitals choose certification through The Joint Commission, this chapter focuses on the interest The Joint Commission has in hospitals developing and sustaining a culture of safety and quality.

The chapter reviews existing empirical evidence on whether or not the mechanisms and orientations associated with compliance programs are effective in producing a culture that promotes appropriate behavior and concludes with recent research that demonstrates the power organizations have to influence behavior.

Law and Ethics

Even though we can think of laws as specifying what we "have to do" or "cannot do" and ethics in terms of what we "should" or "should not" do, law and ethics overlap. The language used in law and ethics is often similar. Both speak of rights, rules, and principles. Both attempt to inform and educate our decisions and activities as to what is acceptable or not. But the law is accompanied by a public sanction. Lombardo (2005) clarifies, "Generally speaking, law represents public social regulation that can be enforced by public officials—police officers and prosecutors. . . . In contrast, when we invoke principles or rules of ethics, we often have in mind aspirational norms that carry no public sanction." Of course, this line is becoming more and more blurred. For example, a physician who violates her ethical proscriptions might be subject to suspension or censure by her professional association, and such actions may lack the publicity of government enforcements. But states maintain databases that are accessible to the public and contain information on any disciplinary action taken against physicians (Public Citizen 2013).

Even though hospitals "voluntarily" seek accreditation from The Joint Commission, and the OIG issues guidance for hospitals to establish "voluntary" compliance programs, in practice, most hospitals think of The Joint Commission's standards and the OIG's guidance in terms of laws that must be obeyed. Moreover, violation of or noncompliance with the standards and the guidance can carry a public sanction—the noncompliant hospital can no longer treat and receive reimbursement from Medicare patients.

But the laws governing hospitals, accreditation standards, and guidance from the OIG cannot cover every situation or every activity in a hospital. In ambiguous situations, rights, rules, and principles can offer guidance. For this reason, most hospitals are serious about developing a culture that explicitly reflects their values. This reason also explains the emphasis that federal authorities and The Joint Commission place on hospitals developing cultures that discourage unethical and illegal conduct and promote safety and quality in healthcare delivery.

Compliance Program Guidance

The mission of the OIG (2011) is "to protect the integrity of Department of Health and Human Services (HHS) programs, as well as the health and welfare of the beneficiaries of those programs."

HHS represents one-quarter of all federal outlays. It administers more grant dollars than all other federal agencies combined. It administers the Medicare program and partners with states to administer Medicaid through its agency, the Centers for Medicare & Medicaid Services (HHS 2011). In 2009, total benefits covered by Medicare were $502 billion (Boards of Trustees, Federal Hospital Insurance and Federal Supplementary Medical Insurance Trust Funds 2010) and expenditures associated with Medicaid were more than $373 billion (CMS 2011). Because of the scope of these programs, HHS has an aggressive interest in preventing fraud, abuse, and waste in its programs—particularly the programs associated with Medicare and Medicaid. One way the OIG prevents fraud, abuse, and waste in Medicare and Medicaid is to insist that various healthcare sectors with which it contracts have effective compliance programs.

For more than a decade, the OIG has been issuing specific compliance program guidance (CPG) covering many of the largest sectors of the healthcare industry (Boese, McClain, and Hernandez-Stern 2009). In its first "Publication of the OIG Compliance Program Guidance for Hospitals," the OIG (1998) stated: "The adaption and implementation of voluntary compliance programs significantly advance the prevention of fraud, abuse, and waste in these health care plans while at the same time furthering the fundamental mission of all hospitals, which is to provide quality care to all patients."

In addition, the CPG states (OIG 1998): "Fundamentally, compliance efforts are designed to establish a culture within a hospital that promotes prevention, detection, and resolution of instances of conduct that do not conform to Federal and State law, and Federal, State, and private payor health care program requirements, as well as the hospital's ethical and business policies."

The CPG continues: "It is incumbent upon a hospital's corporate officers and managers to provide ethical leadership to the organization and to assure that adequate systems are in place to facilitate ethical and legal conduct."

The OIG (1998) insists that the corporate compliance programs must begin with a formal commitment by the hospital's governing body to include seven elements required by the FSG:

1. The development and distribution of written standards of conduct as well as written policies and procedures that promote the hospital's commitment to compliance (e.g., by including adherence to compliance as an element in evaluating managers and employees) and that address specific areas of potential fraud, such as claims development and submission processes, code gaming, and financial relationships with physicians and other healthcare professions

2. The designation of a chief compliance officer and other appropriate bodies (e.g., a corporate compliance committee) charged with the responsibility of operating and monitoring the compliance program and who report directly to the CEO and the governing body

3. The development and implementation of regular, effective education and training programs for all affected employees

4. The maintenance of a process, such as a hotline, to receive complaints, and the adoption of procedures to protect the anonymity of complainants and protect whistleblowers from retaliation

5. The development of a system to respond to allegations of improper or illegal activities and the enforcement of appropriate disciplinary action against employees who have violated internal compliance policies, applicable statutes, regulations, or federal healthcare program requirements

6. The use of audits and other evaluation techniques to monitor compliance and assist in the reduction of identified problem areas

7. The investigation and remediation of identified systemic problems and the development of policies addressing the sanctioned individuals

In 2005 the OIG published its "Supplemental Compliance Program Guidance for Hospitals." This supplementary guidance is not intended to replace the original guidance but rather adds information concerning risk areas in which fraud and abuse of Medicare and Medicaid might arise, such as billing Medicare and Medicaid substantially in excess of usual charges.

The supplementary guidance states, "For those hospitals with existing compliance programs, this document may serve as a benchmark or comparison against which to measure ongoing efforts and as a roadmap for updating or refining their compliance plans" (OIG 2005).

Though OIG efforts are directed at the healthcare sector, and the efforts associated with the FSG are broader, their goals are the same—to promote an organizational culture that increases the likelihood of preventing, identifying, and correcting unlawful and unethical behavior at an early stage. Moreover, the carrot-and-stick approach of the two authorities is the same. Fines for wrongdoing under both OIG and FSG can be lessened if the hospital has a compliance program that can be demonstrated as having the characteristics outlined above.

For example, the OIG (2000) states:

Case Study

A rural hospital in the Southeast self-reported that, while under previous ownership and management, it had submitted claims with information that was falsified to support reimbursement. The hospital uncovered the false claims during the course of an internal audit performed as part of its voluntary compliance program. In the fall of 2000, the hospital agreed to resolve its financial and exclusion liability. The OIG did not impose a CIA because the misconduct was committed by the former management and the new management disclosed its findings to the government as part of a comprehensive preexisting compliance program.

As part of the effort to reduce fraud and abuse in the Federal health care programs, the OIG and the Department of Justice use the False Claims Act (31 U.S.C. 3729-3733) and other authorities to sanction health care providers that have knowingly submitted false claims to Medicare. In addition to the imposition of monetary penalties, the OIG is authorized to exclude providers that violate the False Claims Act from participation in Medicare and other Federal health care programs. Absent a criminal conviction that triggers mandatory exclusion, the OIG may elect not to exclude a health care provider that has engaged in abusive conduct. Where the best interests of the programs are served by allowing continued participation by the provider, the OIG generally requires that the provider adopt specific measures to better ensure its integrity.

> **Case Study**
>
> A Northeast hospital system identified that one of its teaching hospitals had submitted improper claims—they did not have the proper documentation or were upcoded—to federal healthcare programs. The hospital system uncovered the false claims during the course of an internal audit performed as part of its voluntary compliance program. In the summer of 2000, the hospital system agreed to resolve its False Claims Act liability. The OIG did not impose a CIA because the hospital system disclosed the misconduct to the government and the hospital system had a preexisting, comprehensive compliance program.

These measures are set forth in a corporate, institutional or individual integrity agreement (collectively referred to as a CIA).

Corporate, institutional, or individual integrity agreements (CIAs) are subject to extensive negotiations between OIG and the provider. They are expensive and time consuming. They generally require periodic reports to OIG and an independent review organization to verify their accuracy, but they always contain the seven core elements detailed previously. CIAs are generally imposed for five years. But CIAs can be reduced or not imposed at all if the hospital can demonstrate that its compliance program is effective. The case studies provide examples from an informal OIG (2000) review.

> **Corporate, institutional, or individual integrity agreement (CIA)** An agreement between the Office of Inspector General and a healthcare provider that has submitted false claims to Medicare that allows the provider to participate in Medicare programs if it adopts and can demonstrate specific improvement measures in its compliance program.

Incentives to Develop Effective Compliance Programs

The incentives supplied by the FSG and OIG guidelines are powerful. The existence of an effective ethics and compliance program will downgrade sentencing if the organization is indicted for and convicted of wrongdoing perpetrated by one of its agents. But the existence of an effective ethics and compliance program may preclude the indictment altogether.

In 1999, the US Department of Justice issued a set of guidelines, called the **Holder Memo**, to federal prosecutors that they were instructed to consider before filing charges against an organization. One of the guidelines is "the existence/adequacy of the compliance program" (Holder 1999). These guidelines have gone through several iterations (Filip 2008; Thompson 2003) and court challenges (*United States v. Stein* 2006), but whether an organization has a well-designed, effective compliance program or not remains one of the issues that US attorneys have been instructed to consider before indicting an organization.

> **Holder Memo** A set of guidelines issued by the US Department of Justice in 1999 to federal prosecutors that they were instructed to consider before filing charges against an organization.

In spite of the incentives offered by the FSG and the OIG in regard to compliance programs, the following section shows that doubt exists about whether they can be effective in creating a culture that discourages unlawful as well as unethical conduct.

Barriers to Creating an Appropriate Culture Through Compliance Programs

Both the FSG and the OIG stress that organizations should pay attention to how ethics is reflected in their cultures. But when asked why compliance programs do not work better, the American Health Lawyers Association gives a number of reasons, including, "Compliance is widely viewed as a matter for lawyers, not a business priority" and "Few organizations stress the importance of compliance and commitment to doing the right thing" (Coffey 2009).

Following the FSG, OIG guidance for compliance programs originated to detect and deter criminal wrongdoing, particularly fraud in hospitals. Thus, programs tend to be designed and implemented by legal personnel working in the area of compliance (Roberts 2009; Wellner 2005). However, a legal focus is of limited help in resolving issues associated with competing ethical values or commitments (Alfieri 2006). Compliance programs are often led by lawyers or managers who tend to have a bias toward "command and control" rather than a focus on values (Tyler 2005). Moreover, the Sarbanes-Oxley Act of 2002 (which was passed in response to the accounting scandals in the previous decade) is also mandatory to all Security and Exchange Commission (SEC) registrants (Hoffman 2004). Many hospitals are registrants of the SEC because any publicly owned company is subject to detailed disclosure laws about its financial condition, operating results, management compensation, and other areas of their business.

Section 404 of Sarbanes-Oxley requires management's assessment of internal controls (Hoffman 2004), thus reinforcing a legal and management bias to a command-and-control approach toward motivation and behavior of organization employees (Hess 2007).

Accreditation Standards and The Joint Commission

Recent changes in The Joint Commission's Leadership Standards insist the hospital develop an appropriate culture—one that emphases safety and quality.

In 1995, The Joint Commission (then the Joint Commission on Accreditation of Healthcare Organizations) expanded the "Patient Rights" chapter of its accreditation manual for hospitals to include a requirement that hospitals conduct their business and patient care practices in an "honest, decent, and proper manner"; this mandate is called "Organization Ethics" (Joint Commission 1995).

"Honest, decent, and proper manner" refers to way in which a hospital carries out its missions. Thus, this mandate was directed at a hospital's culture. The mandate covered issues associated with marketing, making sure the patient understood any charges incurred as a result of treatment, ensuring that care was effective and safe regardless of the ability of the patient to pay, and other matters.

This specific mandate survived several reiterations in The Joint Commission's accreditation manual for hospitals, but until recently it was located in the manual's chapter on patient rights. And assuredly, it was a misfit with other standards contained in the chapter. The chapter on patient rights (now called "Patient Rights and Responsibilities") was and is mostly concerned with standards concerning clinical issues, specifically clinical ethics issues. So the mandate implied that clinical ethicists might in some way contribute more robustly to the hospital's organizational culture.

Even though academics took the organization ethics mandate to heart and discussed the possible ramifications of it (Spencer et al. 2000), in day-to-day practice, clinical ethicists mostly ignored it. Although clinical ethics issues can arise because of institutional demands, the issues covered by the mandate are not issues that most clinical ethicists understand or want to understand. In hospitals, clinical ethics activities are generally implemented by volunteers. These volunteers are clinicians, chaplains, social workers, or others whose time is limited. Even if clinical ethicists wanted to tackle issues associated with this mandate, in an era of increased pressure to generate revenue, they would not likely be allowed the time. Nor is it within their scope or expertise.

In 2009, The Joint Commission removed this mandate from the "Patient Rights and Responsibilities" chapter and moved it, dropping the term *organization ethics*, to its chapter on leadership.

The chapter on leadership is driven by The Joint Commission's desire to see leadership develop and sustain a culture of safety and quality of care. The standard LD.02.01.01 states, "The mission, vision, and goals of the hospital support the safety and quality of care, treatment and services" (Joint Commission 2013).

Standard LD.03.01.01. states, "Leaders create and maintain a culture of safety throughout the hospital." In its "Introduction to Hospital Culture and System Performance Expectations," The Joint Commission (2013) states: "A hospital's culture reflects the beliefs, attitudes, and priorities of its members, and it influences the effectiveness of performance." The rationale given for Standard LD.04.02.03—"Ethical principles guide the hospital's business practices" (previously called *organization ethics*)—is: "Although some leaders many not be involved in the day-to-day, hands-on operations of the hospital, their decisions and work affect either directly or indirectly, every aspect of the operations. They are the driving force behind the culture of the hospital. Leaders establish the ethical framework in which the hospital operates, create policies and procedures, and secure resources and services that support patient safety and quality care, treatment, and services. Policies, procedures, resources, and services are all influenced by the culture of the hospital and, in turn, influence the culture."

The Joint Commission has made the responsibility for creating and maintaining an appropriate culture of safety and quality a leadership function. This approach parallels the approaches of both the FSG and OIG, which also insist that high-level personnel oversee the development of an organization's culture through compliance programs. Leadership is now directly responsible as well as accountable for ensuring that the hospital reflects a culture of safety and quality of care.

This responsibility means that leadership must develop the knowledge, skills, and abilities to develop and manage such a culture. It must secure the resources to do so, and it must also find ways of knowing when a gap exists. It also must find ways of allowing voices to be heard that might have positive implications for moral distress issues, which often arise because of concerns associated with quality of care (see Chapter 12).

The Joint Commission approach to ensuring that hospitals create and sustain an appropriate culture is more value driven than the approach of the USSC or the OIG, which, in spite of using the language of ethics in their guidelines, seem more interested in preventing and detecting unlawful behavior. Although The Joint Commission does not preclude the hospital endorsing other values, it is clearly focused on the hospital embracing the values of safety and quality and having them reflected in the organization's culture. The following section addresses the available evidence on what has succeeded (or not) in developing and sustaining an organizational culture that goes beyond adherence to the law.

The Evidence

Treviño, Weaver, and Reynolds (2006) undertook a review of behavioral ethics using the following parameters: "For the purposes of this review, behavioral ethics refers to individual behavior that is subject to or judged according to generally accepted moral norms of behavior. Thus, research on behavioral ethics is primarily concerned with explaining individual behavior in the context of larger social prescriptions." This includes research on organizations' ethical infrastructures (ethics and compliance programs) and individual ethical behavior.

They found little "empirical research on the workings and outcomes of these ethical infrastructures." Their results are reviewed below.

Paine (1994) found that ethics and compliance programs could have two different orientations. They can emphasize values, counseling, and responsible conduct, or they can emphasize legal compliance, control, and discipline. She argued that those programs that took the former approach were more likely to have more desirable and long-lasting impacts than those focused on rule compliance.

Weaver, Treviño, and Cochran (1999) confirmed in a wider study that ethics and compliance programs could have the two different orientations, though they noted that values and compliance orientations need not be mutually exclusive. They observed that while external pressures (such as the FSG and OIG) appear able to push organizations into formalizing ethics, internal pressure—for instance, how committed management is to fostering ethical behavior—affects the orientation of these programs. Later, Weaver and Treviño (1999) showed that these different but not mutually exclusive approaches have different impacts on the ethically relevant behavior of individuals in organizations. Their study of both types of programs indicate that, all things being equal, "a focus on monitoring and discipline in an ethics program is more likely to engender a contractual employee attitude toward the organization, rather than a perception of organizational support and trust, or increased salience for one's ethical obligation as an organizational member" (Weaver and Treviño 1999). Their research showed that an approach that sought to propagate a set of values that was eventually reflected in the organization's culture had the stronger and more positive impact—especially in terms of communication. They state: "A values-orientation, in particular, appears to add distinctive and desirable outcomes that cannot be achieved by a perceived focus on behavioral compliance. Moreover, a values-orientation appears important to fully realizing the potential benefits of compliance activities such as reporting misconduct" (Weaver and Treviño 1999).

However, in a more recent study, Treviño, Weaver, and Brown (2008) found troubling results for leaders interested in developing a culture that reflects an organization's values. In the study, they randomly surveyed senior managers and lower-level employees in a financial services company, an industrial products company, and a public utility. Their goal was to identify and compare two types of employees' perceptions of ethics in their respective organizations. Their results suggest that that different identities and roles may lead to different perceptions of ethics between senior managers and lower-level employees. Senior managers consistently had a more positive view of the role of ethics and ethics infrastructures than did lower-level employees. Trevino, Weaver, and Brown (2008) speculate that if "senior managers believe that the ethical environment is already quite positive, they may do too little—provide too little executive ethical leadership or too few financial resources to support effective ethics management."

If senior management and lower-level employees view the ethical environment of the organization differently, a gap or a misalignment exists between the cultures of these two groups. The potential for such a gap should be particularly troubling for hospital leadership because of the different groups employed with or associated with hospitals—each with its own identities and roles. If hospital leadership is serious about seeing the values the hospital endorses reflected in the culture, it should be aware that the potential exists for senior leadership to have a blind spot when it comes to perceiving the ethical environment of the organization. This awareness is particularly important because recent research shows that organizations have much more of an impact on individual behavior than is currently understood.

Moral Behavior and Organizations

Mental model
A deeply held set of generalizations or beliefs about reality that influence how individuals understand the world.

A **mental model** is a concept described by cognitive scientists that refers to deeply held or ingrained assumptions or generalizations about external reality that can take the form of patterns or images that in turn frame and focus how we understand the world (Senge 1990). Because mental models refer to deeply held assumptions, they influence our automatic decision-making processes, which in turn affect our behavior, including our moral behavior.

Mental models hold our implicit associations—associations between concepts. Related concepts can activate each other and trigger behavior or decision making. For instance, a mental model might contain an implicit association between "work" and "prestige." An individual might see a task (work) as one way of achieving prestige, and so the individual who wants prestige might embrace the task or actively seek other opportunities to advance and gain prestige.

Automatic cognitive process
Implicit assumptions and generalizations that represent our understanding of the world and are used in our day-to-day behavior and decision making, including moral decision making.

Implicit associations can also help us become experts. For example, a doctor, seeing patients with similar symptoms, will begin to associate these symptoms with a specific illness. The doctor will begin to know what symptoms to look for when told a patient has this specific illness. The two ideas or concepts are related in the doctor's mind—specific illness and specific symptoms—and when the doctor sees either the illness or the symptoms, she associates the other in her mind and knows what action to take.

We take for granted our mental models, with their implicit assumptions. They represent our understanding of the world, which allows day-to-day behavior and decision making, including moral decision making. As such we can think of mental models as an **automatic cognitive process**.

A **contextual cue** refers to a message, hint, or signal that can be found in a discernable element of the environment. In an organization, contextual cues often reveal the truth about what is really going on or what is really believed by the organization. For instance, if one is interested in "gender equity" in an organization, a contextual cue might be the number of women employed by the organization or how many women have leadership positions in the organization. Contextual cues from our environment inform us about what we can expect; if they trigger our implicit assumptions, they can lead directly to changes in our behavior and decision making.

Contextual cues are found throughout an organization. They may be contained in the slogans of an organization, which may be prominently displayed; in the design of the workplace; in how people dress; or in an organization's newsletter. They are also found in the culture of the organization. Contextual cues, such as how persons in an organization interact together, reflect the culture of the organization. These cues let us know how things are done in a specific organization.

Contextual cue
A message, hint, or signal that can be found in a discernible element of the environment. In an organization, contextual cues often reveal the truth about what is really going on or what is really believed by the organization.

But until recently, little or no empirical evidence examined how individual behavior might be a product of the interaction between automatic cognitive processes and environmental factors that contain contextual clues.

Reynolds, Leavitt, and DeCelles (2010) empirically tested the relationship between mental models (automatic cognitive processes), contextual cues, and moral behavior. They found that mental models *do* interact with contextual cues to shape moral behavior.

While this research seems straightforward—one would expect mental models to interact with contextual clues, to shape behavior both moral and immoral—the research suggests that ". . . perhaps organizations bear more responsibility for the actions of their members than is currently understood" (Reynolds, Leavitt, and DeCelles 2010). Organizations, knowingly or unknowingly, supply contextual cues that can trigger automatic cognitive processes, which may or may not change our moral behavior and decision making. For instance, a person could believe that business is an inherently moral enterprise. He then might associate that belief with the value of acting competitively. These two concepts are linked in his mind. If the organization stressed the value of competitiveness and provided a contextual cue—for instance, in compensation—that person who believes business is inherently moral and associates this belief with competitiveness might act ultracompetitively, even going so far as to break the law (Reynolds, Leavitt, and DeCelles 2010). Or a clinician might believe that a hospital is an inherently moral enterprise. The clinician associates a hospital with the value of delivering care. If the hospital stressed the value of delivering care and provided a contextual cue that emphasized this value—for instance, by stressing the number and range of services it offered—the result might well be overtreatment. Thus, it is in the best interests of organizations to be clear about their values and *what those values mean* and to be wary about supplying contextual cues without explanation.

Conclusion

Hospitals are required by various judicial authorities to develop and sustain cultures that promote ethical behavior and compliance with the law. Hospitals are required by regulators to develop a culture that promotes safety and quality.

Programs designed to promote these cultures can have various orientations ranging from a compliance orientation to a values orientation. Compliance-oriented ethics programs emphasize rules, monitor employee behavior, and discipline misconduct. Values-oriented programs emphasize support for employees' ethical aspirations and the development of shared values. While no reason exists why a program designed to affect the culture of an organization cannot incorporate elements of each, limited but persuasive evidence shows that values-oriented programs produce more positive outcomes for the organization.

Evidence shows that contextual cues supplied by an organization can activate the implicit assumptions embedded in the mental model of an individual, which then might trigger changes in behavior or decision making that may have moral consequences. This connection suggests that an organization bears some responsibility for an individual's behavior.

Hospital leadership is required to develop and sustain an appropriate culture. Moreover, they are accountable if such a culture is not developed. They must find ways of listening to their stakeholders, embedding appropriate contextual cues in the culture for which they are responsible, identifying gaps or misalignments, and not allowing themselves to be blinded by their roles and identities into believing that their ethical infrastructure and organizational culture—including its important component, the ethical climate—is better than it is.

Points to Remember

- Effective ethics and compliance programs are required by both the USSC and OIG. If convicted of wrongdoing, the existence of such a program can result in a sentence downgrade. Moreover, the existence of such a program can preclude indictment of an organization.

- Creating a safety and quality culture is required by The Joint Commission. Hospital leadership is responsible for its development and sustainability.
- The orientation of ethics and compliance programs can vary between a rules or compliance approach and a values approach. Evidence suggests that, all things being equal, a more values-oriented approach produces more positive outcomes for the organization.
- Different identities and roles between senior managers and lower level employees may lead to different perceptions of ethics and ethics infrastructures in an organization.
- Contextual cues are found in all aspects of an organization. Research has demonstrated that contextual cues may trigger the implicit associations found in mental models, which may lead to change in an individual's moral behavior or decision making.

References

Alfieri, A. V. 2006. "The Fall of Legal Ethics and the Rise of Risk Management." *Georgetown Law Journal* 94 (6): 1909.

Boards of Trustees, Federal Hospital Insurance and Federal Supplementary Medical Insurance Trust Funds. 2010. "Annual Report of the Boards of Trustees of the Federal Hospital Insurance and Federal Supplementary Medical Insurance Trust Funds." Accessed April 24, 2013. www.cms.gov/ReportsTrustFunds /downloads/tr2010.pdf.

Boese, J. T., B. C. McClain, and B. Hernandez-Stern. 2009. "Healthcare Behind Bars: The Use of Criminal Prosecutions in Forcing Corporate Compliance." *Journal of Health & Life Sciences Law* 3 (1): 91–131.

Centers for Medicare & Medicaid Services (CMS). 2011. "National Health Expenditure Data." Accessed April 24, 2013. www.cms.gov/NationalHealthExpendData /02_NationalHealthAccountsHistorical.asp.

Coffey, P. S. 2009. "The Reasons Compliance Programs Fail to Protect Against Whistleblower and Enforcement Risk." AHLA 2009 In-House Counsel Program. Published June 28. www.healthlawyers.org/Events/Programs/Materials /Documents/IHC09/coffey_slides.pdf.

Filip, M. R. 2008. "Principles of Federal Prosecution of Business Organizations, Memorandum from Mark R. Filip, Deputy Attorney General, to Heads of Department Components and United States Attorneys." Accessed April 24, 2013. www.usdoj.gov/opa/documents/corp-charging-guidelines.pdf.

Griffith, J. R., and K. R. White. 2010. *The Well-Managed Healthcare Organization*. Chicago: Health Administration Press.

Hess, D. 2007. "A Business Ethics Perspective on Sarbanes-Oxley and the Organizational Sentencing Guidelines." *Michigan Law Review* 105 (8): 1781–816.

Hoffman, T. 2004. "Section 404 of the Sarbanes-Oxley Act: Where the Knee Jerk Bruises Shareholders and Lifts the External Auditor." *Brandeis Law Journal* 240: 239–59.

Holder, E. 1999. "Memorandum from Eric Holder, Jr., Deputy Attorney General, to Heads of Department Components and All United States Attorneys, Bringing Charges Against Corporations." Accessed April 24, 2013. http://federalevidence.com/pdf/Corp_Prosec/Holder_Memo_6_16_99.pdf.

Joint Commission. 2013. *Comprehensive Accreditation Manual for Hospitals.* Oakbrook Terrace, IL: The Joint Commission.

———. 1995. "Patient Rights and Organization Ethics." *Comprehensive Manual for Hospitals.* Oakbrook Terrace, IL: The Joint Commission.

Lombardo, P. A. 2005. "Law and Ethics: An On-going Conversation." In *Fletcher's Introduction to Clinical Ethics,* edited by J. C. Fletcher, E. M. Spencer, and P. A. Lombardo. Hagerstown, MD: University Publishing Group.

Office of Inspector General. 2011. "About Us." Accessed April 24, 2013. http://oig.hhs.gov/organization.asp.

———. 2005. "OIG Supplemental Compliance Program Guidance for Hospitals." *Federal Register* 70 (19): 4858, 4876. Accessed April 24, 2013. http://oig.hhs.gov/fraud/docs/complianceguidance/012705HospSupplementalGuidance.pdf.

———. 2000. "Self-Disclosure of Provider Misconduct: Assessment of CIA Modifications." Accessed April 24, 2013. Office of Inspector General www.hortyspringer.com/Data/misc/Self-Disclosure_Provider.htm.

———. 1998. "Publication of the OIG Compliance Program Guidance for Hospitals." *Federal Register* 63 (35): 8987–98. Accessed April 24, 2013. http://oig.hhs.gov/authorities/docs/cpghosp.pdf.

Paine, L. S. 1994. "Managing for Organizational Integrity." *Harvard Business Review* 72 (2): 106–17.

Public Citizen. 2013. "Physician Accountability." Accessed May 8. www.citizen.org/physicianaccountability.

Reynolds, S., K. Leavitt, and K. DeCelles. 2010. "Automatic Ethics: The Effects of Implicit Assumptions and Contextual Cues on Moral Behavior." *Journal of Applied Psychology* 95 (4): 752–60.

Roberts, R. 2009. "The Rise of Compliance-Based Ethics Management." *Public Integrity* 11 (3): 261–77.

Sarbanes-Oxley Act of 2002, Pub. L. 107-204, 116 Stat. 745 (2002). www.sec.gov/about/laws/soa2002.pdf.

Senge, P. 1990. *The Fifth Discipline: The Art and Practice of the Learning Organization.* New York: Doubleday.

Spencer, E., A. Mills, M. Rorty, and P. Werhane. 2000. *Organization Ethics in Health Care*. New York: Oxford University Press.

Thompson, L. D. 2003. "Memorandum from Deputy Attorney General Larry Thompson to Heads of Department Components and U.S. Attorneys, Principles of Federal Prosecution of Business Organizations." Accessed April 24, 2013. http://federalevidence.com/pdf/Corp_Prosec/Thompson_Memo_1-20-03.pdf.

Treviño, L. K., G. R. Weaver, and M. Brown. 2008. "It's Lovely at the Top: Hierarchical Levels, Identities, and Perceptions of Organizational Ethics." *Business Ethics* 18 (2): 233–52.

Treviño, L. K., G. R. Weaver, and S. J. Reynolds. 2006. "Behavioral Ethics in Organizations: A Review." *Journal of Management* 32 (6): 951–90.

Tyler, T. R. 2005. "Promoting Employee Policy Adherence and Rule Following in Work Settings: The Value of Self-Regulatory Approaches." *Brooklyn Law Review* 70 (4): 1287–321.

United States v. Stein, 435 F. Supp. 2d 330 (SDNY 2006).

US Department of Health and Human Services (HHS). 2011. "About HHS." Accessed April 24, 2013. www.hhs.gov/about/.

United States Sentencing Commission (USSC). 2010. *Federal Sentencing Guidelines Manual*. Accessed April 24, 2013. www.ussc.gov/Guidelines/2010_guidelines/ToC_HTML.cfm.

Weaver, G. R., and L. K. Treviño. 1999. "Compliance and Values Oriented Ethics Programs: Influences on Employees' Attitudes and Behavior." *Business Ethics Quarterly* 9 (2): 315–35.

Weaver, G. R., L. K. Treviño, and P. Cochran. 1999. "Corporate Ethics Programs as Control Systems: Influences of Executive Commitments and Environmental Factors." *Academy of Management Journal* 42 (1): 41–57.

Wellner, P. 2005. "Note: Effective Compliance Programs and Corporate Criminal Prosecutions." *Cardozo Law Review* 27: 497–514.

HEALTHCARE ETHICS, PUBLIC POLICY, AND THE HEALTHCARE ORGANIZATION

Katherine L. Acuff

This chapter is relevant to the following competencies identified in the ACHE Competencies Assessment Tool (see p. xxv):

Communication and Relationship Management
- Facilitate conflict and alternative dispute resolution

Professionalism
- Contribute to professional knowledge and evidence

Knowledge of the Healthcare Environment
- The interrelationships among access, quality, cost, resource allocation, accountability, and community
- Socioeconomic environment in which the organization functions

Business Skills and Knowledge
- Organizational dynamics, political realities and culture
- Organizational mission, vision, objectives, and priorities

Learning Objectives

After completing this chapter, the reader will be able to understand

- the foundations of public health policy,
- the complexity of health and healthcare policymaking,
- how public policies affect healthcare organizations both directly (e.g., Medicare reimbursement rates, the uninsured) and indirectly (e.g., emergency preparedness),
- that health and healthcare public policies might have unintended consequences,

- the ethical tensions that arise as healthcare organizations implement health and healthcare policies, and
- the ethical mandate for healthcare organization leadership to be involved in shaping and critiquing public policies.

Introduction

Public policy
The tools—including statutes, regulations, guidelines, recommendations, executive orders, and court decisions—that federal, state, and local governments use to achieve a particular goal.

Utilitarianism
The principle of achieving the greatest good for the greatest number.

Many textbooks discussing ethics and **public policy** address the macro-ethical issues involved. Public policies are often justified on the basis of **utilitarianism**, or the principle of achieving the greatest good for the greatest number. An example is the mandatory vaccination of children prior to entering school. In policymaking, the fair distribution of scarce resources is often a key issue. Concerns about justice and equity in the healthcare system are frequently central largely because of the high numbers of persons who lack insurance or have inadequate coverage. The contrast of the high numbers of persons without health insurance and the access of others to some of the most sophisticated medical services in the world has led to some ranking the US healthcare system very low compared with those of other developed countries (Murray and Frenk 2010). Additionally, justice and equity concerns are often raised by health policymakers given the health disparities of minorities associated with both poorer access and healthcare outcomes. Such concerns led to the establishment of the National Institute on Minority Health and Health Disparities in 2010 to better focus the National Institute of Health's research agenda concerning health disparities (AHA 2011).

These ethical issues of fairness and justice are discussed in other chapters. The focus of this chapter is on how public policy and the intersection of different public policies sometimes challenge the ethical mission of healthcare organizations.

Public policy is a driving force in shaping how healthcare organizations achieve their missions. Health policies are not static. With healthcare expenditures making up a large percentage of the gross domestic product (GDP), the growing costs of Medicare and Medicaid, the challenges of addressing the needs of the growing numbers of uninsured, continuing concerns about potential large-scale health hazards, and other issues, health and healthcare policy is a frequent focus of policymakers. As a result, persons in leadership roles must be involved in the policymaking process and must monitor the changing policy landscape.

Although some policies are straightforward, this chapter documents that, however well intentioned, public policies may place significant burdens on healthcare organizations that affect how well their missions can be executed. Sometimes policies outline significant new requirements for healthcare organizations without providing financial resources that enable compliance. Healthcare organizations are faced with unanticipated costs that may undermine their financial viability. Public policies may also provide only the broad outlines of new requirements, leaving the interpretation of vague or unresolved issues to the healthcare organization and its professionals. A policy may also have unintended (and unforeseen) consequences. Unanticipated costs, vagueness, unresolved issues, and unintended consequences in public policy can all contribute ethical tensions within the healthcare organization.

Health and Healthcare Policies

Public policy is what federal, state, and local governments do—through statutes, regulations, guidelines and recommendations, executive orders, and court decisions—to achieve a particular goal. These policies are often aimed at either encouraging or discouraging behaviors. For example, placing high taxes on cigarettes or prohibiting advertising of smoking products to children are public policies clearly designed to discourage smoking.

Public policy itself should be an expression of societally accepted values and mores. Public policies concerned with the delivery and financing of care are aimed at promoting the health and well-being of the general society. Hospitals have, as one of their missions, the promotion of the health of the community they serve. Ideally, these policies and the missions of healthcare organizations will support and align with each other. But as this chapter makes clear, this is not always the case.

A distinction is often made between **health policy** and **healthcare policy**, although the distinction sometimes blurs. Health policies may be tailored broadly to either promote or protect the population's health. Such policies include laws promoting lead-paint abatement programs, removing soft drink and candy machines from public schools, or fostering clean air and water. Health*care* policies are crafted to address how healthcare is delivered and financed. Although healthcare organizations may be more interested in the latter, both types of policies impact their operations.

Healthcare policies have three primary concerns:

1. Access to care
2. Quality of care
3. Cost of care

The first, access to care, usually addresses how healthcare is financed. That is, who pays for the health services? Issues surrounding employer-sponsored health insurance, Medicare, and Medicaid are key, but access policy

Health policy
Policy that is tailored broadly to either promote or protect the population's health.

Healthcare policy
Policy that addresses access to healthcare services, the scope and quality of healthcare delivery, and healthcare costs.

concerns also include how best to address the numbers of uninsured, which clearly affects the bottom line of healthcare organizations. Access concerns also include nonfinancial issues, such as geographical barriers, the poor distribution of providers, and language and cultural barriers.

The second major healthcare policy concern is quality of care. Since 1999, several landmark Institute of Medicine (IOM 2001, 1999) reports based on hundreds of studies documented significant problems in the level of medical errors in hospitals as well as the overall quality of care. These reports, as well as reports of substantial variations in the frequency of procedures in different parts of the country not linked to differences in outcomes, have led to incentives for reducing errors, promoting evidence-based medicine, and implementing incentives for high-performance hospitals.

The third concern is healthcare costs. Healthcare costs in the United States exceeded $2.5 trillion in 2009, more than triple the $714 billion spent in 1990 (Kaiser Family Foundation 2011). The United States spends more on healthcare than China spends on everything (Mendonca and Tyson 2011). The United States not only spends more in total but it spends more per capita than any other country, without producing better health outcomes. In 2008, US healthcare spending was $7,681 per capita, more than double that of the next highest country (Kaiser Family Foundation 2011).

Clearly, these three healthcare policy concerns are interrelated. One could cut costs by further restricting access. Improving quality of care might also reduce costs if redundant testing was eliminated or the frequency of hospital-acquired infections was reduced. Improving access might initially increase total healthcare costs—although some debate exists about this assertion—but could improve the quality of care and reduce costs in the long run. People without health insurance tend to have poorer controlled chronic conditions, such as diabetes and high blood pressure, leading to costly emergency department visits and hospital stays. Public policies addressing access, quality, and costs all have direct effects on healthcare organizations.

Health Policy and the Ethical Context of Leadership

Health administrators and policymakers understand that health policies affect the ability of healthcare organizations to achieve their mission of providing quality care while surviving as viable businesses. Many ethical tensions arise as administrators try to implement sometimes costly policies, while still preserving their unique missions. Moreover, health and healthcare policies are in constant flux. For instance, Medicare legislation and rules have been amended dozens of times since the program went into effect in 1966, changing the conditions of participation, the services and procedures covered, and reimbursement rates for hospitals, physicians, and laboratories. These changes variously affect a hospital's operating margin and may positively or adversely affect the hospital's mission. The Disproportionate Share Hospital (DSH) legislation, for example, acknowledged that some hospitals serve larger numbers of the uninsured and Medicaid patients than do other hospitals in their communities and needed additional revenues to offset these losses. As a result, federal law provides annual DSH payments to cover the costs of uncompensated or undercompensated care (CMS 2013; HHS 2013). Other amendments have either cut reimbursement rates to hospitals or providers or imposed sometimes costly additional requirements, for example, in how providers must protect patient information (discussed later in this chapter).

Public policy, no matter how well intentioned or crafted, is a blunt instrument. Not all healthcare organizations are similarly positioned and, as a result, the effectiveness and burdens of a particular policy may affect them differently. For example, initiating electronic patient records is costly for all healthcare organizations. However, sharply different economies of scale may exist when comparing the experiences of a large for-profit urban hospital chain with that of a rural community hospital. So the burden of initiating electronic record keeping for the rural community hospital may jeopardize or compete with the hospital's mission to provide quality care to its community.

In addition, because of the complexity of the health and healthcare policies and the many competing interests, unintended consequences adverse to the healthcare organization often occur. As discussed later in this chapter, the **Emergency Medical Treatment and Active Labor Act (EMTALA)**, which ensures that patients coming to emergency departments are screened and stabilized before being sent away or transferred, also played a role in emergency department closings and exacerbated emergency department crowding and so may have compromised the service mission of these hospitals (CMS 2012).

Healthcare organizations are major stakeholders in public health policy, and through either their own government affairs offices or the efforts of advocacy organizations—such as the American Hospital Association (AHA), the American Medical Association (AMA), and the American College of Emergency Physicians, to name a few—their views are made known to policymakers (Columbia University Medical Center 2011). The range of stakeholders in health policy is diverse, and leaders of healthcare organizations must be aware that their interests and other stakeholders' interests may be quite different.

Emergency Medical Treatment and Active Labor Act (EMTALA)
A 1986 law requiring hospital emergency departments to treat all individuals who show up at their facilities regardless of their ability to pay.

Examples of Health and Healthcare Policies Affecting Healthcare Organizations

This section reviews two federal healthcare policies as examples of how policies may affect the ethical environment of healthcare organizations. These policies address how healthcare organizations must respond to persons presenting to their emergency departments and what measures organizations must take to protect the privacy of patient information. The final section of this chapter discusses some aspects of federal policy regarding emergency preparedness and disaster planning and how it interacts with the emergency department and patient privacy legislation as well as creates additional obligations for healthcare organizations. Together these policies illustrate the complexity of the regulatory environment in which healthcare organizations must operate, the way in which policies can have unintended consequences, and how policies might require review to balance their requirements with the healthcare organization's missions. As a result, leaders in healthcare organizations must involve themselves in public policy formulation.

The Emergency Medical Treatment and Active Labor Act

In 1986, amid reports that many hospitals' emergency departments refused to provide care or diverted persons without health insurance or on Medicaid to other hospitals before they were stabilized, Congress passed EMTALA, sometimes referred to as the "Patient Anti-Dumping Law," as an amendment to Medicare.

EMTALA specifies how covered hospitals must deal with individuals presenting at their facilities in potential emergency situations. Covered hospitals are defined as those having dedicated emergency departments and accepting patients with Medicare coverage.

Generally, EMTALA requires hospital emergency departments to treat all individuals who show up at their facilities regardless of their ability to pay (OSHA 2011a, 2005). Specifically, EMTALA

- requires hospitals with emergency departments to medically screen individuals who come to their facilities in an apparent emergency situation and women in active labor,
- prohibits hospitals from refusing to examine or treat individuals with an emergency medical condition,
- applies to all hospitals with a dedicated emergency department, and
- applies to critical access hospitals.

Some, such as the American College of Emergency Physicians (2013), have called EMTALA an unfunded mandate. Both hospitals and physicians have criticized EMTALA for legislating an ethical standard of care for persons in emergencies without providing a source of payment if those persons are without health insurance. This requirement has put stress on hospitals that often have a problem with emergency department overcrowding and where caring for the uninsured jeopardizes the financial soundness of the operation.

> **Case Study**
>
> You are an administrator of a not-for-profit hospital in a community where a for-profit hospital has just merged with the other hospital in town. The for-profit has closed its emergency department to avoid the financial risk of having to care for uninsured patients. You anticipate that use of your emergency department will triple as a result. Your emergency department is already losing money, but you know this service is vital to meet community needs. What should you do?

Physician staffing of emergency departments is particularly affected. According to a 2010 study on emergency room use (Pitts et al. 2010), Americans are increasingly getting their acute care at hospital emergency departments. Although emergency physicians make up less than 5 percent of physicians, they treat 28 percent of persons needing acute care (Pitts et al. 2010). Emergency department physicians are estimated to "provide more acute care to Medicaid beneficiaries and the uninsured than the rest of US physicians combined" (Hsia, Kellerman, and Shen 2011). EMTALA's requirements place a significant financial burden on hospitals and emergency department physicians.

One unintended consequence of EMTALA is that some private hospital emergency rooms have closed rather than being obligated to treat patients without health insurance. Between 1990 and 2009, the number of hospital-based emergency departments in nonrural areas declined 27 percent (Hsia, Kellerman, and Shen 2011). An analysis of the factors associated with these closures shows that hospitals with for-profit ownership, locations in competitive markets, safety-net status (defined as a hospital that provides more than double the Medicaid share compared with other hospitals within a 15-mile radius), and low profit margins were at the highest risk of closing. In these instances, one could argue that in response to EMTALA, these hospitals have had to compromise their community service mission by closing their emergency departments.

Health Insurance Portability and Accountability Act

The **Health Insurance Portability and Accountability Act (HIPAA)**, another Medicare amendment, contains rules for the coverage and availability

Health Insurance Portability and Accountability Act (HIPAA)
Legislation that provides for the portability of health insurance coverage when workers change or lose their jobs, implements programs to reduce healthcare fraud and abuse, establishes standards for the use and security of health information in electronic health records, and requires the protection and confidential handling of protected health information.

of group health plans, programs to control fraud and abuse, and establishing standards for the use and security of health information (HHS 2011a).

HIPAA's Privacy Rule, which took effect in 2003, was designed to protect individuals' private health information. The unauthorized disclosures of a person's medical status—well documented in cases of HIV infection, for example—has caused job loss, housing discrimination, the loss of health insurance, and personal distress. The Privacy Rule was intended to strictly limit the disclosure of medical information only to those with legitimate interests in the patient's care (HHS 2011a).

HIPAA's Privacy Rule applies only to "covered entities"—individuals and institutions providing healthcare, health plans and other healthcare payers, and health clearinghouses that may process health claims. Under the Privacy Rule, a covered entity may use and disclose an individual's private health information without obtaining the individual's authorization when the information is used for treatment, payment, healthcare operations, or persons otherwise authorized to have access to it, such as a parent or guardian.

Covered entities are required to adhere to strict regulations governing the use and disclosure of protected health information, which is any information about health status, the provision of healthcare, or payments that can be linked to the individual. Information that might link the individual and his health information include 18 potential identifiers, such as Social Security information, insurance identifiers, phone numbers, and addresses. Healthcare organizations must provide patients with notice of their HIPAA privacy rights, and patients are asked to sign waivers if such information is to be shared with other providers involved with their care. Healthcare organizations must also develop policies and procedures about the Privacy Rule's requirements.

Covered entities must keep track of disclosures, designate a privacy official, and monitor complaints involving unauthorized disclosures. The Office for Civil Rights in the US Department of Health and Human Services (HHS) has responsibility for enforcing the Privacy Rule, with authority to levy penalties for violations. In 2009, the Health Information Technology for Economic and Clinical Health (HITECH) Act increased penalties and added categories of violations. The HITECH Act established four categories of violations to address increasing levels of culpability on the part of covered entities. It also increases civil monetary penalties and requires that HHS base penalties on the nature and extent of the violation and of the resulting harm. The HITECH Act's penalty structure substantially increases the potential liability of covered entities and eliminates certain defenses.

Enforcement of HITECH has been significant. In February 2011, HHS assessed $4.3 million in fines against Cignet Health of Prince George's County, Maryland, for failing to comply with the HIPAA Privacy Rule and for failing to cooperate with the investigation (Kauppila 2011). HHS also disclosed a $1 million settlement with Massachusetts General Hospital to resolve a HIPAA privacy complaint (Kauppila 2011).

Most healthcare organizations and physicians are in compliance with HIPAA. But although many healthcare organizations understand the ethical concerns that arise when unauthorized disclosures of health information occur, addressing these concerns comes at a high cost. Many healthcare organizations have complained about HIPAA's compliance burdens, which are expensive and time consuming. Moreover, organizations' fear of financial penalties has often translated into stricter application of privacy controls (and thus more costs) than is required by law (Social Security Administration 2011; Wilson 2006).

Pandemic and All-Hazards Preparedness Act

The responses of healthcare organizations to the requirements of EMTALA and HIPAA illustrate how complex compliance may be and how uncertainty about a policy's requirements sometimes generates inappropriate and resource-consuming procedures. The responses also show how the impact of meeting the financial consequences of a policy may have unintended consequences, as with the closing of emergency departments after EMTALA's enactment. Leaders of healthcare organizations may struggle to assess the genuine requirements of a policy and adjust or implement organizational responses to its requirements in a cost-effective manner.

Specific challenges include orchestrating how the requirements of different policies interact or clarifying a new policy that is either vague or apparently in conflict with existing policies. Such a case is illustrated by legislation addressing national emergencies.

The federal **Pandemic and All-Hazards Preparedness Act of 2006 (PAHPA)** is designed to improve the nation's public health and medical preparedness and response capabilities for emergencies, whether deliberate, accidental, or natural (HHS 2011c). This section briefly describes some sections of PAHPA and how it intersects with other public policies that may cause confusion and uncertainty for those responsible for the health and safety of their communities. It also illustrates how funding for implementing public policy mandates is often absent and how the burden to fill the gap falls on healthcare organizations. Few disagree that healthcare organizations have an ethical obligation, as well as a legal one under PAPHA, to provide aid when their community is in emergency situations. The challenge is to identify the extent of the obligations as well as how to implement them, both in the planning stages and in actual emergencies, without compromising the care of existing patients, putting its staff at risk, and jeopardizing the organization's financial viability.

Pandemic and All-Hazards Preparedness Act of 2006 (PAHPA)
A law designed to improve the nation's public health and medical preparedness and response capabilities for emergencies, whether deliberate, accidental, or natural.

Section 302: Enhancing Medical Surge Capacity. This section enhances medical surge capacity and includes amendments to the Public Health Service Act to direct an assessment of the surge capacities of local communities, the acquisition of mobile medical assets, and signing memoranda of understanding with federal facilities, as appropriate. It also amends the requirements of EMTALA to include medical screening of persons who come to a covered hospital's emergency department because of a state emergency preparedness plan or in a public health emergency that involves an infectious disease.

Section 303: Encouraging Health Professional Volunteers. This section encourages health professional volunteers to be available in disasters as part of increasing medical surge capacity. PAHPA authorizes HHS oversight of federal health personnel and volunteers through the Emergency System for Advance Registration of Volunteer Health Professionals and the Medical Reserve Corps. Identifying volunteer health professionals before an emergency is critical to a rapid response. However, challenges remain both in how such volunteers might be deployed as well as in getting the volunteers in the first place.

First, although HHS has a national qualification and verification system, no national management to respond to disasters crosses state lines. Many disasters fail to recognize state boundaries and require interstate coop-

Medical liability
Occurs when a patient is harmed by a breach of the standard of care established by a professional group or regulatory standards. Also called *medical malpractice.*

eration. However, the licensing of health professionals and **medical liability** laws vary by state, generating confusion and caution among those professionals. Second, the issue of medical liability under declared emergencies remains unresolved. In the aftermath of Hurricane Katrina, the fear of liability of both intrastate and interstate medical personnel prevented many from volunteering (Hodge, Gostin, and Vernick 2007). However, PAHPA was reauthorized in March 2013 without expanding liability coverage for medical personnel (GovTrack 2013).

Section 305: Partnerships for State and Regional Hospital Preparedness to Improve Surge Capacity. This section authorizes the Secretary of Health and Human Services to award competitive grants "to improve surge capacity and enhance community and hospital preparedness for public health emergencies" (HHS 2011b). This Hospital Preparedness Program (HPP) funding is targeted in three areas: enhanced planning, strengthening integration of public and private-sector planning and assets, and improving infrastructure. States might look to model memoranda of understanding for specifying their responsibilities and interactions with other organizations (Hodge et al. 2009) or review professional guidance for planning (Joint Commission 2005).

To be eligible, the application must be from a partnership that includes specified participants (e.g., one or more hospitals, at least one of which is a designated trauma center, and other health resources as well as political subdivisions and one or more states). According to a 2008 evaluation of the HPP, one of its most significant achievements is the emergence of healthcare coalitions, which have involved collaboration and networking among hospitals and between hospitals, public health departments, and emergency management and response agencies (Center for Biosecurity 2009).

HPP funding was reduced by 10 percent in 2012, and healthcare organizations should plan to assume an increasing financial burden for their participation in these community partnerships in the future (HHS 2012). The question for healthcare organizations is how many resources they are ethically obligated to devote to emergency preparedness. These resources include the time it takes to train personnel, participate in community-wide planning, and ensure reasonable levels of medical supplies are available. What is the appropriate ethical balance of planning for future events such as emergencies versus directing resources that could be used immediately in a low-income clinic?

PAHPA has been criticized in other ways. For instance, in a situation of overwhelming emergency, a hospital will be unlikely to acquire all the assets it needs, even if it has memoranda of understanding with federal facilities. And except for vaccines, HHS has not fully considered how to allocate resources for non-pharmacologic resources (e.g., ventilators, hospital beds, quarantine facilities, nonfederal supplies) during emergencies (Hodge, Gostin, and Vernick 2007). Thus, unless the

Case Study

You, the hospital administrator, are appointed to a committee with a mandate to ensure that the hospital has the appropriate planning and communication mechanisms in place to allow the hospital to respond to an emergency or a disaster, either manmade or natural. Although you have worked to meet the guidelines issued by The Joint Commission and the requirements associated with EMTALA, HIPAA, and other policies, in the event of a disaster, you know that if the hospital is overwhelmed, it must resort to rationing. So in addition to reviewing existing guidelines, you want to be in a position to justify any decisions the hospital and its staff must make in a time of crisis.

Moreover, you know that response to an emergency will involve partnerships between the hospital and other entities, including other hospitals. The community will expect the hospital to have the resources it will need to respond to an emergency. But who will pay for these resources? What is the ethical obligation of a healthcare organization to stockpile resources? Under what circumstances is a healthcare organization ethically obligated to make its ventilators, drugs, vehicles, and other resources available to others in the community? What about more distant communities?

Case Study

You are on the emergency preparedness committee of your hospital, a midsized not-for-profit facility with two competing hospitals in the area. You are given the task of developing a plan to coordinate care with these competing hospitals in the event of a natural disaster or an emergency. Your hospital already takes a disproportionate share of the uninsured and Medicaid patients in your community and is in a more precarious financial situation than your competitors. What are your concerns about entering into agreements with these facilities?

state has offered detailed guidance, hospitals must draw up their own plans that can withstand the scrutiny of the community and do their best to reconcile them with appropriate principles like distributive justice and transparency.

Crisis Standards of Care and Medical Liability

Crisis standards of care
A substantial change in usual operations and the level of care a healthcare organization is able to deliver because of a pervasive (e.g., pandemic influenza) or catastrophic (e.g., earthquake, hurricane) disaster.

As noted previously, the issues of **crisis standards of care** and medical liability in emergencies have not been clarified. Because of the importance of this issue, this chapter concludes with a discussion of medical liability and the effort of the Institute of Medicine (IOM) to offer guidance to hospitals that must have policies in place to deal with an emergency.

Healthcare organizations and the professionals within them operate according to standards of care set either by professional groups—such as the American Academy of Pediatrics—or regulations—such as those set by The Joint Commission and similar organizations. When these professional standards are breached, tort law may determine whether medical negligence has occurred and liability exists.

Medical tort liability is of great concern to healthcare organizations and health professionals in normal circumstances, but it is of particular concern in situations of natural disasters or emergencies. Broadly, healthcare providers have an ethical obligation to provide the best care possible in accordance with professional and regulatory standards. However, what should be the standard of care in natural disasters or other emergencies? Should the healthcare organization and the professionals who work there be held to the prevailing practice standards when the number of patients surges, supplies dwindle, and the facility itself may be compromised? Should the standards be adjusted? Who decides?

Some states have addressed this potential problem by passing legislation waiving liability during declared emergencies for what might be considered negligent conduct in normal circumstances (Hodge, Gostin, and Vernick 2007). An alternative to waiving liability is developing new practice standards with the major stakeholders from the community for medical entities to follow in the case of a declared emergency (Kinney et al. 2009). Following these protocols or crisis standards would serve as a defense if medical conduct were challenged. The latter approach is one examined by the IOM.

To help aid healthcare organizations and professionals in determining what the standards of care should be in cases of natural disaster or emergency, a special advisory group of the IOM (2009) issued a report documenting the potential for medical standards of care being challenged in disasters. It also issued guidance for establishing crisis standards of care. In its report, the IOM defined crisis standards of care as "a substantial change in usual health care operations and the level of care it is possible to deliver, which is made necessary by a pervasive (e.g., pandemic influenza) or catastrophic (e.g., earthquake, hurricane) disaster. This change in the level of care delivered is justified by specific circumstances and is formally declared by a state government, in recognition that crisis operations will be in effect for a sustained period. The formal declaration that crisis standards of care are in operation enables specific legal/regulatory powers and protections for healthcare providers in the necessary tasks of allocating and using scarce medical resources and implementing alternate care facility operations."

The IOM's report includes both a vision statement of the characteristics such standards should meet and specific guidance about how the standards should be developed. The IOM's vision, which provides the grounding for an ethical development of crisis standards, sets out the following:

In order to ensure that patients receive the best possible care in a catastrophic event, the nation needs a robust system to guide the public, healthcare professionals and institutions, and governmental entities at all levels. To achieve such a system of just care, the committee sets forth the following vision for crisis standards of care:

- Fairness—standards that are, to the highest degree possible, recognized as fair by all those affected by them (including the members of affected communities, practitioners, and provider organizations); evidence-based; and responsive to specific needs of individuals and the population focused on a duty of compassion and care, a duty to steward resources, and a goal of maintaining the trust of patients and the community

- Equitable processes—processes and procedures for ensuring that decisions and implementation of standards are made equitably
  - Transparency—in design and decision making
  - Consistency—in application across populations and among individuals regardless of their human condition (e.g., race, age, disability, ethnicity, ability to pay, socioeconomic status, preexisting health conditions, social worth, perceived obstacles to treatment, past use of resources)
  - Proportionality—public and individual requirements must be commensurate with the scale of the emergency and degree of scarce resources
  - Accountability—of individuals deciding and implementing standards, and of governments for ensuring appropriate protections and just allocation of available resources

- Community and provider engagement, education, and communication—active collaboration with the public and stakeholders for their input is essential through formalized processes

- The rule of law
  - Authority—to empower necessary and appropriate actions and interventions in response to emergencies
  - Environment—to facilitate implementation through laws that support standards and create appropriate incentives

The IOM's (2009) guidance recommendations for establishing the crisis standards of care are designed to provide a consistent and ethical framework, while not prescribing what the standards should be.

Recommendation 1: Develop Consistent State Crisis Standards of Care

Protocols with Five Key Elements

State departments of health, and other relevant state agencies, in partnership with localities should develop crisis standards of care protocols that include the key elements—and associated components—detailed in this report:

- A strong ethical grounding;

- Integrated and ongoing community and provider engagement, education, and communication;

- Assurances regarding legal authority and environment;

- Clear indicators, triggers, and lines of responsibility; and

- Evidence-based clinical processes and operations.

Recommendation 2: Seek Community and Provider Engagement

State, local, and tribal governments should partner with and work to ensure strong public engagement of community and provider stakeholders, with particular attention given to the needs of vulnerable populations and those with medical special needs, in:

- Developing and refining crisis standards of care protocols and implementation guidance;

- Creating and disseminating educational tools and messages to both the public and health professionals;

- Developing and implementing crisis communication strategies;

- Developing and implementing community resilience strategies; and

- Learning from and improving crisis standards of care response situations.

Recommendation 3: Adhere to Ethical Norms During Crisis Standards of Care

When crisis standards of care prevail, as when ordinary standards are in effect, healthcare practitioners must adhere to ethical norms. Conditions of overwhelming scarcity limit autonomous choices for both patients and practitioners regarding the allocation of scarce healthcare resources, but do not permit actions that violate ethical norms.

Recommendation 4: Provide Necessary Legal Protections for Healthcare Practitioners and Institutions Implementing Crisis Standards of Care

In disaster situations, tribal or state governments should authorize appropriate agencies to institute crisis standards of care in affected areas, adjust scopes of practice for licensed or certified healthcare practitioners, and alter licensure and credentialing practices as needed in declared emergencies to create incentives to provide care needed for the health of individuals and the public.

Recommendation 5: Ensure Consistency in Crisis Standards of Care Implementation

State departments of health, and other relevant state agencies, in partnership with localities, should ensure consistent implementation of crisis standards of care in response to a disaster event. These efforts should include:

- Using "clinical care committees," "triage teams," and a state-level "disaster medical advisory committee" that will evaluate evidence-based, peer-reviewed critical care and other decision tools and recommend and implement decision-making algorithms to be used when specific life-sustaining resources become scarce;

- Providing palliative care services for all patients, including the provision of comfort, compassion, and maintenance of dignity;

- Mobilizing mental health support to manage the effects of crisis standards of care on providers and communities;

- Developing specific response measures for vulnerable populations and those with medical special needs, including pediatrics, geriatrics, and persons with disabilities; and

- Implementing robust situational awareness capabili-

> ### Case Study
>
> You are the CEO of a large academic medical center. It is the largest provider in your community and, as a result, also has the highest number of medical liability suits, which cost time and resources.
>
> The governor has asked you to chair a committee to develop crisis standards of care as part of the state's emergency preparedness efforts. Although you agree to chair this committee, you are concerned about the liability implications of crisis standards of care for your organization. Your state has not enacted any legislation either reimbursing health providers for liability suits in declared emergencies or limiting those suits in such situations.
>
> Who else would you like to participate as part of the crisis standards of care committee—within your organization, in your community, in your state? What other entities—local or national— might you consult with to develop these standards? Do you think you should use this opportunity to lobby for legislative changes to the medical liability law?

ties to allow for real-time information sharing across affected communities and with the "disaster medical advisory committee."

Recommendation 6: Ensure Intrastate and Interstate Consistency Among Neighboring Jurisdictions

States, in partnership with the federal government, tribes, and localities, should initiate communications and develop processes to ensure intrastate and interstate consistency in the implementation of crisis standards of care. Specific efforts are needed to ensure that the Department of Defense, Veterans Health Administration, and Indian Health Services medical facilities are integrated into planning and response efforts.

Conclusion

The US healthcare system is complex and constantly changing. With more than 5,000 hospitals, 800,000 physicians, and hundreds of pharmaceutical and medical device manufacturers, healthcare's impact on the US economy is enormous. The $2.7 trillion in healthcare expenditures 2011 makes the US healthcare system the eighth largest economy in the world—larger than that of France (US Census Bureau 2011). Its share of the US GDP reached 17.9 percent in 2011 (HHS 2012).

In addition, because healthcare costs are increasing faster than inflation, the numbers of uninsured have reached nearly 50 million, many societal needs are competing for public dollars, and health and healthcare policies are a favorite target of lawmakers. Although many of these efforts target healthcare costs—particularly reimbursements to hospitals and physicians—others are increasingly focused on access and quality of care. Layered over those policies directly targeting healthcare organizations are broader public policies, such as emergency preparedness, that have significant impacts on how healthcare organizations operate.

Public health and healthcare policies challenge administrators to find the

---

Case Study

In 2005, Hurricane Katrina flooded New Orleans, wiping out electricity (including back-up generators), communications, and escape routes and essentially leaving Charity Hospital to manage for five days with dwindling medical supplies and food, inoperable equipment, and exhausted healthcare personnel, some of whom had to hand-ventilate critical care patients for prolonged periods. Communications were spotty, evacuation plans had not anticipated being surrounded by waist-high water, and hospital personnel did not know the landing coordinates to give helicopter pilots. Several patients died during this disaster, and some medical personnel were prosecuted for alleged substandard care (Gray and Hebert 2006).

What standards of care should apply in such situations? How should they be developed? What is the best way to educate your staff on the potential need for relaxing the standards of care or rationing equipment or supplies?

resources and foster the leadership needed to comply with policy requirements, train personnel, and forge partnerships with other healthcare and community organizations in the context of furthering the healthcare organization's mission. Sometimes public policies make it difficult to adhere to the hospital's mission while also ensuring its business viability. Health administrators must keep a close eye on changing healthcare policies and have an active role in shaping them.

Point to Remember

- Public policies can affect healthcare organizations both directly and indirectly. Although some policies are straightforward, sometimes public policy can be vague or costly and have unintended consequences. Because health and healthcare policies affect the missions of healthcare organizations, administrators have an ethical obligation to involve themselves in policy formulation and implementation.

References

American Hospital Association (AHA). 2011. "Eliminating Racial and Ethnic Disparities: Eliminating Disparities in Health Outcomes." Accessed April 26, 2013. www.aha.org/aha_app/issues/Disparities/index.jsp.

American College of Emergency Physicians. 2013. "EMTALA." Accessed May 14. www.acep.org/content.aspx?id=25936.

Center for Biosecurity of University of Pittsburgh Medical Center. 2009. "Hospitals Rising to the Challenge: The First Five Years of the U.S. Hospital Preparedness Program and Priorities Going Forward." Accessed April 26, 2013. www.upmc-biosecurity.org/website/resources/publications/2009/2009-04-16-hppreport.html.

Centers for Medicare & Medicaid Services (CMS). 2013. "Medicaid Disproportionate Share Hospital (DSH) Payments." Accessed May 14. www.medicaid.gov/Medicaid-CHIP-Program-Information/By-Topics/Financing-and-Reimbursement/Medicaid-Disproportionate-Share-Hospital-DSH-Payments.html.

———. 2012. "Emergency Medical Treatment and Labor Act (EMTALA)." Published March 26. www.cms.gov/Regulations-and-Guidance/Legislation/EMTALA/index.html?redirect=/emtala/.

———. 2011. "National Health Expenditure Projections 2011–2021." Accessed May 14, 2013. www.cms.gov/Research-Statistics-Data-and-Systems

/Statistics-Trends-and-Reports/NationalHealthExpendData/Downloads
/Proj2011PDF.pdf.

Columbia University Medical Center. 2011. "About the GCA Team." Accessed April 26, 2013. www.cumc.columbia.edu/dept/gc/aboutus.html.

GovTrack. 2013. "H.R. 307: Pandemic and All-Hazards Preparedness Reauthorization Act of 2013." Accessed May 14. www.govtrack.us/congress/bills/113/hr307.

Gray, B., and K. Hebert. 2006. "Hospitals in Hurricane Katrina: Challenges Facing Custodial Institutions in a Disaster." *The Urban Institute*. Published July 14. www.urban.org/publications/411348.html.

Hodge, J. G., E. Anderson, S. P. Teret, J. S. Vernick, T. D. Kirsch, and G. Kelen. 2009. *PACER: Model Memorandum of Understanding Between Hospitals During Declared Emergencies*. Accessed April 26, 2013. www.premierinc.com/safety/topics/disaster_readiness/downloads/11-PACER_Model_MOU.pdf.

Hodge, J. G., L. O. Gostin, and J. S. Vernick. 2007. "The Pandemic and All-Hazards Preparedness Act: Improving Public Health Emergency Response." *Journal of the American Medical Association* 297 (15): 1708–11.

Hsia, R. Y., A. L. Kellerman, and Y. C. Shen. 2011. "Factors Associated with Closures of Emergency Departments in the United States." *Journal of the American Medical Association* 305 (19): 1978–84.

Institute of Medicine (IOM). 2009. *Guidance for Establishing Crisis Standards of Care for Use in Disaster Situations*. Accessed April 26, 2013. www.iom.edu/Reports/2009/DisasterCareStandards.aspx.

———. 2001. *Crossing the Quality Chasm: A New Health System for the 21st Century*. Washington DC: National Academies Press.

———. 1999. *To Err Is Human: Building a Safer Health Care System*. Washington DC: National Academies Press.

Joint Commission. 2005. *Standing Together: An Emergency Planning Guide for America's Communities*. Accessed April 26, 2013. www.jointcommission.org/assets/1/18/planning_guide.pdf.

Kaiser Family Foundation. 2011. "U.S. Health Care Costs." Accessed April 26, 2013. www.kaiseredu.org/Issue-Modules/US-Health-Care-Costs/Background-Brief.aspx.

Kauppila, A. 2011. "Recent HIPAA Enforcement Actions: Strong Medicine for Health Care Employers." *Washington Workplace Law*. Published March 28. www.washingtonworkplacelaw.com/private-employers/recent-hipaa-enforcement-actions-strong-medicine-for-health-care-employers/.

Kinney, E. D., H. A. McCabe, A. L. Gilbert, and J. J. Shisler. 2009. "Altered States of Care for Healthcare Providers in the Pandemic Influenza." *Indiana Health Law Review* 6 (1): 1–16.

Mendonca, L., and L. D. Tyson. 2011. "Reducing the Drag on the American Economy." McKinsey and Company. Accessed April 26, 2013. www.mckinsey.com/insights/americas/reducing_the_drag_on_the_american_economy.

Murray, C. J. L., and J. Frenk. 2010. "Ranking 37th—Measuring the Performance of the U.S. Health Care System." *New England Journal of Medicine* 362: 98–99.

Occupational Safety and Health Administration (OSHA). 2011a. "Hospital E-Tool." Accessed April 26, 2013. www.osha.gov/SLTC/etools/hospital/index.html .www.osha.gov/dts/osta/bestpractices/html/hospital_firstreceivers.html.

———. 2011b. "Emergency Preparedness Planning and Response." Accessed May 14, 2013. www.hhs.gov/ocr/privacy/hipaa/understanding/special/ emergency/index.html.

———. 2005. *OSHA Best Practices for Hospital-Based First Receivers of Victims from Mass Casualty Incidents Involving the Release of Hazardous Substances.* Accessed April 26, 2013. www.osha.gov/dts/osta/bestpractices/html/ hospital_firstreceivers.html.

Pitts, S. R., E. R. Carrier, E. C. Rich, and A. L. Kellerman. 2010. "Where Americans Get Acute Care: Increasingly, It's Not at Their Doctor's Office." *Health Affairs* 29 (9): 1620–29.

Social Security Administration. 2011. "Authority to Waive Requirements During National Emergencies." *Compilation of Social Security Laws.* Accessed April 26, 2013. www.ssa.gov/OP_Home/ssact/title11/1135.htm.

US Census Bureau. 2011. "Table 130: National Health Expenditures—Summary, 1960 to 2008, and Projections, 2009 to 2019." Accessed May 14, 2013. www.census.gov/compendia/statab/2011/tables/11s0130.pdf.

US Department of Health and Human Services (HHS). 2013. *Medicare Disproportionate Care Hospitals.* Centers for Medicare & Medicaid Services. Accessed February 15. www.cms.gov/MLNProducts/downloads/Disproportionate_ Share_Hospital.pdf.

———. 2012. "Public Health Emergency: Funding and Grant Opportunities." Published July 6. www.phe.gov/Preparedness/planning/hpp/Pages/funding .aspx.

———. 2011a. "Health Information Privacy." Accessed April 26, 2013. www.hhs .gov/ocr/privacy/.

———. 2011b. "Hospital Preparedness Program Overview." Accessed April 26, 2013. www.phe.gov/Preparedness/planning/hpp/Pages/overview.aspx.

———. 2011c. "Pandemic and All Hazards Preparedness Act." *Office of the Assistant Secretary for Preparedness and Response.* Accessed April 26, 2013. www.phe .gov/preparedness/legal/pahpa/pages/default.aspx.

Wilson, J. F. 2006. "Health Insurance Portability and Accountability Act Privacy Rule Causes Ongoing Concerns Among Clinicians and Researchers." *Annals of Internal Medicine* 145 (4): 313–16.

HEALTHCARE ETHICS AND A CHANGING HEALTHCARE SYSTEM

Carolyn Long Engelhard

> This chapter is relevant to the following competencies identified in the ACHE Competencies Assessment Tool (see p. xxv):
>
> **Communication and Relationship Management**
> - Identify stakeholder needs/expectations
>
> **Professionalism**
> - Adhere to ethical business principles
>
> **Knowledge of the Healthcare Environment**
> - The interrelationships among access, quality, cost, resource allocation, accountability, and community
> - Socioeconomic environment in which the organization functions
>
> **Business Skills and Knowledge**
> - Provide stewardship of financial resources
> - Potential impacts and consequences of financial decision making on operations, healthcare, human resources and quality of care
> - Marketing principles and tools

Learning Objectives

After completing this chapter, the reader will be able to

- understand the ethical implications of the financial relationship between hospitals and insurers,
- discuss the ethics surrounding how hospitals attempt to equalize revenues from different payers,

- identify how shifting financial risk to providers may cause ethical challenges,
- understand the ethical implications of healthcare reform for healthcare organizations,
- identify the ethical challenges for healthcare organizations under the Patient Protection and Affordable Care Act, and
- discuss how hospitals can maintain their ethical mission in a new era of reform.

Introduction

This chapter begins with a brief historical overview of the growth of healthcare spending over the past 30 years and the strategies of both government and private regulators to constrain the growth—strategies that brought in the potential to challenge hospitals' ethical missions. During the last attempt to manage health spending through payment changes—the managed care era—expenditures were indeed reduced, but at the cost of limiting both necessary as well as unnecessary care, thus sparking ethical tensions around accusations of rationing. In response to the backlash among patients and physicians, health plans relaxed the rigid utilization management techniques and health spending growth resumed. The **Patient Protection and Affordable Care Act** (ACA) of 2010 once again attempts to implement payment and service delivery reforms to "bend the cost curve" of health spending, and once again the potential of ethical challenges arises as healthcare organizations attempt to remain faithful to their mission while reducing spending. This chapter explores the new healthcare reform legislation and the ethical challenges and opportunities it ushers in for hospitals and healthcare organizations.

Patient Protection and Affordable Care Act
A national healthcare reform law designed to expand affordable health coverage for Americans who were uninsured or underinsured, slow the growth of health spending, and improve the healthcare delivery system to ensure more efficient, higher-quality healthcare.

Margin Versus Mission: Historical Overview

Communities place a high degree of trust in their hospitals, and hospitals, because they are a community asset, have a responsibility to be trustworthy and accountable to those they serve. The introduction of private and particularly public health insurance in the middle of the twentieth century made access to hospital-based health services available to larger segments of the US population. This demand spawned an increase in the number of hospitals in the United States, and by 1980 the country had reached 4.5 community hospital beds per 1,000 population (National Center for Health Statistics 2002). Along with expanded health coverage and the concomitant increase in hospital capacity, healthcare spending soared during the 1970s. For example, in the Medicare program alone, spending doubled every four years from its enactment in the mid-1960s to 1980 (Frum 2000).

Ethical Implications of Public and Private Attempts to Slow Health Spending

In 1983, the US government responded to the runaway Medicare spending through the enactment of a hospital-based **prospective payment system** (PPS), which reimbursed hospitals on the basis of **diagnosis-related groups** (DRGs). Under the DRG method, hospitals received a standardized fixed rate per admission based on a patient's diagnosis. This change was a departure from the traditional fee-for-service payment model that reimbursed hospitals for each discrete service provided. Moving to a "bundled" PPS payment system reduced revenues for hospitals and forced them to trim their operating costs, often by becoming more efficient, to remain economically viable.

> **Prospective payment system**
> A payment method that reimburses hospitals on the basis of diagnosis-related groups.

Around the time of the development of the public DRG system in the Medicare program, health maintenance organizations (HMOs), proposed in the 1960s by Dr. Paul Elwood and promoted by the Nixon Administration (Starr 1982), were established to keep medical spending in check in the private sector. The first HMOs were networks of hospitals and salaried physicians that received a fixed amount of money every year for taking care of the medical needs of patient members, regardless of how many procedures and tests were performed. This type of payment system, like Medicare's inpatient DRGs, gave healthcare providers direct financial incentives to provide all the necessary medical care, but no more, because a finite pool of dollars was available to pay for the care.

> **Diagnosis-related group**
> A payment method under which hospitals received a standardized fixed rate per admission based on a patient's diagnosis.

The HMO concept was broadened during the 1990s experiment with managed care, in which employers contracted with health insurance companies to manage the healthcare of their employees to hold down costs. These managed care organizations (MCOs) were more open types of insurance arrangements in which the customer, usually the employer, was free to mix and match doctors and hospitals. MCOs mimicked the payment structure of traditional HMOs and were financed through prepaid capitated allotments. Strictly applied utilization management tools, such as requiring permissions and preapprovals for referrals to specialists or for certain higher cost procedures, were also employed to constrain spending. Under this capitated financial regime, hospitals and doctors effectively became their own insurance company because they bore the financial risk of paying for an unpredictable amount of healthcare. The tension between providing necessary patient care while protecting the bottom line made many providers feel like "double agents," an ethically troubling identity that pitted patients against profits (Angell 1993). Although the managed care experiment worked—health spending was held down and health insurance premiums stabilized—physicians and their patients grew weary of having to seek approval from unknown entities at the other end of the telephone. By the late 1990s, the managed care revolution gave way to a less rigid payment and oversight system in which providers had more autonomy in the practice of medicine and patients had more choices about their care. As might be expected, when managed care's one-time savings were exhausted and its utilization management tools were relaxed, the growth in health spending once again escalated to a rate far outpacing general inflation (Wilson 2011).

As seen in the examples above, hospital payment structures can present ethical challenges for hospitals and may test their moral responsibility to provide appropriate clinical care. Providing too much care through a fee-for-service system or constraining appropriate care under a capitated system each carry ethical challenges because both overuse and underuse of medical services may be problematic. However, hospitals can maintain their fidelity to patient-centered care and uphold their fiduciary and ethical obligations to the community at large by employing strategies that use resources wisely, such as putting together teams of providers with less costly physician extenders (such as advanced practice nurses and physician assistants), streamlining processes, and leveraging reimbursements between private and public payers to maintain profits (Dobson, DaVanzo, and Sen 2006).

The passage of the ACA brings renewed opportunities and threats to the ethical roles of healthcare organizations. By introducing new payment models that encourage hospitals to serve whole communities while doing more with less, hospitals once again will have explicit incentives to reduce utilization to realize savings. But the new payment models will also reward hospitals for coordinating the care of a patient population both in and out of the hospital. Some fear that this financial balancing act will, once again, present renewed ethical challenges to hospitals and other providers. But the system-based model of care envisioned under the ACA also brings new opportunities for hospitals to reaffirm and extend their ethical values and their missions.

The Costs of Caring

Spending Drivers for Hospital Care and the Resulting Ethical Challenges

Hospital care remains the largest single category of health spending. In part, this is a testament to the advances in medical care that have helped people live longer, more productive lives. From 1960 to 2000, half of the improvement in survival among heart attack patients was attributable to technological advances such as cardiac catheterizations, coronary artery bypass, and angioplasties with stents (Cutler, Rosen, and Vijan 2006). However, these advances, while yielding many benefits, add to the demand for medical services and to the cost of providing the service. The average spending per heart attack case rose from $12,083 in 1984 to $21,714 in 1998, a 3.4 percent annual growth in real terms (Cutler and McClellan 2001). Today, approximately 50 percent of the rise in health expenditures over the past several decades is due to advances in technology (CBO 2008).

Demographic shifts are also leading to increased utilization of medical services. The US population is estimated to grow from 310 million in 2010 to 439 million in 2050, with the number of people over the age of 65 more than doubling, from 40 million to 88 million (US Census Bureau 2008). As people age they consume more medical services because they have more health problems. In 2007, mean annual health spending for individuals over the age of 65 was more than three times the amount used by 18- to 44-year-olds, and 50 percent more than the amount used by 45- to 64-year-olds (Centers for Disease Control and Prevention and National Center for Health Statistics 2011). Health spending is particularly high during the last year of life for aging Americans, mostly as a result of services received while hospitalized. Medicare patients spend about six times more in their last year of life than in other years, consuming 10 percent of overall health expenditures and 30 percent of the total Medicare budget (Garson and Engelhard 2007).

The growing prevalence of chronic illness across all age groups and the increasing percentages of American adults and children who are overweight or obese significantly contribute to higher hospital costs. Hospital care spending increases by 11 percent for patients with two chronic conditions and by 46 percent for those with seven or more chronic conditions (Friedman, Jiang, and Elixhauser 2008). Hospitalizations with a diagnosis of obesity jumped by 75 percent between 2001 and 2005 among children who were hospitalized, with the attendant cost of care for these children doubling from $126 million to more than $237 million over that time (Trasande et al. 2009). Part of this increase in spending relates to the use of more services, but a sicker population also requires more intensive care.

In addition to increased spending in hospitals as a result of technological advances, rising rates of chronic illness, and an aging population, hospitals also face a growing burden of uncompensated care costs from uninsured and underinsured patients and shortfalls from public programs. From 2000 to 2007, hospital uncompensated care costs rose from $22 billion to $34 billion, as the number of Americans without health coverage rose from 39 million to 47 million over the same time. From the beginning of the recession in 2007 Medicaid enrollment increased by 6 million individuals through 2010 (Kaiser Family Foundation 2010), and Medicare enrollment is projected to grow significantly because baby boomers became eligible for the program beginning in 2011. Medicaid and Medicare payment rates often fall short of hospitals' costs. Combined underpayments from Medicare and Medicaid rose from $3.8 billion in 2000 to $36 billion in 2009 (AHA 2010b). Although hospital participation in Medicare and Medicaid is technically voluntary, opting out of the governmental health programs is difficult as the two programs account for more than half of all care provided by hospitals (AHA 2010b).

At the same time that the demand for hospital care is rising and public program payments are declining, the cost to provide that care continues to rise. New devices and pharmaceuticals add to hospital expenses, nursing and physician shortages drive up wage rates, and investments in health information technology and other quality-related improvements all contribute to increased spending by hospitals. These factors create fiscal stress and therefore create ethical challenges for healthcare organizations as they seek to fulfill their missions with diminishing resources.

Balancing Expenditures and Revenues: The Ethics of Hospital Cost-Shifting

Hospitals and private insurance companies wrangle annually over how much hospital rates and, by extension, insurance reimbursements will go up each year. For government health programs, however, predetermined fee schedules and reimbursement rates are set by federal and state governments. But as mentioned in the previous section, Medicare and Medicaid payments are lower than their private counterparts. This disparity may lead hospitals to cost-shift, charging private payers more to compensate for shortfalls in payments from public programs. Although documentation of hospital cost-shifting has accumulated in the academic literature over the past 25 years, other variables, such as hospitals' market power, may also explain differential pricing structures (Frakt 2011).

No one disputes, however, that medical spending has outpaced economic growth for at least 30 years (Wilson 2011) and that some payers react to the increased spending by reducing their payments relative to costs. In turn, providers, particularly hospitals, attempt to mitigate the burden of under- and uncompensated healthcare costs by raising their prices to other payers with less market power. As mentioned previously, public payers and the uninsured are the drivers of under- and uncompensated hospital care, and so they benefit from this cost shift, while private insurers typically pay for it. The ability to cost-shift ensures that the uninsured and underinsured have some coverage for their medical needs (Dobson, DaVanzo, and Sen 2006).

However, as public payers continue to pay hospitals less to hold down spending and compensate for more expensive medical services, and private insurers are able to use market leverage and contractual agreements to temper widespread cost-shifting, the financial pressure on hospitals will force them to use other mechanisms to cut costs. This pressure raises the specter of possibly denying some patients access to certain types of expensive but useful services to control spending. Certainly this was the case in the managed care era of tightly constrained spending in which HMOs, under increasing pressure to remain competitively priced, reduced their hospital length of stay by using administrative efficiencies and restricting patient access to some expensive services (Schwartz and Mendelson 1992). Today, as healthcare spending continues unabated and now accounts for almost 18 percent of the entire US economy (Martin et al. 2012), hospitals are under increasing pressure to reduce their spending. This pressure for cost control—either internally because of reduced provider payments or externally from public or private regulators that tie reimbursements to practice guidelines or cost-effective metrics—will present renewed ethical challenges for healthcare organizations (Butler 2010).

Health Reform and Healthcare Organizations

In March 2010, President Obama signed into law the Patient Protection and Affordable Care Act of 2010 (HR 3590, Pub. L. No. 111-148) and the accompanying Healthcare and Education Reconciliation Act of 2010 (HR 4872, Pub. L. No. 111-152). The two acts are collectively referred to as the ACA. The goals of the national health reform effort centered on expanding affordable health coverage for Americans who were uninsured or underinsured, slowing the growth of health spending, and improving the healthcare delivery system to ensure more efficient, higher-quality healthcare.

In the early discussions about health reform, shortly after President Obama's inauguration in January 2009, the hospital industry, along with other health industry stakeholders, worked with the President and members of Congress to shape a national policy. Hospital leaders believed that cuts in Medicare reimbursements were inevitable, and so representatives from the hospital industry successfully advocated for some offsetting benefits, including: inclusion of insurance coverage mandates; expanded eligibility through exchange programs; and defeat of the single-payer and public-option proposals. In this way, hospitals hoped that any reductions in the level of Medicare payments would be mitigated by greater numbers of patients with better paying private health coverage, although the cuts also held the potential ethical challenge of limiting access for those who still lacked public or private health coverage.

Despite hospitals' early successes in helping to define the law, the ACA will affect them in potentially detrimental ways. Whether the law will provide sufficient insurance coverage for the diversity of patients cared for in hospitals is unclear, particularly because almost 12 million undocumented immigrants were excluded from the insurance mandates and from receiving federal subsidies to purchase health coverage. Although having newly insured patients will bring new revenues to hospitals, continuing to treat uninsured and underinsured patients will exacerbate some hospitals' current financial challenges.

In addition, under the ACA, the Centers for Medicare & Medicaid Services (CMS) will launch new payment mechanisms that may bring reduced revenues to hospitals. Over the next few years, CMS, through payments in the Medicare and Medicaid programs, will reward healthcare organizations for high performing, efficient care but also penalize them for quality gaps. Various demonstrations reflecting new payment models will be implemented to test whether changes in payment design can improve hospital efficiency and quality of care. By rewarding better performance and linking or denying payments on the basis of adherence to quality protocols and value-based metrics, hospitals and other providers will be reimbursed on the basis of the quality of the care provided rather than for simply providing a volume of services. The funding and reimbursement changes under the ACA will require concomitant changes in clinical operations for hospitals to remain successful, and, as such, the statute also provides incentives for new organizational structures (Main and Starry 2010). Both of these changes are discussed in the following section.

Funding and Reimbursement Changes

Insurance coverage expansion. The ACA requires all US citizens and legal immigrants (with a few exceptions) to obtain health insurance by 2014, and those who do not will face a penalty. The Congressional Budget Office (2012) projects that the combination of new subsidies for health insurance alongside the Medicaid expansion in states that opt into the new program will enable 14 million uninsured people to gain coverage in 2014 and 27 million by 2021. In addition, the law establishes a mandate for employers with more than 50 employees to offer affordable health coverage or pay a penalty. To help individuals and companies comply with the insurance coverage mandates, the ACA requires each state to establish a health benefits exchange that makes affordable health insurance available to individuals and companies with fewer than 100 employees. Tax credits, premium subsidies, and cost-sharing credits are available to small businesses and low-income individuals and families to help them buy health coverage on the state-based exchanges. The insurance coverage expansion requirements should benefit hospitals by increasing admissions while reducing the amount of uncompensated care, although 30 million Americans are projected to remain uninsured (CBO 2012).

Bundled payments for episodes of care. In 2013 Medicare established a five-year voluntary pilot program in which a bundled payment will be shared across hospitals, physicians, and post–acute care providers during an episode of care that begins three days prior to a hospitalization and extends to 30 days after discharge. If the program is successful, the ACA allows for its expansion in 2016. A similar demonstration project for Medicaid began in 2012. These new payment models encourage hospital and physician alignment as they become partners in payment; the models will prompt a movement away from traditional private practice models for physicians as hospitals move to employ more physicians. In addition, participating hospitals will need to have, or create, robust discharge-planning procedures for patients moving from the hospital to post–acute care settings, thereby encouraging hospitals to create community-based links to overcome the fragmentation currently seen in the system as patients transition from one care setting to another.

Pay for performance. Treatment costs caused by errors, adverse events, or inefficiencies are generally paid for by private and public payers or by patients and their families. In 2008, Medicare adopted a nonpayment strategy whereby it would not provide additional payment to hospitals for those services that reflected adverse events (for example, surgery performed on the wrong site) unless the events were present on admission (AHRQ 2011b). Building on and extending beyond penalizing providers for adverse events, the ACA establishes a value-based purchasing (VBP) initiative within Medicare to pay hospitals on the basis of meeting quality of care thresholds for certain conditions. Beginning in 2013, payments to hospitals are tied to a hospital's performance on a number of quality, efficiency, and patient satisfaction measures for acute myocardial infarction, heart failure, pneumonia, surgeries, and healthcare-associated infections. Successful hospital performance will bring an enhanced DRG payment; failure to meet quality metrics will bring an attendant penalty. The **pay-for-performance** initiatives under the ACA hold the promise of improved coordination, efficiency, and productivity in patient care, leading to enhanced patient outcomes and experiences. However, the accompanying reporting requirements associated with the new payment reforms are also likely to increase hospital administrative costs. Many hospital leaders fear that the changes will be too burdensome; among 284 hospitals and health systems CEOs who said healthcare reform was a top concern, most ranked pressure on operating costs as the ACA's biggest challenge to them (Carlson 2011).

Pay for performance
A payment system in which payments are tied to a hospital's performance on a number of quality, efficiency, and patient satisfaction measures.

Expansion of Medicaid. The federal Medicaid program will be significantly expanded under the ACA, although the level of expansion will be dictated by the 2012 Supreme Court decision that states could opt in or out of the expanded Medicaid program. Moving away from its traditional structure as a health coverage program for categories of low-income individuals (e.g., children, pregnant women, the frail elderly, people with disabilities), in 2014 Medicaid will cover those individuals whose income is equal to or less than 133 percent of the federal poverty level in states that choose to participate in the Medicaid expansion. The Medicaid expansion is estimated to provide an additional 10 million to 11 million people by 2019, 6 million fewer than original estimates that included all state programs (CBO 2012). The Medicaid expansion will defray much of the uncompensated care hospitals currently provide to the uninsured and underinsured in those states that embrace the expanded Medicaid program (NHLP 2012). Despite the increase in Medicaid reimbursements, hospitals remain concerned (Main and Starry 2010) that the increase in insured individuals will not make up for decreasingly available uncompensated care payments because at least 23 million Americans are estimated to remain uninsured after the implementation of the ACA, 22 percent of whom are undocumented immigrants and not eligible for the Medicaid expansion (Buettgens and Hall 2011).

Primary care funding. To improve the focus on primary care, the ACA increases reimbursement for primary care services in several ways. Payment rates in the Medicaid program will be increased to 100 percent of Medicare rates from 2013 to 2014. In addition, physicians in health professional shortage areas with 60 percent of their Medicare billing in primary care will experience a 10 percent bonus for a four-year period beginning in 2011.

Independent Payment Advisory Board. The ACA establishes a 15-member **Independent Payment Advisory Board** (IPAB) that makes recommendations to Congress for reducing per capita growth in the Medicare program and slowing the growth in national health expenditures when spending exceeds a target growth rate. The ACA explicitly restricts IPAB from making recommendations that would increase beneficiary cost-sharing, change eligibility criteria, or restrict benefits in the Medicare program. Congress can override or amend the board's recommendations only with a supermajority vote in both houses, and it has a limited time to pass legislation with alternative cuts that would meet the spending targets. The IPAB under the ACA is controversial and under attack from patients, providers, and elected officials because any reduction in per capita growth in the Medicare program will necessitate fewer services and reimbursements for patients and their providers (Kaiser Health News 2011).

Independent Payment Advisory Board
A 15-member panel established by the ACA that makes recommendations to Congress for reducing per capita growth in the Medicare program and slowing the growth in national health expenditures when spending exceeds a target growth rate.

These funding and reimbursement changes brought under the ACA will challenge healthcare organizations and compel both the governance and medical leadership bodies within organizations to become more fully engaged in how to manage limited and reduced revenues while staying true to their ethical obligations to patients and their communities. This challenge will require leaders to become more involved in helping to shape the policies that affect patient care and to work with larger governmental policymakers to ensure proper stewardship of resources for patients, communities, and the larger society.

Clinical Operations Changes for Hospitals

Accountable care organizations. As of 2012, healthcare organizations may participate in the Medicare program as **accountable care organizations** (ACOs), which were established by the ACA and are administered under CMS's Center for Medicare & Medicaid Innovation. ACOs are integrated healthcare delivery systems that combine a multidisciplinary set of medical practitioners and hospitals and are accountable for the overall care of patients. If ACOs meet quality thresholds—such as having an adequate number of primary care physicians, defining processes to provide evidence-based care, publicly reporting their performance in the areas of cost and quality, and demonstrating improved coordination of patient care—they will be eligible for sharing in any Medicare cost savings that accrue. According to CMS, Medicare could save up to $960 million over three years as a result of the ACO shared savings model (Evans 2011) and the Congressional Budget Office (CBO) estimates those savings could reach almost $5 billion by 2019 (Berenson and Zuckerman 2010). Becoming an ACO presents many structural challenges as well as mission-driven opportunities for healthcare organizations: developing networks that include physicians, hospitals, and other providers to address the full continuum of healthcare needs; providing the infrastructure for clinical information systems to support quality reporting and data management; and developing an overarching patient-centered culture so that the ACO can function as a unified organization. But ACOs hold the promise of moving healthcare organizations from individualized silos of care to partners in an integrated system of care with the goal of improving care for patients.

> **Accountable care organization**
> An integrated healthcare delivery system that combines a multidisciplinary set of medical practitioners and hospitals and is accountable for the overall care of patients.

Hospital-acquired conditions. Based on estimates from the Centers for Disease Control and Prevention (CDC), nearly 2 million hospital-acquired conditions occur each year in hospitals, which contribute to almost 100,000 deaths and cost our healthcare system between $28 billion and $33 billion annually (CDC 2011). In accordance with new regulations that support the ethical obligations for all hospitals to be transparent about their patient care, hospitals must now report their catheter-associated urinary tract infections, central line–associated bloodstream infections, and surgical site infection rate if they want full Medicare reimbursement. Under the ACA, beginning in 2015, hospitals will receive a 1 percent Medicare payment reduction for high levels of hospital-acquired conditions. The purpose of the new reporting requirements is to motivate hospitals to improve their infection control programs; the requirements will provide opportunities for hospital board and leadership bodies to invest in quality improvements in their organizations, thus exercising a primary ethical principle. Although the new requirements and penalties may present fears of losing market share and stigmatizing low-performing hospitals (Varney 2011), other hospitals that have already embarked on programs to reduce hospital-acquired conditions will use their successes to promote their hospital care programs as examples of transparency and accountability. One such example is the Keystone Intensive Care Unit Project in Michigan hospitals, in which they have stopped central line–associated bloodstream infections in intensive care units for up to two years (AHRQ 2011a).

Preventable readmissions. As of 2013, Medicare payments are reduced for hospitals with high rates of potentially preventable readmissions, initially for three conditions: acute myocardial infarction, heart failure, and pneumonia. Preventable hospital readmissions are a significant burden on the US healthcare system, costing an estimated $25 billion annually (PricewaterhouseCoopers' Health Research Institute 2008). Driven largely by suboptimal discharge procedures and inadequate follow-up care, nearly one in every five Medicare patients discharged from the hospital is readmitted within 30 days (Jencks, Williams, and Coleman 2009). The National Priorities Partnership (2010) estimates that total hospital readmissions could be reduced by up to 12 percent by improving procedures for discharging patients, providing better follow-up care, and using health information technology in the coordination of care. Echoing a basic value of healthcare organizations' mission statements, public reporting on readmission rates is required of hospitals and provided to the public. The CBO estimates that this Medicare payment penalty will save $7.1 billion over ten years. Endorsing the ethical principle of disclosure but fearful of repercussions of the new policy, hospitals worry that they will not only lose revenues as readmissions are not reimbursed, but also that they will be penalized for readmissions whose causes may be out of their control such as when patients do not follow physician or hospital orders (Gilbert 2007).

Healthcare Organizations: Ethical Challenges and Opportunities

On the Horizon: Fiscal Stress for Healthcare Organizations

Hospitals are still recovering from the effects of the severe recession in the United States. Many patients continue to forgo care because of financial hardship, and, because of high fixed costs, decreased utilization translates into lower revenues for hospitals. About 70 percent of hospitals reported decreased overall patient volume in 2010, and 72 percent reported a decline in elective procedures (AHA 2010a). As a result, many hospitals are reducing administrative costs and delaying capital investments to economize, while some are consolidating with other hospitals to increase market share and reduce costs or enhance revenues.

Hospitals' financial and ethical obligations will soon extend beyond their four walls as they will increasingly be accountable for the care of patient populations in a community. In response to the ACA's changes in payment models that reward and penalize hospitals for their performance in providing quality and coordination across the continuum of care in a community, hospitals will have to align more directly with physicians and other types of providers in outpatient care settings to meet quality thresholds for reimbursement. The financial risk for hospitals is significant: beginning in 2015, a 300-bed hospital with poor quality metrics could be penalized by more than $1.3 million per year (PricewaterhouseCoopers' Health Research Institute 2010).

In addition, hospitals face other financial challenges. Under the coverage expansions in Medicaid outlined in the ACA, the number of Medicaid recipients will increase by 40 percent over the next ten years. Traditionally, Medicaid rates have not covered all costs. According to the American Hospital Association (AHA 2010b), hospitals received 89 cents for every dollar spent on caring for Medicaid patients in 2008. Although increases in the number of Americans with private insurance under the ACA may compensate somewhat for the greater proportion of low-paying Medicaid patients, hospitals should be prepared for a shift in their payer mix.

In sum, this triumvirate of complex financial variables—the recent recession with its lowered utilization, new performance-based payment models under the ACA, and an increasing volume of inadequate reimbursements through the Medicaid program—will predispose hospitals to severe financial stress unless they find ways to control their fixed costs, continuously improve quality of care, and take advantage of opportunities to gain market share. As Helen Darling, president of the National Business Group on Health, states, "Hospitals are now going to be forced to make changes they've avoided for years. If they don't become more effective and efficient, they won't be paid" (Pearlstein 2011).

The Ethical Healthcare Organization

Hospitals and other healthcare organizations define themselves to their stakeholders (including the communities they serve) through their mission, values statements, and other documents, such as their codes of ethics. The overriding mission of any hospital is to offer the best, most affordable healthcare in an ethical manner with compassion and empathy to its patients. As stewards of societal resources, hospitals and other healthcare organizations that practice ethical behavior will conserve limited healthcare resources by using them efficiently, responsibly, and cost-effectively, yet will devote a portion of their budget to funding uncompensated care for those patients without adequate health coverage. At the community level, an ethical healthcare organization will identify public healthcare needs and build alliances to work with community organizations to promote public health and safety (ACHE 2011). (See Chapter 2 for a detailed discussion of a hospital's missions and values.)

Through their pledge, healthcare organizations promise to respect the religious, spiritual, cultural, and psychological values of their patients and to consider patient care preferences, including decisions to discontinue treatment. An ethical healthcare organization will protect patient information and consider that protection a central part of patient care, educating staff about patient disclosure rules and the need to maintain patient confidentiality. An ethical healthcare organization will disclose financial conflicts of interest and will ensure that both clinical and nonclinical staff will be involved in ethical decision making without fear of reprisals for contrary opinions.

Hospital boards will have new roles and ethical responsibilities under the ACA, which promotes a clinically integrated, systems-based approach to healthcare. Traditionally, hospital boards have focused their activities on financial issues and operating margins. The hospital board of the future will have to be educated about the quality of care provided in their institution and, along with the medical staff, be accountable for valid measurement and accurate reporting of quality outcomes (Goeschel, Wachter, and Pronovost 2010). The ACA's emphasis on integrated, systems-based medicine within a continuum of care in a community may challenge a hospital's traditional individualized approach but nonetheless supports and extends core ethical values of transparency, stewardship of resources, and primacy of patient care.

Ethical Challenges

Just as in the managed care era of the 1990s, the current sweep of new reimbursement models for healthcare organizations—value-based purchasing, readmission penalties, bundled payments, and shared savings programs—reflects a risk shift from the financers of healthcare (public and private insurers) to the providers of care. As in the past, the ACA's emphasis on cost-sensitive health insurance reform involves financial incentives and changes in organizational structures to increase the integration of healthcare while enhancing efficiency. Similarly, in a déjà vu moment for healthcare organizations, the current reforms in healthcare financing and delivery also present ethical challenges.

Medicare and Medicaid payments. The ACA calls for reduced Medicare payments to hospitals, thereby discounting Medicare rates for inpatient care. The volume of Medicaid patients will increase significantly after 2014, when the eligibility criteria expand to include an additional 10 to 11 million Americans. The influx of newly insured patients will help make up the revenue dislocations brought on by Medicaid, but more likely, the reduced Medicare and "disproportionate share" payments hospitals previously received to help offset uncompensated care, alongside more than 23 million Americans still uninsured and needing care, will force healthcare organizations to consider new strategies to make up for lost revenue. They can do this in two ways: either by charging private payers more to compensate for shortfalls in payments from public programs, otherwise known as cost-shifting; or by cutting costs. As both private and public payers move toward a more bundled or global payment system, cost-shifting, a strategy that has been used in the industry for decades, becomes less feasible. Therefore, the more likely scenario is that hospitals will try to cut costs through reduction in services, increased efficiencies, or market consolidation so as to have greater power in negotiations with payers (Frakt 2011).

The ethical tensions for hospitals during this time of transition to new payment and accountable care models will be to continue to provide access to care for those populations that are poorer and sicker and to continue to offer services that communities count on but that do not support themselves, such as burn units. Those health systems that have forged alliances with primary care physicians in the ambulatory sector may be tempted to limit their exposure to uninsured and Medicaid patients. In the inpatient environment, with the advent of public reporting of patient outcomes and Medicare penalties for preventable readmissions, financial incentives exist for hospitals to avoid the sickest patients. Reducing access for patients because they cannot pay or because they are sicker or more difficult to treat would undermine the ethical tenets of healthcare organizations, particularly the covenant between hospitals and the communities they serve.

Paying for quality. Although few would argue with the assertion that those who pay for health services should be assured of receiving quality care, pay-for-performance programs in healthcare have the potential to introduce ethical challenges for physicians and healthcare organizations. Many critics of such programs argue that by selecting only certain health services whose outcomes can be measured (and thus rewarded) will crowd out or marginalize those services not tied to incentives. For instance, patient care that reflects treatments for older patients with complex chronic illnesses and multiple comorbidities may not be eligible for pay-for-performance bonuses because rewarded adherence to specific clinical practice guidelines generally align with discrete diagnoses (Boyd et al. 2005). Another concern is that safety-net hospitals that care for a disproportionate share of low-income and often medically difficult patients may not meet quality thresholds and have limited support or resources to make the necessary system changes. This could create a two-tiered healthcare system where hospitals with more resources or less complicated patients could invest in quality improvement programs and benefit from payment structures that reward that investment (Werner 2010).

Opportunities to Maintain the Ethical Mission

Given the economic and ethical challenges facing healthcare organizations under healthcare reform, how can today's leaders ensure their organizations continue to live up to their moral missions? First and foremost, healthcare organizational leaders need to have an ethical framework in place and instill a culture within their organizations that unethical behavior will not be tolerated. Ethical leadership can make a significant impact—for example, the Veterans Affairs hospital in Lexington, Kentucky, adopted an ethical framework within a humanistic risk-management organizational policy of full transparency regarding disclosure of adverse events after a medical error; the facility believed it had a duty to remain in the role of caregiver and notify the patient of the findings (Kraman and Hamm 1999). An ethical culture begins with effective leadership and filters through an organization through open communication, adherence to shared values, respect for others, and making decisions based on long-term goals that fulfill the organization's mission and vision. In this way, decisions can be made that support and improve the well-being of patients, their caregivers, and the communities in which they live, all the while creating a more equitable, accessible, effective, and efficient healthcare system (Squazzo 2011).

The ACA will present economic and ethical challenges for organizations, but it also contains numerous mechanisms and incentives designed to improve health outcomes and delivery systems. Embedded in the legislation are opportunities for healthcare organizations to reinterpret and reinforce their ethical missions, particularly in the area of transparency and disclosure. Disclosure of financial relationships between health entities (including hospitals, physicians, pharmacists, and others) and distributors of covered drugs, devices, biologicals, and medical supplies must be publicly reported. This transparency will keep organizations accountable for any real or perceived conflicts of interest. In addition, several sections within the ACA require information dissemination via websites and other communication mechanisms summarizing data on clinical performance and other quality measures. By complying with these new disclosure regulations, healthcare organizations support patient education and choice and demonstrate their trustworthiness and dedication to continuously improving the care they provide.

Conclusion

The demand for healthcare is rising because of advances in medicine, an aging population, and a rising burden of chronic disease. With this increased demand comes rising expenditures in healthcare because of a confluence of factors: the cost of developing and providing new medical discoveries, increased personnel costs because of workforce shortages, infrastructure improvements in health information technology, investments in quality tracking systems, and compliance with public and private regulations. The passage of the ACA will continue to bring many changes to healthcare organizations, some of which, in the short term, will challenge existing business models and practice patterns. Almost every aspect of the financing, organization, and delivery of healthcare will be affected: opening up the "black box" of healthcare through disclosure and transparency; changing how medical care is reimbursed so as to be more accountable and value-based; and reconfiguring physicians, hospitals, and communities to seamlessly provide services through the continuum of healthcare. Healthcare organizations will almost certainly have to do more with less in the short term, as payments are tied to performance and additional regulatory and reporting requirements develop.

Yet these changes have the potential to reaffirm and strengthen healthcare organizations' core ethical values and mission. The fundamental ethical principles of trust, stewardship, transparency, and disclosure, peppered throughout health reform legislation, are the same principles institutionalized in every healthcare organization's missions. Shifting from an individualized ethical perspective to one that encompasses the coordination of care across a community-based continuum will require healthcare leaders to act in new ways that will continue to merit the trust, confidence, and respect of their staff, patients, and the general public. The ACA's full reach into medical care and hospital administration is significant and not yet fully knowable, but healthcare organizations have the opportunity to meet the challenges within the law and live up to their ethical obligations to provide high quality, measurable, and cost-effective care in their communities.

Points to Remember

- Healthcare spending in the United States has outpaced general inflation by 2 to 3 percent for the past 30 years. Hospital care is the largest category of health spending. Medical inflation, particularly in the federal Medicare and Medicaid programs, is considered to be unsustainable for the federal budget, particularly as baby boomers age.
- To make up for lower reimbursements in the Medicare and Medicaid programs, healthcare organizations often charge private payers more to compensate for shortfalls in payments from public programs, a practice known as cost-shifting.
- During the 1990s employers forged relationships with private insurers to hold down health spending to stabilize escalating health insurance premiums. Managed care organizations used strict utilization controls

and capitated prepayments to hospitals and physicians to reduce overall use of health services, thereby interjecting ethical tensions for healthcare organizations trying to balance their moral missions with their need to survive financially.

- The Patient Protection and Affordable Care Act (ACA), a federal health reform bill, was signed into law by President Obama in March 2010. While the law carries the promise of almost universal health coverage in the United States, the law is controversial because it contains a mandate that all US citizens obtain health coverage, is considered too costly by critics, and places new regulations on insurance companies, hospitals, and other health industry stakeholders.

- The ACA brings changes to funding and clinical operations for healthcare organizations. The new payment models shift greater financial risk onto hospitals and reward or punish them based on meeting defined quality and efficiency metrics. These changes will reduce overall revenues for hospitals in the short term and challenge hospitals to maintain their ethical missions while remaining fiscally solvent.

References

Agency for Healthcare Research and Quality (AHRQ). 2011a. "ICUs in Michigan Sustain Zero Blood Stream Infections for Up to 2 Years." Accessed May 1, 2013. www.ahrq.gov/news/press/pr2011/clabsiicupr.htm.

———. 2011b. "Never Events." Accessed May 1, 2013. http://psnet.ahrq.gov/primer.aspx?primerID=3.

American College of Healthcare Executives (ACHE). 2011. "Code of Ethics." Accessed May 1, 2013. www.ache.org/ABT_ACHE/ACHECodeofEthics-2011.pdf.

American Hospital Association (AHA). 2011. "The Work Ahead: Activities and Costs to Develop an Accountable Care Organization." Accessed June 13. www.aha.org/aha/content/2011/pdf/aco-white-paper-cost-dev-aco.pdf.

———. 2010a. "Hospitals Continue to Feel Lingering Effects of the Economic Recession." Accessed June 13, 2013. www.aha.org/aha/press-release/2010/100623-pr-recessionimpact.html.

———. 2010b. "Underpayment by Medicare and Medicaid Fact Sheet." Accessed May 20, 2013. www.aha.org/content/00-10/10medunderpayment.pdf.

Angell, M. 1993. "The Doctor as Double Agent." *Kennedy Institute of Ethics Journal* 3 (3): 279–86. Accessed May 1, 2013. http://muse.jhu.edu/login?auth=0&type=summary&url=/journals/kennedy_institute_of_ethics_journal/v003/3.3.angell.html.

Berenson, R., and S. Zuckerman. 2010. "How Will Hospitals Be Affected by Healthcare Reform?" *The Urban Institute*. Accessed May 1, 2013. www.urban.org/publications/412155.html.

Boyd, C. M., J. Darer, C. Boult, L. P. Fried, L. Boult, and A. W. Wu. 2005. "Clinical Practice Guidelines and Quality of Care for Older Patients with Multiple Comorbid Diseases." *Journal of the American Medical Association* 294 (5): 716–24.

Buettgens, M., and M. Hall. 2011. "Who Will Be Uninsured After Health Insurance Reform?" *Robert Wood Johnson Foundation*. Accessed May 1, 2013. www.rwjf.org/en/research-publications/find-rwjf-research/2011/03/who-will-be-uninsured-after-health-insurance-reform-.html.

Butler, S. 2010. "Concerns Presented by the New Health Legislation." *Cancer Journal* 16 (6): 629–34.

Carlson, J. 2011. "What Really Matters to the CEO." *Modern Healthcare*. Published January 24. www.modernhealthcare.com/article/20110124/MAGAZINE/110129991.

Centers for Disease Control and Prevention and National Center for Health Statistics. 2011. "Health, United States, 2010: In Brief." Accessed May 1, 2013. www.cdc.gov/nchs/data/hus/hus10_InBrief.pdf.

Centers for Disease Control and Prevention. 2011. "Healthcare Associated Infections: The Burden." Accessed May 1, 2013. www.cdc.gov/HAI/burden.html.

Congressional Budget Office (CBO). 2012. "Estimates for the Insurance Coverage Provisions of the Affordable Care Act Updated for the Recent Supreme Court Decision." Accessed May 20, 2013. www.cbo.gov/sites/default/files/cbofiles/attachments/43472-07-24-2012-CoverageEstimates.pdf.

————. 2008. "Technological Change and the Growth of Healthcare Spending." Accessed May 1, 2013. www.cbo.gov/ftpdocs/89xx/doc8947/01-31-TechHealth.pdf.

Cutler, D., and M. McClellan. 2001. "Is Technological Change in Medicine Worth It?" *Health Affairs* 20 (5): 11–29.

Cutler, D. M., A. B. Rosen, and S. Vijan. 2006. "The Value of Medical Spending in the United States, 1960–2000." *New England Journal of Medicine* 355: 920–27.

Dobson, A., J. DaVanzo, and N. Sen. 2006. "The Cost-Shift Payment 'Hydraulic': Foundation, History, and Implications." *Health Affairs* 25 (1): 22–33.

Evans, M. 2011. "Hell No, We Won't ACO." *Modern Healthcare*. Published June 6. www.modernhealthcare.com/article/20110606/MAGAZINE/306069950#.

Frakt, A. B. 2011. "How Much Do Hospitals Cost-Shift? A Review of the Evidence." *Milbank Quarterly* 89 (1): 90–130.

Friedman, B., H. J. Jiang, and A. Elixhauser. 2008. "Costly Hospital Readmisisons and Complex Chronic Illness." *Inquiry* 45: 408–21.

Frum, D. 2000. *How We Got Here: The '70s.* New York: Basic Books.

Garson, A., and C. Engelhard. 2007. *Health Care Half-Truths: Too Many Myths, Not Enough Reality.* Lanham, MD: Rowman & Littlefield.

Gilbert, J. A. 2007. *Strengthening Ethical Wisdom: Tools for Transforming Your Health Care Organization.* Chicago: American Hospital Association.

Goeschel, C. A., R. M. Wachter, and P. J. Pronovost. 2010. "Responsibility for Quality Improvement and Patient Safety." *Chest* 138 (1): 171–78.

Jencks, S. F., M. V. Williams, and E. A. Coleman. 2009. "Rehospitalizations Among Patients in the Medicare Fee-for-Service Program." *New England Journal of Medicine* 360 (14): 1418–28.

Kaiser Family Foundation. 2010. "State Fiscal Conditions and Medicaid." Accessed May 1, 2013. www.kff.org/medicaid/upload/7580-07.pdf.

Kaiser Health News. 2011. "IPAB Under Attack from All Sides." Published June 10. www.kaiserhealthnews.org/daily-reports/2011/june/10/ipab .aspx?referrer=search.

Kraman, S. S., and G. M. Hamm. 1999. "Risk Management: Extreme Honesty May Be the Best Policy." *Annals of Internal Medicine* 131 (12): 963–67.

Main, D. C., and M. M. Starry. 2010. "The Effect of Health Care Reform on Hospitals: A Summary Overview." *Pillsbury Winthrop Shaw Pittman LLP.* Accessed May 1, 2013. www.pillsburylaw.com/siteFiles/Publications/2C9547A6BFC BB37D8366EA2272190123.pdf.

Martin, A. B., D. Lassman, B. Washington, A. Catlin, and the National Health Expenditure Accounts Team. 2012. "Growth in US Health Spending Remained Slow in 2010; Health Share of Gross Domestic Product Was Unchanged from 2009." *Health Affairs* 31 (1): 208–19.

National Center for Health Statistics. 2002. *Health, United States, 2002.* Hyatttsville, MD: National Center for Health Statistics.

National Health Law Program (NHLP). 2012. "Q & A: Disproportionate Share Hospital Payments and the Medicaid Expansion." Accessed May 20, 2013. www.apha .org/NR/rdonlyres/328D24F3-9C75-4CC5-9494-7F1532EE828A/0 /NHELP_DSH_QA_final.pdf.

National Priorities Partnership. 2010. "Preventing Hospital Readmissions: A $25 Billion Opportunity." *National Quality Forum.* Accessed May 1, 2013. www .noplacelikehomeaz.com/Docs/NPP_Preventing_Hospital_Readmissions .pdf

Pearlstein, S. 2011. "Real World Making Health-Care Reforms." *Washington Post* May 21.

PricewaterhouseCoopers' Health Research Institute. 2010. "Health Reform: Prospering in a Post-Reform World." Accessed May 1, 2013. www.pwc.com/us/en /health-industries/publications/prospering-in-a-post-reform-world.jhtml.

———. 2008. "The Price of Excess: Identifying Waste in Healthcare Spending." Accessed May 1, 2013. www.pwc.com/us/en/healthcare/publications/the-price-of-excess.jhtml.

Schwartz, W. B., and D. N. Mendelson. 1992. "Why Managed Care Cannot Contain Hospital Costs Without Rationing." *Health Affairs* 11: 100–107.

Squazzo, J. D. 2011. "Ethical Wisdom." *Healthcare Executive* 26 (3): 31–35.

Starr, P. 1982. *The Social Transformation of American Medicine.* New York: Basic Books.

Trasande, L., Y. Liu, G. Fryer, and M. Weitzman. 2009. "Effects of Childhood Obesity on Hospital Care and Costs, 1999–2005." *Health Affairs* 28 (4): 751–60.

US Census Bureau. 2008. "Projections of the Population by Selected Age Groups and Sex for the United States: 2010–2050." Accessed May 1, 2013. www.census.gov/population/projections/#.

Varney, S. 2011. "Hospitals Face New Pressure to Cut Infection Rates." *National Public Radio.* Accessed May 1, 2013. www.npr.org/2011/05/28/136712657/hospitals-face-new-pressure-to-cut-infection-rates.

Werner, R. M. 2010. "Does Pay-for-Performance Steal from the Poor and Give to the Rich?" *Annals of Internal Medicine* 153 (5): 340–41.

Wilson, K. B. 2011. "Health Care Costs 101." *California HealthCare Foundation.* Accessed May 1, 2013. www.chcf.org/publications/2011/05/health-care-costs-101.

LEADERSHIP AND THE HEALTHCARE ORGANIZATION

Gary L. Filerman, Ann E. Mills, and Paul M. Schyve

This chapter is relevant to the following competencies identified in the ACHE Competencies Assessment Tool (see p. xxv):

Communication and Relationship Management
- Communicate organizational mission, vision, objectives, and priorities
- Facilitate conflict and alternative dispute resolution

Leadership
- Potential impacts and consequences of decision making in situations both internal and external
- Foster an environment of mutual trust
- Assess the organization, including corporate values and culture, business processes, and impact of systems on operation

Professionalism
- Consequences of unethical actions
- Professional roles, responsibility, and accountability
- Conduct self-assessments
- Serve as the ethical guide for the organization
- Mentor, advise, and coach

Business Skills and Knowledge
- Potential impacts and consequences of financial decision making on operations, healthcare, human resources, and quality of care
- Principles and practices of management and organizational behavior

Learning Objectives

After completing this chapter, the reader will be able to

- identify the two primary ethical responsibilities of leaders;
- understand how mental models, which incorporate narratives, social roles, and role relationships, can blind leaders into misperceptions of reality;
- understand moral imagination;
- understand practical moral reasoning; and
- understand how the use of moral imagination and practical moral reasoning can help leaders devise novel solutions to troublesome moral or ethical situations, conflicts, or events.

Introduction

Healthcare organization leaders have two fundamental ethical responsibilities. The first is to recognize and understand the moral complexities and consequences embedded in events, situations, or decisions, and act accordingly. The second is to nurture and maintain an organizational culture that ensures that others in their institutions recognize and understand the moral complexities and consequences embedded in the events or situations they confront and the decisions they must make.

The focus of this chapter is on how persons aspiring to leadership roles in hospitals or other healthcare organizations can best prepare themselves to recognize and understand the moral complexities and consequences embedded in events, situations, or decisions. The chapter also discusses the related question of how persons in leadership roles can best prepare themselves to lead and manage when the event, situation, or decision is morally problematic.

Blinded leader
A leader who is not able to recognize a morally problematic situation or decision.

A **blinded leader** is a leader who does not recognize or understand the moral complexities or consequences before her. Consequently, a blinded leader is incapable of fulfilling these two fundamental ethical responsibilities. Leaders can become blinded in several ways. The concept of mental models was introduced in Chapter 10. This chapter begins with a more detailed discussion of mental models and how they can blind a leader. A mental model that is often seen in persons working in healthcare organizations is one that

Separation thesis
The idea that business decisions and moral or ethical decisions are distinct.

incorporates the belief that value-creating activities, such as business, can be separated from ethics or morality; consequently one can use sentences such as "*x* is a business decision, not an ethical decision" and "*y* is an ethical decision, not a business decision" (Freeman 1994). Freeman calls this belief the **separation thesis**.

This chapter also introduces the idea of **moral imagination**. Moral imagination is a three-step process that, if used appropriately, can help a leader reduce blindness and envision a solution to a morally problematic event, situation, or decision. Moral imagination is not the same as moral reasoning. Both are needed to identify and develop morally justifiable solutions.

Practical moral reasoning is a framework or guide composed of a series of questions that can help an individual work through a morally problematic event or situation. Each profession may develop its own guides. Because people in different professions confront dissimilar events or situations, these guides offer differing sorts of questions aimed at helping people work through profession-specific or situation-specific morally troubling events or situations—although common themes are often reflected in the various guides (see Chapter 6).

Healthcare administrators make decisions that affect organizations. The healthcare organization itself is a system composed of multiple subsystems. A decision that affects one subsystem will usually affect other subsystems within the organization. And most of these decisions and the changes incurred as a result of them will have moral consequences, not just in the subsystem that is the focus of change. In addition, these moral consequences may affect the ethical culture of the institution as a whole. Therefore, the moral reasoning framework presented here is based on thinking about systems. **Systems thinking** describes thinking about the system as a whole, which is distinct from thinking about parts of a system. For instance, one could think about the whole of a payroll managing system and how its parts interact and function together. Or one could think about time keeping, that part of the payroll managing system concerned about employee hours. This framework includes questions a leader should ask when making a decision that might affect the culture of her institution. Systems thinking offers a beginning point for a practical moral framework. It helps identify the questions that students, administrators, or executives should ask themselves when considering system changes.

The concepts introduced in this chapter are tools that future healthcare administrators should master and become adept at using. However, these tools will not be effective if future leaders do not develop and reflect on the positive values they themselves consider important.

Even the most thoughtful leader cannot know everything about her organization or what is going on everywhere in the organization. Nor can she know what everyone is thinking or doing and, therefore, she can neither identify nor resolve every morally or ethically problematic event or situation that arises in the organization. She must acknowledge this, find ways of

Moral imagination
The ability in a particular circumstance to consider and evaluate possibilities not determined by that circumstance, or limited by its operative mental models, or framed by a set of rules or rule-governed concerns.

Practical moral reasoning
A framework or guide composed of a series of questions that can help an individual work through a morally problematic event or situation.

Systems thinking
Describes thinking about the system as a whole as distinct from thinking about the parts of a system.

listening to voices throughout the organization, and fulfill her second fundamental ethical responsibility by being supportive of an organizational culture that helps all its members see the moral complexities and consequences embedded in the situations and events they face and the decisions they make every day.

Leadership Blindness

Mental Models

A mental model, also known as a mind-set, refers to deeply held or ingrained assumptions or generalizations that influence how we perceive and understand the world (Werhane 1999). Peter Senge (1990) and other theorists use the concept of mental models to explain the human component of organizational and systems change (see Chapter 11 for more discussion).

Mental models are formed on the basis of knowledge, experience, or history or a combination thereof. They are the lenses through which we understand the present. Mental models can be simple or complex. For instance, a person's mental model might be that people are inherently good. Consequently, his interactions with people will be different than those of a person whose mental model is that people are inherently self-serving. Or a healthcare administrator, whose mental model is that her hospital is adequately serving the needs of the community, may not listen objectively to ideas for service changes that would respond to changes in the community.

Mental models are powerful because they affect what we see, how we make sense of what we see, and, therefore, what we do. Depending on their mental models, two people can observe the same event and interpret it quite differently (Werhane 1999).

Mental models both shape and influence how we experience the world—situations, interpersonal relationships, the behavior of others, and so on. We cannot experience except through mental models. They frame the ways in which we make sense of our experiences, including the ways by which our brains store, manage, and retrieve data selectively.

Mental models have advantages and disadvantages. For instance, once embedded, mental models become implicit and can be recalled and applied rapidly and repeatedly. Ralph Stacey (2003) notes that this advantage occurs during the process of becoming an expert. Another advantage of mental models is that they are socially learned, so they can be shared by others in a group, whether a family, a society, a nation, a political party, a profession, or a social group. When mental models are shared, they become part of the culture of the group, and the efficiency of communication is increased before a decision is made or action is taken. (Of course, too often a leader may assume that a mental model is shared when, in fact, it is not.)

However, the advantages of mental models are coupled with potential disadvantages. The assumptions or generalizations that comprise a mental model are usually either too narrow, too focused, too broad, or too general to accurately and fully represent the real world. Moreover, when mental models become deeply ingrained, they are relied on without question (Senge 1990). Thus, individuals may make decisions or take actions on the basis of incomplete information or an incomplete picture

Case Study

For some years, a longtime chairman of the board of a large urban hospital maintained a friendly relationship with the CEO. The chairman had been instrumental in the CEO's appointment and often praised the CEO as a "doer," not just a "thinker." The CEO in turn relied on the board chairman for advice and support.

The chairman was interested in expanding the hospital's clinical services. The CEO concurred. Over time, other members of the board became increasingly dubious about the direction of the hospital, believing these additional services were ill-matched with the needs of the community. The CEO dismissed these concerns. He continued to have full faith in the leadership direction supplied by the chairman of the board.

What mental models do you observe in this case?

Are they having a positive effect on the direction of the hospital?

of what is occurring. This risk is increased if the environment or situation has changed since the mental model was first developed. In these cases, mental models may limit our ability to recognize and adapt to what may be important to a given situation. In this way, mental models may also limit our effectiveness as leaders and managers.

Mental Models and the Separation Thesis

In 1994, frustrated by the fact that in business schools "business" and "business ethics" were perceived as autonomous, Freeman articulated the separation thesis (Freeman 1994). The idea that "business" and "morality" (or "ethics") are somehow separate from each other is still alive and well in healthcare when doctors want to practice medicine based on the ethics of the Hippocratic Oath, not make business decisions, and administrators want to make business decisions, not decisions about care. But because hospitals are businesses in which every clinical decision has resource implications and every resource decision has clinical implications, any decision made by a doctor is a business decision (e.g., cost) as well as a healthcare decision. And if we believe that healthcare delivery has a moral core, then any decision made on behalf of a hospital or other healthcare organization by an administrator has moral or ethical implications.

Embedding this separation between business, morality, and ethics in our mental models is dangerous because it directs us into what Werhane

Case Study

Any situation in which patient safety can be improved and is not can be considered morally problematic.

A physician noticed that the rate of urinary tract infections was increasing in the hospital. Urinary catheters often cause urinary tract infections, especially if removing them is delayed. The physician asked that reminder stickers be put in patients' charts so that busy staff can remember when to remove the catheter.

Rates of urinary tract infections decreased. Because the average cost per patient without a urinary tract infection is about $10,000 while average costs for patients with urinary tract infections are more than $40,000, the hospital ended up saving tens of thousands of dollars. What is the business thinking in this case? What is the medical thinking? What is the end result?

(1999) calls a "false dilemma" or "an illusion that business can either be morally good or profitable" but not both. This separation is dangerous because it leads us to believe that somehow doing "good" is incompatible with doing "well."

When embedded in our mental models, the separation thesis drives us into making inappropriate or inaccurate judgments. For instance, this mental model may direct us toward assuming that a for-profit hospital will somehow not provide quality care to its patients. Or that a for-profit hospital is not as caring as a nonprofit. Or that a wealthy board member is incapable of understanding the needs of a community. If a person's mental model of the relationship between business and morality or ethics is the separation thesis, it can prevent the person from seeing that a business organization, such as a hospital, can both embrace a normative core (standards and values which the hospital aspires to in achieving its mission) and flourish economically. Moreover, this mental model will often limit a person's ability to envision what can be done to improve a morally problematic situation or dilemma.

The case study illustrates that a hospital can identify a morally problematic situation and do something about it while simultaneously saving precious resources.

Narratives

Narratives
Stories that individuals and organizations use to communicate their identity and values that help to frame their mental models.

Individuals as well as organizations have **narratives,** or stories, that help frame and shape their mental models (Werhane and Moriarty 2009). Organizations have mission statements, values statements, and other documents that communicate the identity and purpose of the organization. These statements are the formal narrative of the organization. Narratives told by individuals about life in the organization can be thought of as informal narratives. These informal narratives can reaffirm or reject the formal narrative of the organization. Ideally, of course, formal and informal narratives should align with and support each other.

Having a robust organizational narrative, in which both formal and informal narratives are consistent and synergistic, is an advantage to leadership because it helps develop and sustain an organizational culture. It can help leaders look for opportunities and make decisions that reflect the purpose, principles, and values of the organization. But a robust organizational narrative also has disadvantages. It can blind the mental models of individuals and organizations to reality. For instance, an organization with a long and proud narrative of being committed to its values and principles can be blinded when individuals make decisions and act outside of the narrative. An organization whose narrative insists that it does not act immorally can blind responsible individuals

> ### Case Study
>
> Despite a difficult financial outlook, 75-year-old Able Hospital has continued to merit its reputation for adhering to its mission of responsiveness to community needs.
>
> The members of the highly visible, self-perpetuating board take pride in their role protecting the hospital's assets and traditions. Their efforts to find the support necessary to maintain high-quality services are well known and are appreciated by the community.
>
> When a community hospital in a nearby town announced that it was facing bankruptcy, the Able board and CEO moved quickly, despite some risk, to arrange a merger for operational synergies that would benefit both institutions.
>
> The CEO ordered the purchase of five Chevrolet Suburbans so that he and other executives could commute in comfort between the two hospitals. He was angered when the purchasing agent advised him against it, arguing that smaller and more fuel-efficient vehicles would be more appropriate given the financial situation and the negative impression of high-cost vehicles. The CEO insisted that his order be followed, and the cars were purchased. The board did not inquire about the purchase, feeling that the CEO's decisions are always in alignment with their values.
>
> Do you think the mental models of the CEO and the board members are blinded? Why?

in the organization from seeing that people in the organization are making immoral decisions. If an executive cannot step outside the organizational narrative, or recognize it for what it is, she will be trapped by the logic of the narrative and be unable to see where it diverges with reality or where reality has changed and a new narrative or changed behaviors are needed (Werhane and Moriarty 2009). (If the executive recognizes that the organizational narrative does not align with organization reality and is not in a position to do anything about it, he might experience moral distress. See Chapter 7.)

Social Roles

Everyone in an organization has a number of roles. These **social roles** define what that person does, what relationships that person has, and what outcomes that person is expected to produce. In addition, social roles define the relationship of the individual to the organization and the layers of an

Social roles
A person's responsibilities, functions, and relationships that in turn define the organization and the layers of an organization.

organization. The social roles needed by an organization to fulfill its mission define the organization itself (Werhane and Moriarty 2009). As such, social roles are instrumental in helping to shape individual mental models.

Social roles provide a certain amount of predictability in organizational life, as most people understand their roles and adhere to them. But if roles are understood too rigidly, if they are blindly adhered to, roles can fail to empower individuals to confront and deal with unanticipated situations (Werhane and Moriarty 2009).

For example, in a study designed to ascertain why mortality rates for patients with acute myocardial infarction vary substantially across hospitals, even when adjusted for severity, Curry and colleagues (2011) found that, among other factors, lower-performing hospitals had roles that were narrowly circumscribed, particularly nurse and pharmacist roles. (This may also have contributed to the lack of communication that study authors found in the lower-performing hospitals.)

In the lower-performing hospitals, the roles of nurses and pharmacists may have been rigidly defined. But the nurses and pharmacists in those hospitals may also have had a circumscribed view of their *own* roles. Werhane and colleagues (2011) state, "Identification with a particular role, then, can blind one from challenging what is demanded from that role, particularly in difficult or stressful situations."

Leaders may become blinded if their mental models are shaped and influenced by their social roles and the expectations associated with those roles. When this occurs, leaders are not likely to clearly see what is going on. They are seeing what their mental models predispose them to see. For instance, Chapter 10 presents evidence that people in senior positions in various organizations have a different perspective on the ethical environments of their

---

Case Study

When asked why one hospital performed better than another, one physician said people in the hospital were encouraged to pay attention to the roles of others and to speak up if they believed something was or might be wrong. "If the nurse only knows the nursing role and the tech only knows the tech role, and the RT [radiology technician] only knows the RT role, there may not be additional pairs of eyes backing me up. But here, our people are encouraged to speak up and not confine themselves to their prescribed roles. And it happens a lot that they find something, observe something, read something, hear something that helps me avoid trouble when I am working with a patient."

You will be an administrator, not a physician. However, you will receive information from a variety of roles. You will be asked to make decisions based on this information. Should your subordinates (and the roles they represent) be encouraged to speak up if they believe that something is wrong? Or do you think that it encourages greater efficiency and promotes greater harmony for persons not to criticize or question the information you receive from other roles? Is this an either–or situation?

Adapted from Curry et al. (2011).

organizations than do people lower on the organizational hierarchy. More senior employees consistently have a rosier view of the ethical environments of their organizations than do people lower in the hierarchy. This might be an example of senior personnel being blinded by their social roles, with the result being that they are unable to clearly see what is going on within the organization. This also might be an example of leaders being blinded by the formal narrative of their organizations.

Role Relationships

The relationships between and among roles are important. These relationships come with expectations and contribute to the functioning of any organization. But **role relationships** also help shape mental models, sometimes to the detriment of the organization.

Role relationships
The relationships people form because of their specific roles within an organization. They include expectations for each party's behavior. For instance, a nurse and physician will probably have a role-specific relationship.

Leaders are responsible for inspiring, communicating with, and motivating people—both their peers and their subordinates—to do what the leaders want them to do. This section focuses on the problems that might arise because of a specific relationship—the role relationships between those who hold positions of authority in an organization and those who do not. Some highly regarded research suggests that deference to authority might cause people to act in extreme, immoral, and unlawful ways, even going so far as to cause hurt to strangers.

Dr. Stanley Milgram, a Yale professor in the early 1960s, performed famous experiments on human obedience (Milgram 1974, 1963). His intent was to discover why people acquiesced in or aided in horrific acts during the Holocaust. He found with "numbing regularity" that good people acquiesced to the demands of authority, and consequently "performed actions that were callous and severe" (Milgram 1965, 74). His results have been consistently confirmed in other experiments (Blass 1999).

Explaining his findings, Milgram (1974) stated, "Each individual possesses a conscience, which to a greater or lesser degree serves to restrain the unimpeded flow

Case Study

A newly hired chief compliance officer at a university hospital came across what she thought was a simple billing glitch. The university's computer system inexplicably was configured to charge the maximum possible daily reimbursement rate for all Medicare patients regardless of the actual care provided—essentially overcharging the federal government millions of dollars. As she delved deeper into the problem, she became aware that the glitch had been in place for some time. She became suspicious that the computer error was deliberate.

The chief compliance officer raised the issue in a report to her superior. She was instructed to rewrite her report to make it appear there had been no finding of deliberate overbilling. The chief compliance officer did what she was told.

Why do you think the chief compliance officer did what she was told to do?

of impulses destructive to others. But when he merges his person into an organizational structure, a new creature replaces autonomous man, unhindered by the limitations of individual morality, free of humane inhibition, mindful only of the sanctions of authority."

So, as Werhane and Moriarty point out, it is important to remember that leaders "often fail to recognize that employee obedience usually has little to do with their [the leaders'] own brilliance, values, experience or ability to lead—it is primarily due to their position of recognized authority. The problem is not simply the phenomenon of obedience to authority; it is also an issue of leadership. Leaders can become so involved in their roles and accompanying expectations that their decisions reflect what they perceive to be their own role responsibilities. When this happens, leaders may fail to examine how their directives are being interpreted and implemented several layers down within the organization" (Werhane and Moriarty 2009, 9).

Values and Leaders

An inability to accurately see what is going on is not the only way a leader can be blinded. A leader who does not have well-thought-out positive values may not be able to recognize a morally problematic situation or decision. Therefore, leaders should continually cultivate and question their own set of values, which should align with the values of the healthcare organization.

Moral Imagination

This chapter prepares aspiring leaders in hospitals and other healthcare organizations to recognize and understand the moral complexities and consequences embedded in events, situations, or decisions. But having recognized and understood these complexities and consequences, the question becomes what to do about them.

Werhane's (1999) exploration of this question introduced the world of business ethics to the concept of moral imagination. The concept has been used to better understand the process of moral decision making (Roca 2010).

Building on the work of Johnson (1993, 1985) and Kekes (1991) among others, Werhane (1999) defines moral imagination as "the ability in particular circumstances to discover and evaluate possibilities not merely determined by that circumstance, or limited by its operative mental models, or merely framed by a set of rules or rule-governed concerns."

The process of moral imagination begins with an awareness of the specific event, situation, decision, or conflict. Therefore, leaders must be self-aware; they must be aware of their own mental models, narratives, social roles, role relationships, and values to reduce the possibility that they might be blinded into not seeing the full significance of the particular circumstance that confronts them.

The first stage of moral imagination is to be aware of the mental models, narratives, values, social roles, and role relationships embedded in the situation. This stage begins with an awareness of the possible moral conflicts or dilemmas that might arise in the situation, including the dilemmas created, at least in part, by the dominating narrative, mental model, social roles or role relationships, values, or the situation itself. To be aware of the narrative, mental models, values, and social roles and role relationships in a situation requires awareness of the other stakeholders and their perceptions of the dilemma.

Case Study

The CEO of a large academic medical organization was worried. Grants funded through the National Institutes of Health were drying up. Revenue associated with clinical activities was down, gifts to the organization were down, and the endowment had declined in value because of a downturn in the stock market. The CEO called a meeting of the chairs of all the clinical departments. He told them that their researchers should be bringing in more industry-sponsored grants and that those who had industry grants should be thinking of ways to expand or extend them. The CEO wanted the chairs to know that he had few funds to offer for bridge support for those researchers who were not bringing in their own salaries.

The chairs in turn put pressure on their researchers to find or enlarge industry grants. One clinical investigator, who had a large industry grant to conduct a Phase II clinical trial, had been thinking about pulling the plug because he had not been able to recruit enough subjects that met the eligibility criteria. After listening to his chair, he wondered if he should tell his research coordinator to make the eligibility criteria less rigorous.

The less-rigorous criteria might affect the outcomes of the trial in any number of ways. Do you think this was the intention of the CEO or the chairs?

In the second stage of moral imagination, to be fully aware of the situation and the possible moral conflicts that might arise, effective leaders must try to emotionally disengage from the situation. To do so, a leader must attempt to put aside her own mental model and narrative so that bias is not introduced as she attempts to fully understand the situation or dilemma. One can never completely disengage from either the situation or one's own mental model; both are context driven. Nevertheless, attempting to separate oneself from the situation and being aware of the limitations of one's own mental model allow a leader to begin to work toward a solution that may not have been evident when the process began (Werhane 1999).

These activities lead to the third stage of moral imagination: the development of more creative normative or value-driven perspectives that enable one to find or devise solutions or alternatives that may be novel, morally justifiable, and economically viable.

Case Study

A small community had experienced a large influx of Latino families. The local hospital began seeing an increasing number of Latino children coming to the hospital with severe automobile crash–related injuries. Many of these children had to be transported to a trauma center in a neighboring city to receive specialized care that the local hospital was unable to provide. Because most of these children were uninsured, both hospitals soon felt a negative impact on their operating margins.

The hospital CEO was aware that many board members were angry about the disproportionate amount of services now going to the Latino population. Moreover, she understood that the cause of their anger was that many of these cases could have been avoided if the children had been in child safety seats or wearing seatbelts, but use of safety seats and seatbelts among the Hispanic population was low.

The hospital CEO spoke to the trauma center CEO and together they developed a plan for both organizations to partner with churches in their communities to educate the Latino population about the necessity of children using safety seats and wearing seatbelts. Both CEOs felt that education would reduce these injuries and, consequently, improve their operating margins.

The CEO of the trauma center agreed to supply the staff and most of the resources needed for the outreach effort. He also agreed to outline the plan to the board of the smaller community hospital and ask the board for the remaining resources.

Do you think the plan shows moral imagination? Why or why not?

Why do you think the hospital CEO agreed to let the CEO of the trauma center speak to the local hospital board? Do you think that this decision might affect whether or not the remaining needed resources are allocated? Why?

Moral Reasoning

Moral imagination is not a substitute for moral reasoning. Both are necessary to get to the point of making a decision that is morally justifiable. Moral imagination and moral reasoning should operate in tandem to envision and critique possible solutions.

Moral reasoning can be practical or theoretical—it can be grounded in what is achievable in any given situation or event, or it can appeal to moral principles. The limitation of theoretical moral reasoning is that it starts with a set of general moral principles and then seeks to apply them to specific cases. Werhane (1999) points out, "The result is often a disconnect between theory and practice, a failure of application due to a failure to comprehend how moral theory relates to the relevant practice." Moreover, theoretical moral reasoning might lead to premature conclusions or decision making. Relying on a general principle can blind leaders from appreciating more nuanced aspects of the situation or event.

Practical moral reasoning is often presented as a framework for reasoning through a moral problem or event. For instance, physicians have offered practical moral frameworks as decision guides for managing a moral or ethical problem in the care of a patient. An example of such a guide is shown in Exhibit 14.1.

1. State the problem plainly
2. Gather and organize data
   a. Medical facts
   b. Medical goals
   c. Patient's goals and preferences
   d. Context
3. Ask: Does the problem raise ethical or moral issues?
4. Is more information or dialogue needed?
5. Determine the best course of action and support it with reference to one or more sources of moral or ethical value:

Ethical principles	Beneficence, nonmaleficence, respect for autonomy, justice
Rights	Protections for patients that are independent of the professional's obligations
Consequences	Estimation of the goodness or desirability of likely outcomes
Comparable cases	Reasoning by analogy from prior cases
Professional guidelines	Use various professional guidelines like the American Medical Association's "Code of Medical Ethics"
Conscientious practice	Preserve the personal and professional integrity of clinicians

6. Confirm the adequacy and coherence of the conclusion

EXHIBIT 14.1
A Clinician's Approach to Clinical Ethical/Moral Reasoning

Source: Kaldjian, Weir, and Duffy (2005).

Practical Moral Reasoning for Managing System Changes

Leaders manage hospitals and other healthcare organizations. These organizations are composed of processes, people, materials, and information. Leaders manage these systems to produce appropriate outcomes while simultaneously ensuring these systems reflect the desired culture of the institution. Moreover, leaders must ensure that these systems do not impede the proper functioning and the culture of other systems with which they intersect.

A decision that affects one part of a system—or subsystem—may have unintended consequences in another part of the system and even in other systems with which it intersects. Any system change may affect the culture of that specific system and may also have ramifications for the culture of the entire institution. Because leaders are responsible for the systems they oversee, thinking about the nature of systems, how systems work, and how to change systems—collectively comprising systems thinking— is an essential perspective in the process of moral decision making.

Theorists have stressed different aspects of systems as they model organizations, groups of organizations, and organizational processes (Berwick 1998; Deming 1982; Donabedian 1978; Kaplan and Norton 1996; Laszlo and Krippner 1998; Plsek 2001; Senge 1990; and Stacey 2003). This section draws from these models to present a framework that leaders can use as they work through an ethically problematic event or situation that requires a modification to a system while simultaneously ensuring that the ethical culture of the organization is maintained or enhanced.

Differing situations require identification of different information and the application of different guidelines. Future leaders should think about how to approach moral decision making through the lens of a system that includes humans—moral agents—that incorporates those elements of moral imagination and moral reasoning essential to an institutional ethical culture.

The important characteristics of a system that is designed and managed by humans are

1. purposes or goals,
2. values,
3. boundaries,
4. resources,
5. interactions,
6. ability to change, and
7. outcomes.

We briefly describe these characteristics and why they are important for a leader to consider in the process of moral decision making (Chen, Mills, and Werhane 2007). For each characteristic, we propose a set of questions that provide a practical moral reasoning in managing and changing systems.

Purposes or goals: A system may be micro, intermediate, or macro. It may be simple or complex. All systems are intended to fulfill one or more purposes or goals. The intended purposes or goals of a system help define its normative (standards and values) dimensions (Werhane 2002), allowing judgments about whether the intended purposes or goals are legitimate and whether the purposes or goals are being achieved by the system under consideration.

People form a system when they work together in such a way that the whole is greater than the sum of individual efforts. This only occurs, though, if they have a common goal and a vision of how the goal is to be achieved (Chen, Mills, and Werhane 2007; Plsek 2001; Senge 1990; Stacey 2003). That is, the people in the system must share the same mental model of the system for it to produce the desired outcomes. The goals of the system and the vision (mental models) of the people in the system support the desired culture of the system.

Leadership must be clear about the primary purpose or goal of a system because systems, as well as individuals, often have more than one purpose or goal; often these can conflict, producing confusion and affecting desired outcomes, thereby affecting the culture of the system. Moreover, as discussed in Chapter 2, actual goals can be different from stated goals. So leaders must differentiate the stated goals of the system from their actual goals, and they must know the relative priorities of the goals.

Questions a leader should ask about the purposes and goals of a system include:

- What are the stated goals of the system?
- Are the stated goals the desired goals?
- Are the stated goals different from the actual goals?
- How are the actual goals of the system prioritized relative to each other?
- Are they aligned with the desired goals of the organization?
- Do they follow the same priorities as those of the organization?

Values: Systems reflect values, which in turn reflect the culture of the system. And as discussed throughout this book, actions taken to achieve one value might compromise the achievement of another value (often referred to as a conflict among values), producing confusion in system participants and possibly harming the system's culture.

Leaders must be clear about what values the system is reflecting, what values the system should reflect, and whether or not these values are appropriate to the system's goals. Leaders must also be clear about their priorities when values conflict.

Questions leaders should ask about the values of a system include:

- What are the stated values of the system?
- Are the stated values the desired values?
- Are the stated values different from the actual values?
- Are the system's actual values aligned with the values of the organization?
- Do the system's values follow the same priority as those of the organization?
- Are these values shared among system members?

Boundaries: Knowing and defining a system's boundaries is important in identifying the system. This process is as not as straightforward as it may seem (Stacey 2003; Werhane 2002). A system may be relatively autonomous or "closed"—it functions independently of other systems, and its boundaries are easy to identify. But more probably, the system is "open"—it intersects with other systems, both horizontally and vertically. Because it affects and is affected by other systems, its boundaries can be difficult to discern. Nevertheless, clarifying boundaries, which often means clarifying role relationships, allows a leader to identify the relationships with other systems that are necessary for an understanding of how the systems work both independently and together. Once leaders have clarified the boundaries of a system, they can ask how systems interact with each other, whether or not the interaction is appropriate, and whether or not the interaction is important in achieving the system's goals and reflecting its values and culture.

Questions that a leader should ask about the boundaries of a system include:

- What are the role relationships in the system?
- Are these relationships helping the system achieve its goals and values?
- Where does the system intersect with other systems?
- What are the role relationships in the intersection?
- Are the goals and values of intersecting systems compatible with those of the system under review?
- Are the relative priorities of the goals and values of the intersecting systems compatible with the system under review?

Resources: The resources of a system include technology, infrastructure, and people with different skills and skill levels (Donabedian 1978). A system cannot achieve its purposes or goals if its resources are not appropriate or sufficient. For instance, clinics need certain equipment, technology, and the requisite number of people possessing certain skills. If any one of these is missing or inappropriate, the clinic will not achieve its purposes or goals. Leaders must be able to assess whether a system has appropriate or sufficient resources to ensure that it is able to fulfill its purposes or goals.

Questions the leader should ask once he determines that a system needs additional (or fewer or a different combination of) resources to achieve its purposes or goals include:

- Is the envisioned change appropriate to the mission and values of the organization?
- Will the change affect the culture of the system?

If the leader determines that the culture of the system will be affected by a change in resources, then he might consider reallocating other resources, such as education, to ensure the desired culture of the system is maintained or enhanced.

Interactions: Interactions between the resources of a system, particularly the interactions of the people in a system, can advance or detract from a system's goals, so interactions are important to consider when determining whether a system can fulfill its purposes or goals (Deming 1982; Kaplan and Norton 1997; Stacey 2003). Interactions that occur both within a system and between systems are, in part, a function of how these systems are designed.

The interactions of a given system range from rigid to entirely flexible. A system can be designed more rigidly if the same outcome is desired again and again and the same interactions are required to produce it. But in some instances achieving the purposes or goals of a system requires greater flexibility (Plsek 2001). A clinic may have multiple goals and multiple desirable outcomes. Moreover, goals cannot always be anticipated; for example, the goals of a patient may well be different than the initial goals of the patient's physician. To address these differences in patient-centered care, interactions between patients and physicians should be allowed to be flexible. A leader must know whether or not a system should be designed rigidly or be allowed flexibility. How a system is designed and how interactions take place are fundamental to whether a system is able to achieve its purposes or goals (Chen, Mills, and Werhane 2007).

Interactions also depend on a person's mental model, which, ideally, aligns with the system's culture. But a person's mental model may not align with the system's culture. For instance, the nurse whose mental model about the unit she works on is that her concerns about the unit will not be addressed will probably not mention them to her supervisor. An administrator who believes that a clinic could be more effective and efficient, but whose mental model of the clinic is that the doctor in charge will not listen, might decide not to mention her ideas.

Questions that a leader should ask about the interactions in or between systems include:

- Is the system designed appropriately for desired outcomes?
- Are the desired outcomes facilitated or inhibited by flexibility or by rigidity in the system design?
- Are role relationships appropriate for needed interactions?
- What is the desired culture of the system?
- What kind of culture is reflected in system participants' interactions?

Ability to change: All systems can and most likely do change over time, either for better or worse (Plsek 2001; Stacey 2003). One reason that systems involving humans change is that the mental models of system participants change over time. For instance, we have all had "a-ha" moments when we realize that something we are doing can be done in a more efficient or effective way. These "a-ha" moments often result from or result in a change in our mental models of the system in which we are working.

The beliefs and values that are incorporated in the mental models of the people working in and with a system can also change, thereby pushing the system toward change. For instance, if a person believes that the goal of a system is inappropriate or unattainable, the interactions of that person may reflect that belief and cause the system to change.

Identifying the multiple stakeholders in a system can be hard for a leader and knowing the mental models of those stakeholders can be harder still. Moreover, a leader cannot expect to know all the ethically troubling events, situations, or decisions that occur within a system. But she can ensure that a system has a mechanism through which stakeholder voices can be heard. This will allow her to determine if the system is changing in ways that align with the values of the organization.

Questions a leader should ask about a system's ability to change include:

- Is a mechanism in place that elicits as well as allows system stakeholders to voice their values and beliefs?
- Is this mechanism appropriately located in the system?
- Is the mechanism used?
- Does use of the mechanism result in recognition of stakeholder voices and feedback?

This mechanism will be ineffective unless system participants are able to trust the leaders responsible for the system.

Outcomes: The actual outcomes produced by a system may be difficult to predict, and in some cases even to identify, because they may be unintended or even produced in another connected system. This is especially true for systems designed to be more flexible (Plsek 2001). For example, the goal of managed care was to reduce costs and

Case Study

A large academic medical center and a community hospital are considering merging. Proponents argued that the merger would result in significant quality improvement as well as efficiencies that could then be passed on to payers and patients. But the CEO of the community hospital wondered how such different systems could function as one.

In spite of the difficulties involved in merging two different systems, what might persuade you to merge?

improve care, not create widespread uncertainty and suspicion. But once the outcomes that a system is producing are identified, they can be used to evaluate whether or not a system is fulfilling its purposes or goals. Moreover, by measuring outcomes against other system expectations, like goals, values, and resources, a leader can determine a system's efficiency and effectiveness.

Questions a leader should ask about the outcomes of a system include:

- What outcomes are being produced by the system?
- Do these outcomes align with the goal or purpose of the system?
- Do these outcomes align with the values of the system?

A leader in a healthcare organization can use this framework in conjunction with moral imagination to help identify how the event or dilemma might be affecting the system under consideration. Or a leader can use it to determine whether or not a system change will align with the goals and values of the institution. This framework can also be used as administrators consider combining systems.

Conclusion

This chapter provides students with tools they will need as future leaders of healthcare organizations that face moral and ethical uncertainties and concerns. It demonstrates how leaders can be blinded by their mental models—which are in part shaped by narratives, social roles, and role relationships—and how this blindness inhibits the use of moral imagination. This chapter also shows how moral imagination, coupled with moral reasoning, might enable a leader to envision novel ways of resolving morally problematic events or situations.

Even the most thoughtful leader cannot know everything that is going on in her organization. She cannot know every change that is occurring, how people are responding, or how they may be changing their mental models. Nevertheless, leaders must ensure that the systems they oversee function productively, that they change in alignment with their purposes and goals, and that individuals have recourse when confronted with an ethical or moral issue they are unsure how to handle.

Edgar Schein (2010), a prominent management theorist and consultant, asserts that the only thing of real importance that leaders do is create and manage culture. A properly managed organizational culture—in which leadership communicates and reflects values—and the values of the organization—which allow other voices to be heard and encourage everyone in the institution to recognize and understand the moral complexities and consequences embedded in their decisions—can provide support to individuals confronted with these issues. A properly managed organizational culture helps frame mental models, and it can give direction to systems as they change.

Points to Remember

- A mental model is a concept that refers to deeply held or ingrained assumptions or generalizations that influence how we perceive and understand the world.
- Moral imagination is the ability in particular circumstances to discover and evaluate possibilities not merely determined by that circumstance, limited by its operative mental models, or framed by a set of rules or rule-governed concerns.
- Narratives, social roles, and role relationships can be incorporated into a mental model and may blind a leader into misperceiving reality.
- Leaders have two fundamental ethical responsibilities: 1) to recognize and understand the moral complexities and consequences embedded in events, situations, or decisions, and 2) to nurture and maintain an organizational culture that ensures that others recognize and understand the moral complexities and consequences embedded in the situations they confront and the decisions they make. To fulfill these responsibilities, leaders must, among other things, listen to other voices.
- Practical moral reasoning is a framework or guide composed of a series of questions that can help an individual work through a morally problematic event or situation.
- Values and beliefs are incorporated into a person's mental model. As a person changes her values and beliefs, she can influence system change.

References

Berwick, D. 1998. "Crossing the Boundary: Changing Mental Models in the Service of Improvement." *International Journal for Quality in Health Care* 10 (5): 435–41.

Blass, T. 1999. "The Milgram Paradigm After 35 Years: Some Things We Now Know About Obedience to Authority." *Journal of Applied Social Psychology* 29 (5): 889–1109.

Chen, D. T., A. E. Mills, and P. H. Werhane. 2007. "Tools for Tomorrow's Healthcare System: A Systems-Informed Mental Model, Moral Imagination, and Physicians' Professionalism." *Academic Medicine* 83 (8): 723–32.

Curry, L. A., E. Spatz, E. Cherlin, J. W. Thompson, D. Berg, H. H. Ting, C. Decker, K. M. Krumholz, and E. H. Bradley. 2011. "What Distinguishes Top-Performing Hospitals in Acute Myocardial Infarction Mortality Rates?" *Annals of Internal Medicine* 154 (6): 384–90.

Deming, W. E. 1982. "Improvement of Quality and Productivity Through Action by Management." *National Productivity Review* 1 (1): 12–22.

Donabedian, A. 1978. "The Quality of Medical Care." *Science* 200 (26): 856–63.

Freeman, R. E. 1994. "The Politics of Stakeholder Theory: Some Future Directions." *Business Ethics Quarterly* 4: 409–22.

Johnson, M. 1993. *Moral Imagination.* Chicago: University of Chicago Press.

———. 1985. "Imagination in Moral Judgment." *Philosophy and Phenomenological Research* 46: 265–80.

Kaldjian, L. C., R. F. Weir, and T. P. Duffy. 2005. "A Clinician's Approach to Clinical Ethical Reasoning." *General Internal Medicine* 20 (3): 306–11.

Kaplan, R. S., and D. P. Norton. 1996. *The Balanced Scorecard: Translating Strategy into Action.* Boston: Harvard Business School Press.

Kekes, J. 1991. "Moral Imagination, Freedom, and the Humanities." *American Philosophical Quarterly* 28: 101–11.

Laszlo, A., and S. Krippner. 1998. "Systems Theories: Their Origins, Foundations and Development." In *Systems Theories and a Priori Aspects of Perception,* edited by J. S. Jordon. Amsterdam, the Netherlands: Elsevier.

Milgram, S. 1974. *Obedience to Authority: An Experimental View.* New York: Harper and Row.

———. 1965. "Some Conditions of Obedience and Disobedience to Authority." *Human Relations* 18 (1): 57–76.

———. 1963. "Behavioral Study of Obedience." *Journal of Abnormal and Social Psychology* 67 (4): 371–78.

Plsek, P. 2001. "Redesigning Health Care with Insights from the Science of Complex Adaptive Systems." In *Crossing the Quality Chasm: A New Health System for the 21st Century,* 309–23. Washington, DC: National Academies Press.

Roca, E. 2010. "The Exercise of Moral Imagination in Stigmatized Work Groups." *Journal of Business Ethics* 96 (1): 135–47.

Senge, P. 1990. *The Fifth Discipline: The Art and Practice of the Learning Organization.* New York: Doubleday.

Schein, E. 2010. *Organizational Culture and Leadership,* 4th ed. San Francisco: Jossey-Bass.

Stacey, R. D. 2003. *Strategic Management and Organizational Dynamics: The Challenge of Complexity.* New York: Prentice Hall.

Werhane, P. H. 2002. "Moral Imagination and Systems Thinking." *Journal of Business Ethics* 38 (1/2): 33–42.

———. 1999. *Moral Imagination and Management Decision Making.* New York: Oxford University Press.

Werhane, P. H., L. P. Hartman, D. Moberg, E. Englehardt, M. Pritchard, and B. Parmar. 2011. "Social Constructivism, Mental Models, and Problems of Obedience." *Journal of Business Ethics* 100 (1): 103–18.

Werhane, P. H., and B. Moriarty. 2009. "Moral Imagination and Management Decision Making." *Business Roundtable Institute for Corporate Ethics.* Accessed May 3, 2013. www.corporate-ethics.org/pdf/moral_imagination.pdf.

TOWARD A NEW PERSPECTIVE

Gary L. Filerman, Ann E. Mills, and Paul M. Schyve

Introduction

From the many perspectives on ethics that are reflected in the preceding chapters, one overarching theme emerges: the new perspective on managerial ethics in healthcare must be built on a commitment to integrity—personal and organizational.

This book is based on our assumption that you are planning a career in healthcare administration to make a positive difference to healthcare, to the organizations you serve, and to their stakeholders. The takeaway is that as a health professional, the most important positive contribution you can make is to protect and enhance the moral core of the healthcare organization. (In the Introduction, we noted that each healthcare organization will have a distinct moral core that depends on its mission and that each healthcare organization has a service mission: to alleviate pain and suffering and help restore the health of its patients. This service mission should be the foundation of the healthcare organization's moral core.) But you cannot make this contribution if your own integrity is weak or compromised. Nor can you make it if the integrity of the organization is weak or compromised. Thus, protecting the moral core of the healthcare organization requires a commitment to your personal integrity and a commitment to the integrity of the organization you serve.

We believe the integrity of healthcare organizations has deteriorated. In spite of carefully constructed mission and value statements, too many cases exist of healthcare organizations "pushing the envelope." As illustrated by the cases in this book, many of which are drawn from actual events, a healthcare organization's integrity has been compromised for short-term gain too many times. This compromise diminishes the trust of stakeholders, it diminishes organization morale, and it diminishes you.

As organizations grow in size and complexity it becomes easier for these slips in integrity to go undetected, and it becomes harder to identify exactly where ethical accountability and responsibility lie. But ultimately *you* are ethically accountable and responsible. You will help shape and guide the healthcare organization. You will prevent or accelerate the slips. This is why you need to incorporate into your thinking this new perspective on managerial ethics in healthcare.

The new perspective recognizes that every decision or activity has the potential to undermine or enhance the moral core of the healthcare organization. But for this perspective to have meaning, for it to be translated into action, depends upon your integrity and the integrity of the organization. Working with colleagues who share this perspective, you will turn the tide and re-earn the trust that the healthcare organization is committed to the values associated with its mission.

Your Moral Core

You have a moral core as well and, as exemplified by your professional code, the foundation of this moral core embodies the service mission of the healthcare organization: to alleviate pain and suffering and help restore the health of your patients.

In the same way that you must protect and enhance the moral core of your organization, you must protect and enhance your own moral core. This cannot be done without a commitment to integrity.

About Integrity

Many dimensions are associated with the concept of integrity. When people say that a person has integrity, that can mean that the person adheres faithfully to her values or moral core. Or it can mean the person is honest, or truthful, or courageous. Integrity can also mean whole or without a flaw. Integrity can mean complete. And in an organizational context, integrity can be and should be associated with leadership. We encourage you to think about the implications of all of these dimensions for the professional healthcare administrator.

Adhering Faithfully to Your Values and Moral Core

The concept of integrity is meaningless without a clear understanding of your moral and ethical values. This book discusses values that should be important to the mission of the healthcare organization and its stakeholders, including its professionals and employees. We hope that you are in a position now to identify, understand, reflect on, crystallize, and internalize the values you believe are important and upon which your role in a healthcare organization will be built. But do not take our word for what should be considered important values. *You* must identify your values and moral core. *You* must determine why you believe these values are important. *You* must figure out why and what gives these values special meaning in a healthcare context. Your values and moral core are distinctive competencies, to be continually developed, reflected on, and refined.

Adhering faithfully to your values and moral core requires that your values and moral core have been crystallized and internalized so that they underlie every decision or action you take. (Recall the discussions of mental models throughout this book.) This means recognizing and understanding that your values and moral core are not relative or situation-specific.

Do not mistake remaining faithful to your values and moral core as rigidity. Your values may change over time but your commitment to adhere to them should not. Remaining faithful to your values and moral core does not mean never compromising. You *will* compromise; sometimes, perhaps more often than you would like to think, compromise is the only way to get something done. But adherence to your values and moral core will provide you with a perspective on the sort of compromise you can make and still live comfortably with yourself.

If integrity requires that your values and moral core are crystallized and internalized, you will have a lens through which viewing all of the complex ethical and moral challenges that you will encounter in a healthcare organization's internal and external environment is possible. Integrity gives power to your values and moral core. It enables you to be consistent in applying them.

Honesty

You cannot have integrity without being honest with yourself, recognizing your biases, proclivities, self-interest, and the limits of your knowledge. You cannot have integrity without being honest in your personal and executive relationships. You cannot have integrity without truthfulness, letting people know where you are coming from and why the place you are coming from is important.

To be honest with yourself, you must ask yourself the hard questions. Do you compromise your values or moral core for personal goals, promotion, pay, status? How do you define your self-interest? What motives drive your self-interest? What kind of compromises are you prepared to make in the context of your self-interest? What kind of compromises are you *not* prepared to make? What are you seeking to bring to the organization you serve and your profession? What do you want to accomplish in addition to what the organization wants you to accomplish?

Courage

You cannot easily adhere to your values and moral core in all complex situations. You will surely be in situations where the values that should guide decision makers are blurred or confused—or appear as something other than they are—as appeals to the future are often used to justify short-term gain. Moreover, standing aside and avoiding uncomfortable situations or conflict is often easier and less risky. But doing so compromises your integrity and will generate moral distress in at least some stakeholders.

As discussed in Chapter 7, moral distress occurs when someone is prevented from doing what he believes is the right thing to do. Moral distress occurs because some kind of impediment exists to a professional making the right decision or performing the right activity. Recognizing moral distress and seeking to alleviate it takes courage.

When you ignore an ethical breach, one that does not concern you because doing the right thing is hard and maybe expensive or risky—even when you recognize the possible adverse consequences—you not only compromise your own integrity, you compromise the integrity of the organization.

You may be overruled in making decisions. However, most stakeholders will understand you are not criticizing if they recognize that your questions reflect your values or moral core. But your integrity will be compromised if you do not try to facilitate the right decision or activity.

Whole and Without Flaw

This dimension of integrity has implications for you as a professional. As a professional you seek to exemplify excellence. You seek to be whole and without a flaw.

Knowledge, competencies, and experience are all needed for excellence. Excellence requires the professional commitment both to continually be well informed and to contribute knowledge and wisdom to the field. Excellence also requires communication skills. This competency is essential for far more than presentations to the executive team and board. Effective communication skills are central to sharing and advocating for personal and organizational integrity.

Professional healthcare administrators share values with the other health professions and have a distinctive code that addresses the place of values in the healthcare organization's decision-making process. As a health professional, you join a community of practice that shares obligations and ethical frameworks—you do not stand apart from them or above them. This community is what distinguishes professionalism. In a healthcare context, general managers often do not recognize the ethical issues described in the foregoing chapters, do not know how to analyze them, and do not know how to resolve them—regardless of their personal integrity or recognition of their leadership responsibility for an ethical culture.

Complete

A balanced, healthy life is fundamental to you in your role as a professional. Completeness requires that you do not permit your work to consume all of your energies and attention to the point that you lose your perspective on what is important or forget why you are doing what you are doing.

Leadership

As you progress with your career, you will assume leadership roles. Integrity is associated with leadership. Integrity inspires confidence in an individual's motivation, judgment, and behavior. It allows colleagues to trust you and trust that the decisions you make are based on clearly articulated values.

We have discussed how important it is for leaders to listen to the various and diverse voices in the healthcare organization. Those voices will not be forthcoming nor will they be truthful if you are not trusted. And if this is the case, you will not be well placed to make the most informed decisions.

Integrity is not an academic exercise. You will carry your integrity into all kinds of situations and relationships, many of which will challenge your comfort zone. The strength of your integrity and the clarity of your values and moral core will allow you to acquire the new perspective on managerial ethics in healthcare. This perspective will enable you to effectively manage these challenges.

Integrity and Your Organization

Hospitals are arguably the most complex organizations in society, embodying the most complex interplay of potentially conflicting personal, professional, community, and philosophical values. This complexity generates tensions that are inherent in the enterprise. Be alert to them. These tensions have the potential to undermine the integrity of the organization.

Know Your Organization

Be alert to the integrity of the people around you and the integrity of the organization. Study your colleagues, your role models, and the leaders in the organization and the field to understand their integrity, what values they advocate and demonstrate, their consistency, and how it contributes to or detracts from the respect for their judgment, especially in ethically complex situations.

To be optimally successful, healthcare organizations must have integrity and fealty to values, explicit or implicit. The key to keeping them vital is consistency. Does the organization consistently make decisions in alignment with its mission and values? Or does the organization test or push ethical financial and legal boundaries? For executives to push the boundaries is easy, confusing their personal interests (e.g., professional and social status) with what is good for the organization or the community. Confusing measures of organizational success (e.g., size, prestige of board members, market share, and scope of services) with the interests of the community is also easy, especially when the C-suite participants do not bother to question the ethics of individual and organizational behaviors.

Conclusion

The chapters in this book repeatedly stress how important it is to manage your organization's culture. How you behave reflects your beliefs and values. How the organization behaves reflects its beliefs and values.

Your integrity is not formed in a vacuum. Integrity cannot be delegated to a committee or to the public relations department. It will be reflected in your daily decisions and activities and those of your peers. It is formed through a continual and dynamic process requiring observation, thought, reflection, and action. Likewise, the integrity of an organization is not formed in a vacuum. Ultimately, the foundation of the healthcare organization's integrity is the cumulative integrities of leaders in the organization. These leaders are the stewards of the organization's culture.

All of the conversations, cases, and vignettes in this book are designed to equip you to manage yourself, and your organization, to help you acquire a new perspective on managerial ethics in healthcare. You cannot do this without integrity.

We have high expectations for you and for your profession.

APPENDIX

Federal Sentencing Guidelines

History

In response to the perception that justice was unevenly applied in sentencing for criminal conduct, Congress passed the Sentencing Reform Act of 1984 (Title II of the Comprehensive Crime Control Act of 1984). This act created the United States Sentencing Commission (USSC), an independent agency in the judicial branch of government. One purpose of the USSC is to establish sentencing policies and practices for the federal criminal justice system that will ensure the ends of justice by promulgating detailed guidelines prescribing the appropriate sentences for offenders convicted of federal crimes. The result of the commission's work is the Federal Sentencing Guidelines (FSG) (USSC 2010).

In 1991, the FSG extended its reach from individuals to organizations found guilty of violating federal law. The overview for Chapter 8, "Sentencing of Organizations," states that an "organization" means "a person other than an individual"—corporations, partnerships, labor unions, pension funds, trusts, nonprofit entities, and government units (USSC 2010). Healthcare organizations, whether nonprofit or for-profit, incorporated or unincorporated, are included under this definition.

Chapter 8 has a twofold purpose: just punishment and deterrence. Its purpose in regard to just punishment is to distinguish different levels of criminal activity and specify the appropriate restitution and punishment associated with that activity.

In terms of deterrence, Chapter 8 acknowledges that, in spite of their best efforts, institutions are vulnerable to the actions of their agents. The chapter states that even though individual agents are responsible for their own criminal conduct, organizations are additionally vicariously liable for offenses committed by their agents and as such can be held culpable for the individual's actions.

The guideline seeks "to alleviate the harshest aspects of this institutional vulnerability by incorporating into the sentencing structure the preventive and deterrent aspects of a systemic compliance program" for the purposes of detecting and preventing criminal conduct, and promoting a culture that encourages ethical conduct and compliance with the law (USSC 2010).

Thus, Chapter 8 offers incentives for organizations to institute programs designed to detect and prevent wrongdoing. If the organization can demonstrate that it has an "effective compliance and ethics program," up to 95 percent of the fine range can be mitigated.

Until 2005, guidelines associated with just punishment were mandatory. The sentencing court had to elect a sentence from within the guideline range, and the court could not depart from a guideline-specified sentence unless a particular case presented atypical features, which had to be specified. Failure to follow the sentencing guidelines could result in an appeal by either the defendant or the government. However, the Supreme Court's decisions in *United States v. Blakely* (2004) and *United States v. Booker* (2005) converted the mandatory sentencing regime of the guidelines to an advisory one.

Even though the sentencing range in the guidelines is advisory, in regard to organizations, little has changed in sentencing practices thus far. Moreover, significant changes are not anticipated in the foreseeable future. That federal judges would ignore the organizational guidelines is doubtful because that would require them to substitute their own definition of "an effective compliance and ethics program" (Fiorelli and Tracey 2007).

Chapter 8, Part B, spells out the purposes and minimum requirements for an effective compliance and ethics program:

§8B2.1. Effective Compliance and Ethics Program

(a) To have an effective compliance and ethics program, for purposes of subsection (f) of §8C2.5 (Culpability Score) and subsection (c)(1) of §8D1.4 (Recommended Conditions of Probation - Organizations), an organization shall—

(1) exercise due diligence to prevent and detect criminal conduct; and

(2) otherwise promote an organizational culture that encourages ethical conduct and a commitment to compliance with the law.

Such compliance and ethics program shall be reasonably designed, implemented, and enforced so that the program is generally effective in preventing and detecting criminal conduct. The failure to prevent or detect the instant offense does not necessarily mean that the program is not generally effective in preventing and detecting criminal conduct.

(b) Due diligence and the promotion of an organizational culture that encourages ethical conduct and a commitment to compliance with the law within the meaning of subsection (a) minimally require the following:

(1) The organization shall establish standards and procedures to prevent and detect criminal conduct.

(2)(A) The organization's governing authority shall be knowledgeable about the content and operation of the compliance and ethics program and shall exercise reasonable oversight with respect to the implementation and effectiveness of the compliance and ethics program.

(B) High-level personnel of the organization shall ensure that the organization has an effective compliance and ethics program, as described in this guideline. Specific individual(s) within high-level personnel shall be assigned overall responsibility for the compliance and ethics program.

(C) Specific individual(s) within the organization shall be delegated day-to-day operational responsibility for the compliance and ethics program. Individual(s) with operational responsibility shall report periodically to high-level personnel and, as appropriate, to the governing authority, or an appropriate subgroup of the governing authority, on the effectiveness of the compliance and ethics program. To carry out such operational responsibility, such individual(s) shall be given adequate resources, appropriate authority, and direct access to the governing authority or an appropriate subgroup of the governing authority.

(3) The organization shall use reasonable efforts not to include within the substantial authority personnel of the organization any individual whom the organization knew, or should have known through the exercise of due diligence, has engaged in illegal activities or other conduct inconsistent with an effective compliance and ethics program.

(4)(A) The organization shall take reasonable steps to communicate periodically and in a practical manner its standards and procedures, and other aspects of the compliance and ethics program, to the individuals referred to in subparagraph (B) by conducting effective training programs and otherwise disseminating information appropriate to such individuals' respective roles and responsibilities.

(B) The individuals referred to in subparagraph (A) are the members of the governing authority, high-level personnel, substantial authority personnel, the organization's employees, and, as appropriate, the organization's agents.

(5) The organization shall take reasonable steps—

(A) to ensure that the organization's compliance and ethics program is followed, including monitoring and auditing to detect criminal conduct;

(B) to evaluate periodically the effectiveness of the organization's compliance and ethics program; and

(C) to have and publicize a system, which may include mechanisms that allow for anonymity or confidentiality, whereby the organization's employees and agents may report or seek guidance regarding potential or actual criminal conduct without fear of retaliation.

(6) The organization's compliance and ethics program shall be promoted and enforced consistently throughout the organization through (A) appropriate incentives to perform in accordance with the compliance and ethics program; and (B) appropriate disciplinary measures for engaging in criminal conduct and for failing to take reasonable steps to prevent or detect criminal conduct.

(7) After criminal conduct has been detected, the organization shall take reasonable steps to respond appropriately to the criminal conduct and to prevent further similar criminal conduct, including making any necessary modifications to the organization's compliance and ethics program.

(c) In implementing subsection (b), the organization shall periodically assess the risk of criminal conduct and shall take appropriate steps to design, implement, or modify each requirement set forth in subsection (b) to reduce the risk of criminal conduct identified through this process.

References

Fiorelli, P., and A. M. Tracey. 2007. "Why Comply? Organizational Guidelines Offer a Safer Harbor in the Storm." *Journal of Corporation Law* 32 (3): 467–90.

United States Sentencing Commission (USSC). 2010. *Federal Sentencing Guidelines Manual.* Accessed April 24, 2013. www.ussc.gov/Guidelines/2010_guidelines/ToC_HTML.cfm.

GLOSSARY

Accountable care organization. An integrated healthcare delivery system that combines a multidisciplinary set of medical practitioners and hospitals and is accountable for the overall care of patients.

American Association of Critical Care Nurses. A professional association focused on providing its members the knowledge, skills, and abilities they need to provide optimal care to critically ill patients.

American Society for Bioethics and Humanities. The leading national organization for professionals in bioethics.

Applied business ethics. The study of an organization's behavior through the lens of ethical or moral principles and values.

Applied ethics. The philosophical evaluation of controversial moral issues or practices.

Automatic cognitive process. Implicit assumptions and generalizations that represent our understanding of the world and are used in our day-to-day behavior and decision making, including moral decision making.

Blinded leader. A leader who is not able to recognize a morally problematic situation or decision.

Burnout. Emotional or physical exhaustion caused by prolonged stress or frustration.

Clinical ethics. Focuses on ethical issues associated with delivery of patient care.

Clinical ethics consult. A model in which the clinical ethics mechanism is provided by an individual or a small group of experts as a consulting service.

Clinical ethics mechanism. An individual or group that grapples with ethical issues confronted by the care of particular patients, with a view toward resolving specific care issues. Sometimes called a clinical ethics service or committee.

Code of Hammurabi. The first recorded set of laws in human history (circa 1772 BCE). These laws included acceptable standards for the practice of medicine.

Community benefit. A wide array of activities nonprofit hospitals are required to provide and account for—and for-profit hospitals may provide—to benefit their community, such as delivering free and discounted services to persons in need, conducting community needs assessments, collaborating with other organizations to improve community health and well-being, providing health promotion programs and information, and engaging in community building activities.

Community Charter of Fundamental Social Rights of Workers. A charter adopted in 1989 by the Commission of the European Community that establishes the major principles on which the European labor law model is based.

Compassion fatigue. The inability to continue to provide help and care in crisis situations because of repeated exposure to these situations.

Complex adaptive system. A system composed of many interconnected parts (e.g., people), each with the freedom to act in ways that are not fully predictable but will affect other parts in the system, resulting in those parts also changing—often in unpredictable ways. As the parts change, the system's functions and outputs adapt, often unpredictably.

Compliance programs. Guidelines designed to promote a culture that pays attention to ethics and encourages compliance with the law. Required by the Federal Sentencing Guidelines and the Office of Inspector General.

Conscientious objection. Refusal to perform a specific legal role, responsibility, or other activity because of moral or other personal beliefs.

Contextual cue. A message, hint, or signal that can be found in a discernible element of the environment. In an organization, contextual cues often reveal the truth about what is really going on or what is really believed by the organization.

Core values. Essential values of an organization; sometimes referred to as "guiding principles."

Corporate, institutional, or individual integrity agreement (CIA). An agreement between the Office of Inspector General and a healthcare provider that has submitted false claims to Medicare that allows the provider to participate in Medicare programs if it adopts and can demonstrate specific improvement measures in its compliance program.

Covenantal workplace. A working environment in which relationships are based on mutual trust, engagement, and care; contrasted with a *transactional* workplace, in which employee skills are applied in order to advance organizational objectives and obtain a return benefit.

Crescendo Effect. A model describing the interaction over time between increasing moral distress in repeated situations and increasing moral residue that lingers in the aftermath of recurring moral distress.

Crisis standards of care. A substantial change in usual operations and the level of care a healthcare organization is able to deliver because of a pervasive (e.g., pandemic influenza) or catastrophic (e.g., earthquake, hurricane) disaster.

Crossing the Quality Chasm: A New Health System for the 21st Century. A 2001 report from the Institute of Medicine detailing quality gaps in healthcare and proposing solutions for improvement.

Culture of safety. A component of the organizational culture that focuses on ensuring safety for patients and their families, staff, and practitioners. It includes a just culture that recognizes the inevitability of human error and yet holds individuals accountable for irresponsible actions. Required by The Joint Commission in healthcare organizations.

Descriptive business ethics. Analyzes the moral development of managers; describes and compares organizations, organizational cultures, the integration of ethics into administrative decision making, the role of codes and other authorities, and the effect of government regulations on organizational activities. Investigates causal relationships between individual moral beliefs and organizational mission statements.

Diagnosis-related group. A payment method under which hospitals received a standardized fixed rate per admission based on a patient's diagnosis.

Directors. Members of a healthcare organization's or system's governing board, which is ultimately responsible for the oversight and direction of the organization or system.

Duty of care. Requirement that directors use independent judgment in the exercise of their responsibilities on behalf of the organization and that they be reasonably well informed.

Duty of loyalty. Requirement that directors exercise their responsibilities in the best interest of the organization, not in their own interest or the interest of other persons or entities.

Emergency Medical Treatment and Active Labor Act (EMTALA). A 1986 law requiring hospital emergency departments to treat all individuals who show up at their facilities regardless of their ability to pay.

Ethical climate. Shared perceptions of how ethical issues should be addressed and what is ethically correct behavior for the organization.

Ethical standards. A belief about how we should behave.

Ethically acceptable minimum wage. A "living wage" that allows a full-time employee to be able to meet the basic needs of himself and a small family. Not the same as the legal minimum wage.

Ethics. The study and analysis of morality.

Facilitation model. The goal of the consultation is to help those involved articulate the ethical issues in conflict and explore how best to resolve those issues.

Florence Nightingale Pledge. The pledge often made by graduating nurses that emphasizes the duty of the nurse to obey the physician as part of the nurse's duty to care for the patient. It calls for responsible obedience, with the needs of the patient being the primary consideration.

Freeman, R. Edward. Philosopher and professor of business administration who first conceptualized the firm as a vehicle whose purpose is to coordinate stakeholder interests.

Health Insurance Portability and Accountability Act (HIPAA). Legislation that provides for the portability of health insurance coverage when workers change or lose their jobs, implements programs to reduce healthcare fraud and abuse, establishes standards for the use and security of health information in electronic health records, and requires the protection and confidential handling of protected health information.

Health policy. Policy that is tailored broadly to either promote or protect the population's health.

Healthcare policy. Policy that addresses access to healthcare services, the scope and quality of healthcare delivery, and healthcare costs.

Healthcare sustainability. Defined by "triple bottom line" practices that minimize environmental impact, fiscal waste, and negative effects on the community. Addressing sustainability issues is ethically consistent with providing safe, quality care.

Hippocratic Oath. Written by Hippocrates and his followers in the fifth century BCE; defined the ethical standard for practicing physicians and spelled out a number of virtues necessary for one to enter the profession. It emphasized the principles of nonmaleficence (do no harm) and beneficence (obligation to help the patient to the extent possible) as defining the duty of physicians toward the individual patient.

Holder Memo. A set of guidelines issued by the US Department of Justice in 1999 to federal prosecutors that they were instructed to consider before filing charges against an organization.

Independent Payment Advisory Board. A 15-member panel established by the ACA that makes recommendations to Congress for reducing per capita growth in the Medicare program and slowing the growth in national health expenditures when spending exceeds a target growth rate.

Informed consent. The right of individuals to decide whether (1) to accept recommended healthcare services, and (2) to receive the information needed to make the decision.

IntegratedEthics Initiative. A comprehensive, systemwide ethics program based on quality improvement principles and strategies for organizational change; developed by the US Department of Veterans Affairs. The initiative has three components: ethics consultation, preventive ethics, and ethical leadership.

Joint Commission, The. An independent, not-for-profit organization that accredits and certifies more than 20,000 healthcare organizations and programs in the United States.

Mediation model. Aims for an answer that comes out of discussion between the involved parties, acknowledges various points of view and concerns, and is acceptable to the parties involved, even if it might not be the first-choice outcome.

Medical ethics. The study and analysis of moral issues (issues of right and wrong) as applied to the fields of medical treatment and research.

Medical liability. Occurs when a patient is harmed by a breach of the standard of care established by a professional group or regulatory standards. Also called *medical malpractice.*

Mental model. A deeply held set of generalizations or beliefs about reality that influence how individuals understand the world.

Microsystem. The team that works together to provide care to the patient.

Mission statement. A public document describing an entity's reason for existence, its purpose, and its specific activities.

Moral climate. Shared perceptions of how ethical issues should be addressed and what is ethically correct behavior for the organization.

Moral conflict. A disagreement or uncertainty about what actions to take when values conflict with each other.

Moral core. The underlying explicit and implicit set of values that the organization or person holds, which drive the organization's or person's attitudes and behavior. Each healthcare organization and healthcare administrator will have a unique moral core, but common to all should be the mission to alleviate pain and suffering and to help restore the health of patients.

Moral distress. Occurs when individuals perceive that they are constrained from taking an ethically appropriate action. As a result, they experience compromised moral agency.

Moral imagination. The ability in a particular circumstance to consider and evaluate possibilities not determined by that circumstance, or limited by its operative mental models, or framed by a set of rules or rule-governed concerns.

Moral minimums. The idea that although people cannot always agree about what is "good," they have almost universal agreement about what is "bad."

Moral residue. Feelings that linger after a morally distressing situation that caused an individual to be seriously compromised.

Morale. The state of an individual's or a group's feelings and willingness to accomplish assigned tasks.

Morality. Focuses on the "good" or "right" answer to a problem or dilemma arising from a conflict involving fundamental human values.

Narratives. Stories that individuals and organizations use to communicate their identity and values that help to frame their mental models.

Normative applied business ethics. Evaluates business practices and decision making in light of standards and codes, develops rules and codes appropriate to the context of management and administration, and offers a framework of moral reasoning to evaluate and solve ethical dilemmas. Seeks to develop and use sets of normative rules of conducts, codes, standards, or principles that govern what one ought to do when well-being, rights, or integrity are at stake.

Normative judgments. Evaluations in moral terms.

Nursing ethics. A subset of applied ethics concerned with the activities and decisions made in the field of nursing.

Organization ethics processes. Processes designed to help leadership, staff, and professionals think through ethical uncertainty or conflicts that can occur when missions and values conflict. They are distinct from clinical ethics processes. Required by The Joint Commission.

Organizational culture. The customary or traditional ways of thinking and doing things, which are shared to a greater or lesser extent by all members of the organization and which new members of the organization must learn and at least partially accept to be accepted into the service of the firm.

Organizational ethics. Focuses on the structure and conduct of the organization that makes the delivery of patient care possible.

Pandemic and All-Hazards Preparedness Act of 2006 (PAHPA). A law designed to improve the nation's public health and medical preparedness and response capabilities for emergencies, whether deliberate, accidental, or natural.

Patient Protection and Affordable Care Act. A national healthcare reform law designed to expand affordable health coverage for Americans who were uninsured or underinsured, slow the growth of health spending, and improve the healthcare delivery system to ensure more efficient, higher-quality healthcare.

Pay for performance. A payment system in which payments are tied to a hospital's performance on a number of quality, efficiency, and patient satisfaction measures.

Percival's *Code of Medical Ethics.* Published in 1803 by Thomas Percival. The code emphasized the Hippocratic tradition and professional etiquette and was written for physicians practicing in hospitals or other medical institutions, thus adding institutional considerations to the patient focus.

Practical moral reasoning. A framework or guide composed of a series of questions that can help an individual work through a morally problematic event or situation.

Professional ethics. Ethics as applied to questions concerning a particular profession.

Professionalism. Behavior characterized by traits that include a high degree of generalized and systematic knowledge; placing community interests over self-interest; self-control through codes of ethics and voluntary associations organized and operated by specialists in the same field; and a system of rewards that is primarily a set of symbols of work achievement rather than ends in themselves.

Prospective payment system. A payment method that reimburses hospitals on the basis of diagnosis-related groups.

Psychological distress. The physical and emotional symptoms that arise in stressful or emotional circumstances.

Public good. Goods made available to everyone (regardless of how they are delivered or financed) so that they benefit individual recipients and, in the aggregate, benefit society as a whole.

Public policy. The tools—including statutes, regulations, guidelines, recommendations, executive orders, and court decisions—that federal, state, and local governments use to achieve a particular goal.

Quality improvement. An approach to managing quality that continuously improves the quality and performance of an organization's internal processes as well as its outputs.

Right answer model. The idea that a good clinical ethics consultation outcome would be the identification and implementation of the right answer.

Role relationships. The relationships people form because of their specific roles within an organization. They include expectations for each party's behavior. For instance, a nurse and physician will probably have a role-specific relationship.

Sarbanes-Oxley Act of 2002. A federal law requiring organizations to place a greater emphasis on corporate responsibility, regulatory compliance, and ethics at all levels of management and governance.

Separation thesis. The idea that business decisions and moral or ethical decisions are distinct.

Social roles. A person's responsibilities, functions, and relationships that in turn define the organization and the layers of an organization.

Stakeholder. Any individual or group, including the community, that is affected by the activities of an organization.

Stakeholder theory. The theory that the goal of any organization and its management is, or should be, the flourishing of the organization and all of the individuals or groups that affect or are affected by the organization.

Stewardship. An understanding that all of the resources of the organization, including financial resources and real property, are held in trust by the organization for the good of others.

Systems thinking. Describes thinking about the system as a whole as distinct from thinking about the parts of a system.

Trustees. Directors who are responsible for protecting and advancing a specific community resource (such as a not-for-profit hospital) in the interest of others.

Tuskegee Experiment. A US Public Health Service clinical study (1932–1972) that tracked the progression of untreated syphilis in black men even after effective treatments had been developed.

United Nations Declaration of Human Rights. Adopted in 1948 by the United Nations General Assembly to articulate the human rights and fundamental freedoms that are applicable to every person, everywhere. The document is meant to serve as a bulwark against oppression and discrimination.

Utilitarianism. The principle of achieving the greatest good for the greatest number.

Values statement. A public statement describing the values endorsed by the entity. Because these statements are public, they allow judgments about the entity. They can also legitimize the entity if societal expectations are reflected.

Willowbrook Hepatitis Study. A clinical study in which a hepatitis B vaccine was tested without proper consent in children housed in an institution for the mentally disabled.

INDEX

Abortion, 99, 100
ACA. *See* Patient Protection and
    Affordable Care Act
Academic medical centers
    relationship with ethics centers, 14
    values conflicts in, 33, 34
Access, to healthcare
    American Medical Association's
      support for, 102
    effect of health insurance coverage
      on, 244
    effect of hospital ownership status
      on, 43–45
    as healthcare policy focus, 225–26
    relationship to healthcare costs, 226
Accountability
    board of directors' promotion of,
      69, 70
    of crisis standards of care, 235
    of healthcare executives, 199–200
    of healthcare professionals, 90–91
    for patient safety, 36, 38
    in stakeholder relationships, 84–91
Accountable care organizations
    (ACOs), 253, 297
Accreditation
    of healthcare professionals, 90
    of hospitals, 25–26, 207, 208
    by Joint Commission, 25–26
Accrediting agencies, influence on
    healthcare organizations, 14
Acculturation, of physicians, 161–62
ACHE. *See* American College of
    Healthcare Executives
Acquired immunodeficiency virus syn-
    drome (AIDS), 42
Act-deontologists, 7

Act-utilitarians, 7
Administrators. *See also* Chief execu-
    tive officers (CEOs); Healthcare
    executives; Managers
    conflict with medical staff, 113
    internal and external challenges to,
      9–10
    role and responsibilities of, 2–3
Advertising, of healthcare, 63–64
Advocacy
    as community benefit, 54
    of healthcare providers, 104,
      114–15
    as leadership role, 149
    moral, 98
Advocacy organizations, 227
Affordable Care Act. *See* Patient Pro-
    tection and Affordable Care Act
African Americans, health status of, 42
Agency for Healthcare Research and
    Quality (AHRQ), 42
American Academy of Pediatrics, 234
American Association of Critical Care
    Nurses, 149
American College of Emergency Phy-
    sicians, 227
American College of Healthcare
    Executives
    Codes of Ethics of, 98, 106–10,
      115
    definition of, 106
    ethical leadership statement of, 58
    ethical policy statements of, 151
    as Healthcare Leadership Alliance
      member, xxv
    professional ethics requirement of,
      166

American College of Healthcare Exec-
    utives Competencies Assessment
    Tool domains, xxiv–xxv
  business skills and knowledge, 1,
    19, 51, 79–80, 95, 121, 177,
    205, 223, 265
  communication and relationship
    management, 1, 19, 79, 177,
    223, 265
  knowledge of the healthcare envi-
    ronment, 1, 19, 177, 205, 223
  leadership, 1, 19, 51, 79, 95, 121,
    177, 205, 265
  professionalism, 79, 121, 223, 265
American College of Physicians, xxv
American Health Lawyers Association,
    212
American Hospital Association, 197,
    227, 255
American Medical Association
  advocacy role of, 227
  Council on Ethical and Judicial
    Affairs (CEJA) of, 111
  "ethical climate" surveys by, 12
  Institute for Ethics of, 11
  Principles of Medical Ethics, 98,
    101–103, 111, 165
  recommendations regarding
    healthcare disparities, 42–43
American Nurses Association
  Code of Ethics for Nurses of,
    104–105
  Online Journal of Nursing of, 106
American Organization of Nurse
    Executives, xxv
American Osteopathic Association, 207
American Society for Bioethics and
    Humanities, 132
Antidiscrimination movement, 184
Applied business ethics, 81
  normative, 81–82, 301
Applied ethics, 8, 297
Aretaic theories, of ethics, 6
Aristotle, 6
Ascension Health Care Network, 45

Assumptions, mental models–based,
    269
Audit and compliance committees,
    65, 71
Authority, obedience to, 273–274
Automatic cognitive process, 216–
    218, 297
Autonomy, of patients, 125, 129

"Baby Doe" regulations, 127
Bankruptcy, of hospitals, 44
Behavior. *See also* Unethical behavior
  cultural factors in, 38
  ethical, examples of, 70
  illegal, 5
  moral, effect of mental models on,
    216–18
Behavioral ethics, definition of,
    214
Beliefs, as mental model component,
    283, 284
Beneficence, 99, 111, 114, 300
Bioethical principlism, 7
Bioethicists, 131
Bioethics, 125
Blinded leaders, 266–67, 268–74
  definition of, 266, 297
  effect of mental models on,
    266–74
Board committees
  audit and compliance committees,
    65, 71
  governance committees, 71
  quality committees, 64–65, 71
Board of directors, 72
  case studies of, 59, 62, 64, 73
  commitment to organizational
    mission, 60, 62, 63, 75
  decision-making process of, 72
  diversity and inclusiveness of, 61,
    75
  duties of, 56–58, 71–72
  effectiveness of, 71–72
  effect of Affordable Care Act on,
    256

executive sessions of, 72
expertise and skills of, 60–61, 75
independence of, 61–62, 75
interactions with managers, 56, 57–58, 74–75
meetings of, 70
membership of, 58–59, 75
mission focus of, 62
as models of ethical behavior, 58
orientation of new members, 71
personal commitment by, 59, 75
recruitment of, 59
roles and responsibilities of, 46–47, 54–58, 62–70, 75
selection of, 59, 75
self-evaluation of, 71, 73, 75
strategic planning involvement, 63–64
time commitments from, 60–61
workplace justice responsibility of, 66–68
Bon Secours Richmond Health Center
growth value of, 34, 44
mission statement of, 22–23, 24
organizational culture of, 35
statement of patients' rights and responsibilities, 29–30, 32
values statement of, 24–25
Bonuses, 70
Bottom line
ethical, 198
triple, 196, 199, 300
Budgets, 68–69
Bundled payment system, 245, 251
Burnout, 140, 145, 297
Business
separation from morality, 266–67, 269–70
social responsibility of, 84
Business ethics, 8, 79–94
applied, 81
case studies of, 87, 91, 92
descriptive, 81, 82, 299

of employee-employer relationships, 184
normative applied, 81–82, 301
relationship with healthcare ethics, 86–91
stakeholder theory and, 82–86
Bylaws, 56, 62

Cancer treatment centers, carcinogen-free, 202
Capital expenditures, budgeting for, 68
Capitation, 245, 246, 259–60
Care, duty of, 57, 58, 66, 75, 299
Care environment, definition of, 202
Caring, as organizational ethic, 60
Catholic healthcare organizations. *See also names of specific healthcare organizations*
mission statements of, 22–23
response to labor unions, 190–91
social justice teaching of, 190–91
treatment guidelines of, 32
Census Bureau, 186
Center for Medicare and Medicaid Innovation, 253
Center for Regulatory Effectiveness, 45
Centers for Disease Control and Prevention (CDC), 253
Centers for Medicare & Medicaid Services (CMS)
hospital payment mechanisms of, 250
role of, 208
Certification
of hospitals, 207
of physicians, 165–66
Change, mental models of, 268
Change management
moral reasoning use in, 277–83
for quality improvement, 169, 172
Charitable mission, 57. *See also* Community benefit
Charity Hospital, New Orleans, 238

Chief executive officers (CEOs)
  compensation for, 187–89
  performance evaluation of, 66–67,
    68
  responsibilities of, 46–47
Children, obesity in, 247
Chronic illness
  in African Americans, 42
  healthcare costs of, 247
  treatment for, 52–53
  in uninsured populations, 226
Cignet Health, 230–31
Clinical ethicists, 125
  expertise of, 131–32
  volunteers as, 213
Clinical ethics
  definition of, 122, 124–25, 136,
    297
  history of, 124–25
  relationship with organizational
    ethics, 121–24, 136
Clinical ethics committees. *See* Clinical
  ethics mechanisms
Clinical ethics consultations, 126–27,
  128, 136, 149
  definition of, 126, 297
  ethicists' expertise in, 131–32
  facilitation model of, 130, 132, 299
  as IntegratedEthics Initiative com-
    ponent, 150–51, 300
  mediation model of, 130–31, 300
  right answer model of, 130, 302
Clinical ethics mechanisms, 126, 132
  case study of, 134–35
  clinical ethics policies component
    of, 127–28
  definition of, 122, 297
  educational component of, 128,
    136
  emergence of, 125–28
  financial support for, 133
  institutional support for, 134–35
  organizational support for, 132–33
  policy formulation component of,
    136
  quality improvement of, 129–32

relationship with senior administration, 123–24, 128–36
Clinical ethics services. *See* Clinical
  ethics mechanisms
CMS. *See* Centers for Medicare and
  Medicaid Services (CMS)
Code of Hammurabi, 98
Code of Medical Ethics (Percival), 100,
  101, 302
Codes of ethics
  case study of, 111–12
  changes to, 110–18
  development of, 98–110
  of healthcare executives, 98, 106–
    10, 115, 165–66
  of non-healthcare professionals,
    105–106
  societal influences on, 110–13
Collective bargaining, 189–91
Collectives, 9, 12
Communication skills, of healthcare
  leaders, 12, 290, 291
Communitarian ethics, 7–8
Community
  as healthcare focus, 53
  moral commitment to, 199
  of practice, 290
  responsibility to, 44, 109
Community benefit, 65–66
  components of, 65–66
  definition of, 54, 297–98
  as hospital boards' focus, 62, 64
  plans for, 75
Community Charter of Fundamental
  Social Rights of Workers, 186,
  303
Community health centers, 42
Community members, as hospital
  board members, 54–55, 61
Compassion, 22–23, 24, 164
Compassion fatigue, 140, 298
Compensation
  for executives, 67–68, 187–89,
    193
  just, 70, 186–89
Competition, free and open, 84

Complex adaptive systems, 170, 298

Complexity
of healthcare organizations and systems, 12, 13, 38, 39, 238, 291
moral, 266–68

Compliance programs, 14
definition of, 207, 298
Federal Sentencing guidelines for, 210, 212, 293–96
legal focus of, 212
Office of Inspector General's guidelines for, 208–11, 212, 214, 215
orientation of, 215, 218, 219

Confidentiality
as defined in codes of ethics, 99, 101
of organizational information, 57
of patient information, 230–31, 299

Conflict management process, 39–41

Conflicts, ethical and moral. *See also* Values conflicts
definition of, 162
in quality improvement, 168–69, 173
resolution of, 39–41, 170–72, 174

Conflicts of interest, 105
disclosure of, 57

Congressional Budget Office (CBO), 250, 253, 254

Conscientious objection, 5, 145, 298

Consequentialist theories, 7

Consolidation, within healthcare system, 114, 116–17
case study of, 44

Consultants, 67–68, 190

Consultation services, in clinical ethics. *See* Clinical ethics consultations

Contextual cues, 217–18, 298

Continuous quality improvement. *See* Quality improvement (QI)

Contract theory, contemporary versions of, 7–8

Contractual agreements, with healthcare organizations, 91

Controversial issues, in healthcare
disparities in healthcare, 41–43, 47, 224
role of for-profit hospitals, 43–46

Core values, definition of, 23, 298

Corporate, institutional, or individual agreements (CIA), 211, 298

Cost containment
under Affordable Care Act, 255
as barrier to organizational culture, 38
as ethical dilemma cause, 43–46
in response to economic recessions, 254–55

Cost-shifting, 248–49

Covenantal ethics, 58

Covenantal workplace, 69–70, 298

Credentialing, of physicians, 65

Crescendo Effect, 142–43, 147, 151, 298

Crisis standards of care, 232–38, 298

Crossing the Quality Chasm: A New Health System for the 21st Century (Institute of Medicine), 36, 162, 165, 166, 170, 226, 298

Cultural factors
in behavior, 38
as health determinants, 201
implication for clinical ethics, 125

Culture
ethical. *See* Ethical culture
organizational. *See* Organizational culture
of quality improvement, 167–68
of systems, 166

Culture of safety, 36–38
characteristics of, 37–38
definition of, 36, 298
regulatory requirements for, 213–14, 218

Customers
as quality improvement focus, 161
as stakeholders, 82–83

Data, use in quality improvement, 150–51

Data Quality Act (DQA), 45

Decision making, ethical, 40–41
based on principles, 276
versus business decision making, 266–67, 269–70
guidelines for, 115–16
mental models-based, 269

Demographic shifts, 247

Deontological theories, of ethics, 7

Descriptive business ethics, 81, 82, 299

Diagnosis-related groups (DRGs), 245, 251, 299

Directors. *See also* Board of directors
comparison with trustees, 55
definition of, 52, 55, 74
responsibilities of, 55

Disaster preparedness and response
case study of, 233
crisis standards of care for, 234–238
Pandemic and All-Hazards Preparedness Act (PAHPA), 231–34, 302

Discharge-planning procedures, 251

Disclosure
of health information, 230–31
of medical errors, 258

Disparity, in healthcare, 41–43, 47, 224

Disproportionate Share Hospital (DSH) legislation, 227, 256–57

Diversity
of board of directors' membership, 61, 75
of hospitals' patients and employees, 38, 39, 125, 256
implication for clinical ethics, 125
respect for, 256

Donated funds, 69

"Do no harm" principle, 90, 170, 181, 199–200, 300

Duty
of board of directors, 56–58
of care, 57, 58, 66, 75, 299
of loyalty, 57, 58, 61, 299

Effectiveness, of healthcare systems, 24
as quality improvement component, 162, 165, 167

Efficiency, of healthcare systems, 24
conflict with other healthcare values, 168–69, 170
as quality improvement component, 162, 165, 167, 168–69, 170

Elderly population, healthcare expenditures for, 247

Emergency departments, closure of, 229

Emergency Medical Treatment and Active Labor Act (EMTALA), 227, 228–29, 229, 233

Emergency preparedness and response. *See* Disaster preparedness and response

Emotional distress, 143

Employee-related polices and issues, of healthcare organizations, 54, 177–94
board of directors' responsibility for, 66–67
employees' privacy, 182–85
fairness, 178, 182, 192
just compensation, 70, 186–89
mandatory influenza vaccinations, 179–82, 185
nonsmoking as a condition of employment, 182–85
union organizing, 189–91, 193

Employees
healthcare organizations' obligations to, 85, 109
as stakeholders, 82–83

Employers, employee health insurance mandate for, 250

End-of-life care
cost of, 247
policies for, 127

Energy conservation, 196, 198–99

Energy costs, of healthcare industry, 197

Engineering, professional relationships in, 90

Engineering ethics, 8

Environmental ethics. *See also* Sustainability, in healthcare
relationship to healthcare ethics, 196–97

Environmental factors, as health determinants, 201

Equality of opportunity, 164

Equity, in healthcare, 24, 224
of crisis standards of care, 235
as quality improvement component, 162, 165, 167

Ethical agents, organizations as, 10–14

Ethical climate
barriers to, 38–39, 47
board of directors' promotion of, 69–70, 75
case study of, 35, 36
definition of, 12, 35, 299
positive, 35–36

Ethical culture. *See also* Organizational culture
board of directors' promotion of, 62
case study of, 39

Ethical dilemmas
comparison with moral distress, 138
cost containment–related, 43–46
healthcare executives' responses to, 115–16
resolution of, 138

"Ethical expertise," 126

Ethical guidelines, development of, 98–110

Ethical language, 1–10
justification for use of, 5–6
non-normative uses of, 4–5
normative uses of, 4

Ethical management, allies in, 14

Ethical standards, 3, 299

Ethical tension, xxii, 33-34, 47. *See also* Conflicts

Ethicists. *See* Clinical ethicists

Ethics
definition of, xxv, 97, 299
differentiated from morality, xxv, 3–4
language of, 1–10
relationship to law, 207–208

Ethics centers, 14

Ethics committees, 112, 115, 116, 169
combined with ethics consulting services, 126–27

Ethics consolidation, 150–51

Ethics programs
compliance-oriented *versus* values-oriented, 215, 218, 219
Federal Sentencing Guidelines for, 207, 210, 293–96

European Union, air pollution-related mortality in, 197

Euthanasia, xxv-xxvi, 99, 100, 125

Evidence-based management, 146

Evidence-based medicine, 37

Evidence-based practice, 162

Excellence, in healthcare leadership, 290

Executives. *See also* Healthcare executives
compensation for, 67–68, 187–89, 193

Executive sessions, 72

Expectations, regarding ethical behavior, 70

Experimental research, 110, 111
in quality improvement, 169, 173

Experts, use of mental models by, 216, 268

External requirements, for ethics in healthcare, 205–21
as barrier to organizational culture, 38
compliance and ethics programs, 14, 207, 208–16, 218, 219, 293–96, 298

Facilitation model, of clinical ethics consults, 130, 132, 299
Fairness
   in employee management, 178, 182, 192
   in resource allocation, 224
   in stakeholder relationships, 86
False Claims Act, 210–11
Federal Sentencing Guidelines, 206–207, 210, 214, 215, 293–96
Fee-for-service payment system, 245, 246
Feminist care ethics, 7–8
Financial stress, on healthcare organizations, 254–60
"First, do no harm" rule, 90, 170, 181, 199–200, 300
Florence Nightingale Pledge, 103–104, 299
For-profit healthcare organizations
   comparison with not-for-profit organizations, 44
   role of, 43–46
Fraud and abuse prevention initiatives
   case study of, 210
   compliance programs for, 208–11
   Health Insurance Portability and Accountability Act-based, 229–30
   in Medicaid and Medicare, 208–209
Freeman, R. Edward, 84, 299

Genetic Information Nondiscrimination Act, 185
Genetic testing, presymptomatic, 185
Goals, 10
   actual *versus* stated, 36, 279
   ethical judgment regarding, 5
   prioritization of, 36
   in sustainability, 196
   as system components, 278–79, 281, 282
   teleological approaches to, 11
Governance. *See also* Board of directors

leadership for, 54–58
Governance committees, 71
"Greenwashing," 199
Gross domestic product, healthcare expenditures as percentage of, 197, 224, 238
Group health plans, 229–30

Hammurabi, Code of, 98, 297
Hazardous situations, 39
HCA (Hospital Corporation of America), 198
Health, determinants of, 201
Health benefits exchange, 250
Healthcare
   moral core of, 46
   as moral obligation, 163–65, 174
   as public good, 164–65
   rationing of, 113–14
   as a right, 164
   as a service, 52–54, 60, 287
   as a social and community good, 53–54
   values-based aims of, 162, 165, 166, 172–73, 174
Healthcare and Education Reconciliation Act, 249. *See also* Patient Protection and Affordable Care Act
Healthcare costs. *See also* Healthcare expenditures
   effect of hospital ownership status on, 43–45
   effect of medical technology on, 246–47
   effect on healthcare access, 226
   as healthcare policy focus, 225, 226, 238
   multiple factors affecting, 258–59
   relationship to inflation, 260
   smoking-related, 184
   spending drivers for, 246–48
Healthcare executives
   codes of ethics of, 98, 106–10, 115, 165–66

most important responsibility of, xxi
quality improvement role of,
    165–68
Healthcare expenditures
    under Affordable Care Act, 244
    cost-shifting approach to, 248–49
    historical overview of, 244–46
    hospital care as percentage of,
        246–48
    international comparison of, 226,
        238
    under managed care, 244, 245–46,
        259–60
    per capita, 226
Healthcare organizations. *See also spe-
    cific healthcare organizations*
    as communities of practice, 54
    comparison with non-healthcare
        organizations, 82
    complexity of, 12, 13, 38, 39,
        291
    conflicts of interest within, 57, 105
    contractual agreements with, 91
    ethical, 255–56
    fundamental purpose of, 36
    healthcare executives' responsibil-
        ity to, 108–109
    structures and processes of, 13–15
Healthcare policy
    definition of, 225, 300
    examples of, 228–234
Healthcare professionals. *See also*
    Nurses; Physicians
    accreditation of, 90
Healthcare systems
    challenges facing, 224
    complexity of, 12, 38, 39, 238,
        291
    development of, 112–13
    international comparison of, 224
    two-tiered, 257
Healthcare utilization
    economic factors affecting, 254–55
    effect of demographic shifts on,
        247

Healthcare workers, mandatory influ-
    enza vaccination of, 179–82, 185
Health Information Technology for
    Economic and Clinical Health
    (HITECH) Act, 230–31
Health insurance
    effect on healthcare access, 244
    premiums of, 245–46
Health Insurance Portability and
    Accountability Act (HIPAA),
    229–31, 299
    Privacy Rule of, 230–31, 299
Health maintenance organizations
    (HMOs), 245, 249
Health policy
    definition of, 225, 300
    ethical tensions associated with,
        226–27
    stakeholders in, 227
Health promotion, 52–53
Health status, of racial/ethnic minor-
    ity groups, 42
Heart attack patients, treatment costs
    for, 246–47
Hepatitis B vaccinations, mandatory,
    110
Hippocrates, 98–99, 170
Hippocratic Oath, 7, 269
    definition of, 99, 124, 300
    "first, do no harm" rule of, 90,
        170, 181, 199–200, 300
    modern version of, 100–101, 110
    original version of, 98–99, 124
Hispanic Americans, healthcare dispar-
    ity among, 42
Holder Memo, 211, 300
Hospital-acquired conditions, 253–54
Hospital care, spending drivers for,
    246–48
Hospital chains, 43–44
Hospital Preparedness Program
    (HPP), 232–33
Hospitals. *See also specific hospitals*
    accreditation of, 25–26, 207, 208
    certification of, 207
    increased demand for, 244

preventable readmissions to, 254
specific purposes of, 20–21, 47
Human subjects research, 110, 111, 169, 173
Hybrid healthcare organizations, 45–46

Immigrants, undocumented, 250, 252
Immigration, 125
Independent Payment Advisory Boards (IPABs), 252, 300
Infant mortality rate, 42
Infectious disease, screening for, 232
Influenza vaccinations, mandatory, 179–82, 185
Informed consent, 125, 130, 180, 300
Institute of Medicine (IOM)
  crisis standards of care report from, 234–38
  Crossing the Quality Chasm: A New Health System for the 21st Century, 36, 162, 165, 166, 170, 226, 298
  To Err Is Human: Building a Safer Health System, 36, 226
  goals and values guidelines of, 11
  recommendations regarding healthcare disparities, 42
  Unequal Treatment: Confronting Racial and Ethnic Disparities in Health Care, 41
  values statement of, 24
Institutional ethics committees, 14
Institutional review boards, 169
IntegratedEthics Initiative, 150–51, 300
Integrated health systems, 55
Integrity, 287–92
  compromises of, 143, 287–88, 290
  organizational, 287, 291–92
  personal, 287, 288–91, 292
Intermediate sanctions committees, 65

Job discrimination, toward smokers, 182–85
Joint Commission
  clinical ethics requirement of, 112, 126

conflict resolution requirement of, 39–40
definition of, 25, 300
hospital accreditation authority of, 25–26, 207, 208
leadership standards of, 12, 36, 96, 212, 213
organizational ethics requirement of, 11, 212–14
patient rights and responsibilities requirement of, 26–32, 212–14
safety and quality culture requirement of, 36, 212–14
standard of care requirement of, 234
Journal of Healthcare Management, 106
Journal of the American Medical Association, 106
Judgment
  categories of, 5–6
  normative, 10
Justice
  as basis for universal healthcare, 164
  in healthcare, 224
  social, 190–91

Kaiser Permanente, 199, 200, 202
Keystone Intensive Care Unit Project, 254

Labor unions, 189–91, 193
Lasagna, Louis, 100–101
Law(s)
  influence on healthcare organizations, 14
  regarding organizational culture, 206–208
  relationship to ethics, 207–208
  relationship to unethical behavior, 5
Leaders, 265–68. *See also* Blinded leaders
  fundamental ethical responsibilities of, 266, 284

promotion of organizational culture by, 167–68
Leadership
American College of Healthcare Executives' statement on, 58
as cultural safety component, 37
ethical, 150–51, 258
fiduciary, 56, 74–75
generative, 56, 74
for governance, 54–58
of integrated health systems, 55
integrity in, 291
Joint Commission's standards for, 12, 36, 96, 212, 213
role of ethics in, 10
strategic, 56, 74
through personal example, 58
transactional, 146
transformational, 62
Leadership ethics councils, 14
Leadership groups, conflict resolution between, 40
Leadership teams, responsibilities of, 46–47
Lean, 169, 172
Learning
as culture of safety characteristic, 37
experiential, quality improvement as, 161
organizational, 56
practice-based, 165
Liability. See Medical liability
Life-sustaining treatment, withholding or withdrawal of, 110, 127, 256
Living wage, 186–89, 192–93
Loyalty, duty of, 57, 58, 61, 299

Macro-level
of organizational ethics, 9, 21
of value conflicts, 21
Malpractice, definition of, 232
Managed care, healthcare expenditures under, 244, 245–46, 259–60
Managed care organizations (MCOs)
contracts with, 91
payment systems of, 245, 246

Managerial ethics
as applied ethics, 8
new perspective on, 287–92
Managers
interactions with board of directors, 56, 57–58, 60, 74–75
responsibilities and roles of, 54, 55
as stakeholders, 82–83
Massachusetts General Hospital
mission statement of, 22, 23, 24
organizational culture of, 35
patients' rights and responsibilities statement of, 26–28, 32
privacy violation complaint against, 231
values statement of, 24
Mediation model, of clinical ethics consults, 130–31, 300
Medicaid
administration of, 208
Affordable Care Act-related expansion of, 250, 251–52, 255, 256–57
Disproportionate Share Hospital (DSH) legislation and, 227, 256–57
enrollment in, 247–248
fraud and abuse prevention in, 208–209
Medicaid beneficiaries, emergency department care for, 229
Medicaid expenditures, 208
Medicaid reimbursement
under Affordable Care Act, 256–57
bundled payment program of, 251
for primary care, 252
as underpayment, 248, 255, 256–57, 259
Medical errors, 226
disclosure of, 258
as mortality cause, 36
Medical ethics, definitions of, 96, 97, 300
Medical liability
definition of, 232, 300

during disasters and emergencies, 232, 234, 237, 238
Medical staff, conflict with administrative staff, 113
Medical surge capacity, 232–33
Medical technology
  healthcare cost effects of, 246–47
  implication for clinical ethics, 124–25
Medicare
  accountable care organizations' participation in, 253
  administration of, 208
  under Affordable Care Act, 250, 251, 252, 253–54
  amendments to, 226–27, 228, 229–31
  Disproportionate Share Hospital (DSH) legislation and, 227
  enrollment in, 247–48
  fraud and abuse prevention in, 208–209
  Independent Payment Advisory Boards (IPABs) of, 252
  prospective payment system of, 245, 302
Medicare expenditures, 208, 244–45, 247
Medicare reimbursement
  under Affordable Care Act, 256–57
  bundled payment system of, 251
  for primary care, 252
  reductions in, 249, 253–54, 254
  requirements for, 28, 207
  as underpayment, 248, 256–57, 259
Mental models
  advantages and disadvantages of, 268–69
  as automatic cognitive process, 216–18
  as blinded leadership cause, 266–74
  case studies of, 269, 270
  definition of, 216, 268, 284, 300
  effect of role relationships on, 273–74
  effect of social roles on, 271–73

  effect on moral behavior, 216–18
  implicit associations component of, 216, 218, 219
  interaction with contextual cues, 217, 218
  misalignment with organizational culture, 281
  moral imagination relationship of, 274–75
  narratives of, 270–71
  separation thesis of, 269–70
  of systems, 278, 281–82
Mergers, 282
Meso-level, of organizational ethics, 9
Meta-ethics, 6–8
Micro-level
  of organizational ethics, 9
  of value conflicts, 21
Microsystems, 278
  culture of, 166–67, 168
  definition of, 300
Mind sets. *See* Mental models
Minimum wage, 67, 186–87, 299
Mission
  alignment with budget, 68–69
  alignment with healthcare marketing, 63–64
  alignment with societal expectations, xix, 23, 43, 46
  board of directors' commitment to, 60, 62, 63, 75
  common purposes of, 47
  conflicts associated with, 21, 33, 35
  confusion regarding, 39
  prioritization of, 36, 39
  relationship to values, xx, 21
Mission statements, 22–23
  advocacy for, 149
  case study of, 26
  definition of, 22, 301
  examples of, 22–23, 24
  as narratives, 270
  purpose of, 22
Modeling, of ethical behavior, 58
Moral agency, moral dilemma-based compromise of, 138

Moral agreement, 130

Moral behavior, effect of mental models on, 216–18

Moral climate, 58, 301

Moral commitment, 128–29

Moral core
  as basis for integrity, 288–89
  definition of, xxi, 301
  individual, xxi
  organizational, xix–xx, 287

Moral distress, 137–57
  adverse effects of, 139, 146
  alternative terminology for, 145
  as barrier to organizational culture and ethical climate, 38
  case studies of, 140–41, 144–45
  causes of, 138, 139–41, 139–46
  comparison with classic ethical dilemmas, 138
  Crescendo Effect of, 142–43, 147, 151, 298
  definition of, xxii, 38, 138, 139–40, 290, 301
  examples of, 141–42, 145–46
  at individual level, 143–45
  leadership responses to, 145–46
  levels of, 141–45
  outcomes of, 145
  strategic responses to, 146–51
  understanding of, 139–42
  unrecognized, 139

Morale, definition of, 187, 301

Moral frameworks, xxii

Moral imagination, 274–75, 283
  case study of, 275
  definition of, 267, 274, 284, 301
  in moral decision making, 274, 278
  relationship to moral reasoning, 267, 276

Morality
  definition of, xxv, 97, 301
  differentiated from ethics, xxv, 3–4
  separation from business, 266–67, 269–70

Moral minimums, 86, 301

Moral reasoning
  case study of, 276
  practical, 267, 276–83, 284, 302
  relationship to moral imagination, 267, 276
  theoretical, 276

Moral residue, 142–43, 301

Narratives
  definition of, 270, 301
  formal and informal, 270–71, 273
  as mental model component, 284
  relationship to moral imagination, 274–75

National Business Group on Health, 255

National Center for Ethics in Health Care, 151

National emergencies, medical preparedness and response capabilities for, 231–34, 302

National Institute on Minority Health and Health Disparities, 224

National Priorities Partnership, 254

Negligence, 57, 234

Neonatal intensive care units, 200

Nightingale, Florence, 103–104, 299

Nightingale Nursing School, London, 103

Nonmaleficence ("do no harm"), 99, 170, 181, 199–200, 300

Nonsmoking, as condition of employment, 182–85

Normativity, 4

Not-for-profit healthcare organizations
  comparison with for-profit organizations, 44
  as hybrid organizations, 45–46

Not-for-profit status, of hospitals, 66

Nurses
  conflicts of interest experienced by, 105
  ethics conversation programs for, 147

as healthcare board members, 60
moral distress in, 148
Nursing, professional ethics of, 103–106, 301
Nursing Home Reform Act, 126, 127

Obama, Barack, 249, 260
Obedience
to authority, 273–74
of nurses to physicians, 104
Ochsner Health System, 30–32
Office of Inspector General (OIG)
compliance program guidance from, 208–11, 214, 215
mission of, 208
organizational culture guidance from, 206, 207
Off-the-job behavior, of employees, 192
Online Journal of Nursing, 106
Opportunity, equality of, 164
Organ donation and transplantation, 111
Organizational culture, 34–39
barriers to, 38–39, 47
benefits of, 34–35
case study of, 39
definition of, 12, 34, 301–302
ethical climate component of, 12, 21, 35–36, 38–39, 47, 69–70, 75, 299
importance of, 283–84
leaders' responsibility for, 266, 267–68, 283–84
regulatory requirements for, 206–207, 218
relationship with mental models, 281, 283–84
safety as component of, 36–38
values-oriented, 215–16
Organizational ethics, 145
definition of, 96, 122–23, 136, 302
as healthcare administrators' responsibility, 8–10
macro-level, 9

meso-level, 9
micro-level, 9
relationship with clinical ethics, 121–24, 136
Organizational ethics committees, 123
Organizational statements, 22–25
Organization ethics processes, 40
Ownership status. *See also* For-profit healthcare organizations; Not-for-profit healthcare organizations
effect on healthcare access and costs, 43–45
effect on healthcare quality, 43–46

Pandemic and All-Hazards Preparedness Act (PAHPA), 231–34, 302
Partners HealthCare, 198–99
Paternalism, of physicians, 102
Patient(s)
autonomy of, 125, 129
healthcare executives' responsibility to, 108
role in sustainability, 200–201
trust in physicians and hospitals, 96
"Patient Anti-Dumping Law." *See* Emergency Medical Treatment and Active Labor Act (EMTALA)
Patient care, as board of directors' responsibility, 62, 64–65
Patient-centered care
conflict with other healthcare values, 168–69
as culture of safety component, 38
as healthcare core value, 24
as quality improvement component, 162, 165, 167, 168–69
Patient-level response, to moral distress, 148, 151
Patient Protection and Affordable Care Act, 249–54
accountable care organizations provision of, 253
definition of, 244, 302
goals of, 249

as healthcare consolidation cause, 114, 116–17
healthcare disparity-specific provisions of, 42
health insurance coverage expansion under, 250
hospital-acquired conditions regulations of, 253–54
impact on healthcare organizations, 249–59, 260
Independent Payment Advisory Boards (IPABs) of, 252, 300
Medicaid expansion under, 251–52, 255, 256–57
payment models of, 246, 251, 256–57, 260
primary care funding provision of, 252
Patient rights, 110–12
American Medical Association's support for, 102
implication for clinical ethics, 125
implication for professional codes of ethics, 110–12
Patient safety. *See* Safety
Patient Self-Determination Act, 126, 127
Patients' rights and responsibilities statements
conflict with organizational culture, 35
examples of, 26–32
Pay-for-performance payment system, 251, 255, 257, 302
Performance evaluations, of chief executive officers, 66–67, 68
Performance improvement. *See* Quality improvement (QI)
Pew Forum on Religion and Public Life, 163–64
Physicians
certification of, 165–66
codes of ethics of, 98, 101–103, 111, 117, 165
conflicts of interest experienced by, 105

credentialing of, 65
as determinants of medical ethics, 96
emergency department, 229
employment of, 65
as healthcare board members, 60
paternalism of, 102
privileges of, 65
role in sustainability, 200
Preventive care, 52–53, 196
Preventive ethics, 150–51
Primary care, 52–53, 252
Principles
as basis for decision making, 276
societal influences on, 110–13
Principles of Medical Ethics (American Medical Association), 98, 102–103, 111, 165
Privacy
of employees' behavior, 182–85, 192
of health information, 229–31, 299
Privileges, of physicians, 65
Product-focused businesses, 53
Professional ethics, 8, 95–119
case study of, 114
of current healthcare system, 113–15
definition of, 302
of nurses, 103–106
of physicians, 98, 101–103, 111, 117, 165
relationship to healthcare system changes, 112–13
threats to, 113–15
Professionalism
attributes of, 165
definition of, 97–98, 302
of healthcare executives, 199
of healthcare providers, 53, 90
Profit and profitability
as goal, 81, 84, 85, 88
prioritization of, 92, 93
as sustainability component, 196
Prognosis committees, 124–26

Prospective payment system, 245, 302
Psychological distress, 140, 302
Public good
definition of, 164, 302
healthcare as, 164–65
Public health
effect of pollution on, 197
emergencies in, 181, 231–32
individual health *versus*, 201
promotion of, 256
sustainability component of, 196
Public health policy, 238–39
Public Health Service Act, 232
Public policy, 223–25
adverse effects of, 224–25
definition of, 224, 225, 302

Quality, of healthcare
under Affordable Care Act, 250,
255, 257
as healthcare organizations' fundamental purpose, 36
as healthcare policy focus, 225, 226
for racial/ethnic minority groups,
41–42
relationship to organizational size,
43–44
Quality assurance programs, 14
Quality committees, 64–65, 71
Quality improvement (QI), 159–76
case studies of, 163, 167, 171, 173
characteristics of, 160–61
of clinical ethics mechanisms,
129–32
as conflict resolution method,
170–72, 174
culture of, 167–68
definition of, 160, 302
ethical challenges to, 168–70
ethical conflicts in, 168–69, 173
harmful consequences of, 170, 173
leaders' role in, 167–68, 173
as moral obligation, 163–66, 173
need for, 162
physicians' resistance to, 161–62

process of, 170–71
professional ethics as basis for, 165
research in, 169, 173
resources for, 168–69
role of, 161–62

Racial/ethnic minority groups, healthcare disparity among, 41–43,
224
Rationing, of healthcare, 113–14
Readmissions, preventable, 254
Recessions, economic, 247, 254–55
Regulations
consolidation-based, 116–17
influence on healthcare organizations, 14
Religiously-affiliated hospitals. *See also*
Catholic healthcare organizations
end-of-life care policies of, 12
moral commitment of, 128–29
Resource allocation, 11
budgeting for, 68
for emergency preparedness,
233–34
ethical practices in, 255–56
fair, 224
government-mandated, 114–15
as healthcare rationing, 113–14
as sustainability issue, 19, 198
Resource limitations, effect on mission
and values, 21, 33
Resources, of systems, 280–81
Respecting the Just Rights of Workers:
Guidance and Options for Catho-
lic Health Care and Unions (US
Council of Catholic Bishops),
191
Reward structures, 69, 70
Right(s)
to die, 110, 125
to form labor unions, 189–91, 193
healthcare as, 164
of patients, 26–32
Right answer model, of clinical ethics
consultations, 130, 302

Rights movements, 110, 113
Risk management, 14
Role obligations, 85
Role relationships, 273–74, 284, 303
Rule-deontologists, 7
Rule-utilitarians, 7

Safety
    accountability for, 36, 38
    conflict with other healthcare val-
        ues, 168–69
    culture of, 36–38, 47, 213–14,
        218
    as healthcare core value, 24
    of healthcare systems, 165
    as quality committees' responsibil-
        ity, 64–65
    as quality improvement compo-
        nent, 167, 170
St. Mary's Hospital, Richmond, Vir-
    ginia, 22–23
Sarbanes-Oxley Act, 146, 212, 303
Security and Exchange Commission
    (SEC), 212
Senior management
    moral leadership role of, 135
    perception of the ethical environ-
        ment, 215–16, 219
    perspective on ethical environ-
        ment, 272–73
    relationship with clinical ethics
        mechanisms, 123–24, 128–36
Separation thesis, 266–67, 269–70,
    303
Service mission, of healthcare organi-
    zations, xix–xx, 52–54, 60, 287
Situation ethics, 7
Six Sigma, 169, 172
Size, organizational, relationship to
    healthcare quality, 43–44
Smoking policies, 182–85, 225
Social environment, influence on ethi-
    cal judgment, 5–6
Social good, healthcare as, 53–54
Social justice, 190–91

Social responsibility, of business, 84
Social roles, 271–73
    case study of, 272
    definition of, 271, 303
    as mental model component, 284
    relationships among, 273–74
Societal expectations, regarding
    healthcare organizations, 23, 43,
    46
Society
    healthcare executives' responsibil-
        ity to, 109
    influence on codes of ethics,
        110–12
    moral obligation to provide health-
        care, 163–65
Socioeconomic factors, as health
    determinants, 201
Specialty certifying boards, 165
Stakeholder map, 89
Stakeholders
    as barrier to organizational culture,
        39
    definition of, xix, 3, 20, 83, 88, 303
    in health policy, 227
    management's fiduciary responsi-
        bility to, 84
    mental models of, 282
    prioritization of, 83–84, 85–86
    quality improvement goals and val-
        ues of, 171, 172, 173, 174
    recognition by board of directors,
        61–62
Stakeholder theory, 82–86, 93
    accountability relationships con-
        cept of, 84–91
    definition of, 83, 303
Standards of care, crisis-related, 232–
    38, 298
Stewardship
    board of directors' commitment
        to, 59
    conflict with healthcare quality, 21
    definition of, 55, 68, 303
    financial, 62, 68–69

Strategic planning, 63–64

Strategy, as healthcare boards' focus, 62

Subcultures, 38, 39

Subsystems, 166, 168, 267

Suicide, assisted, 125

Supply chain, sustainability approach to, 201–202

Sustainability, in healthcare, 195–204
    clinician's role in, 200
    core components of, 196
    cost implications of, 198–199
    definition of, 196, 300
    healthcare administrator's role in, 199–200
    patient's role in, 200
    triple bottom line practices in, 196, 199, 300
    values conflicts associated with, 198

Syphilis, 110

System-level response, to moral distress, 148–51

Systems. *See also* Healthcare systems
    boundaries of, 279–80
    changes to, 281–82
    characteristics of, 278
    closed, 279–80
    culture of, 166
    formation of, 278
    mental models of, 278, 281–82
    normative, dimensions of, 278
    open, 279–80
    outcomes of, 282–83
    purposes and goals of, 278–79, 281, 282
    resources of, 280–81
    values of, 279

Systems approach, to quality improvement, 160–62

Systems-based practice, 165–66

Systems thinking
    definition of, 267, 303
    in moral decision making, 277–83
    in quality improvement, 167, 174

Tax-exempt status, of healthcare organizations, 66, 68

Team discussions, about moral distress, 147–48

Technical expertise, of board of directors, 60–61, 75

Teleological ethical theories, 1, 7

Tenet Healthcare Corporation
    mission statement of, 23, 25, 43
    Ochsner Health System of, 30–32
    organizational culture of, 35
    patients' rights and responsibilities statement of, 30–32

Theories, ethical, 6–8

Timeliness, in provision of healthcare, 24
    as quality improvement component, 162, 165, 167
    values conflicts related to, 168–169

To Err Is Human: Building a Safer Health System (Institute of Medicine), 36, 226

Transactional leadership, 146

Transactional work relationships, 70

Transformational leadership, 62

Transparency
    Affordable Care Act–mandated, 258
    of crisis standards of care, 235
    in decision making, 116, 146
    in governance, 72
    in hospital-community relationship, 46

Trustees. *See also* Board of directors
    comparison with directors, 55
    definition of, 52, 74, 303
    ethical responsibilities and roles of, 54–55
    mission focus of, 62

Tufts University School of Medicine, 100

Tuskegee Experiment, 110, 303

Uncertainty, ethical
    code of ethics-related, 113–16, 118

quality improvement-based resolution of, 170–72, 174
quality improvement-related, 170, 173
Uncompensated care, 44, 247, 248, 252
Underinsured population, 249
Underserved communities, 42
Unequal Treatment: Confronting Racial and Ethnic Disparities in Health Care (Institute of Medicine), 41
Unethical behavior
    context of, 4
    as obedience to authority, 273–74
    organizational, 81
Uninsured population, 224
    under Affordable Care Act, 249–50, 252, 256–57
    emergency department care for, 227, 228–29
    healthcare access policy regarding, 225–26
    size of, 238, 247, 250
    uncompensated healthcare for, 44, 247, 248, 252
Union organizing, 189–91, 193
United Nations Declaration of Human Rights, 186, 303
United States Department of Health and Human Services
    Emergency System for Advance Registration of Volunteer Health Professionals of, 232
    ethics and compliance program requirements of, 206–207, 208–12
    Medical Reserve Corps of, 232
    Office for Civil Rights of, 230
United States Department of Health and Human Services, 208–209. *See also* Office of Inspector General (OIG)
United States Department of Justice, Holder Memo from, 211, 300

United States Department of Veterans Affairs, 12, 238, 258
    IntegratedEthics Initiative of, 150–51, 300
    National Center for Ethics in Health Care, 151
United States Sentencing Commission, 206–207, 210, 214, 215, 293, 296
United States v. Blakely, 294
United States v. Booker, 294
Universal healthcare, 163–64, 260
Utilitarianism, 7, 81, 224, 303
Utilization management, 245, 246

Vaccinations
    mandatory, 179–82, 185, 224
    Willowbrook hepatitis B vaccination study, 110
Value-based purchasing, 251
Value-creating activities, *versus* ethical activities, 266–67, 269–70
Values
    adherence to, 288–289
    alignment of, 13–14, 15
    as basis for integrity, 288–289
    as clinical ethics consultation issue, 131
    compromise of, 289
    confusion regarding, 39
    ethical, 11
    ethical judgment regarding, 5
    of leaders, 274
    as mental model component, 282, 284
    misalignment of, 13, 24
    prioritization of, 13, 39
    relationship to mission, 21
    sustainability-related, 202
    as system components, 279, 282
Values-based aims, of healthcare, 162, 165, 166, 172–73, 174
Values conflicts, 11–12, 15, 33–34, 35
    in academic medical centers, 33, 34

adverse effects of, 279
priorities of values in, 279
in quality improvement, 168–69
sustainability-related, 198
Values statements, 47
advocacy for, 149
definition of, 23, 303
examples of, 24–25
purposes of, 23–24
Value-theories, 6
Veterans Health Administration. *See*
United States Department of
Veterans Affairs
Vision, prioritization of, 36
Vision statements, 32–33, 270
Volatile organic compounds (VOCs),
202
Volunteers
clinical ethicists as, 213
in disaster and emergency
responses, 232

Wages, fair and just, 186–89, 192–93
Waste, healthcare industry-related,
197
Waste-reduction strategies, 197. *See
also* Sustainability, in healthcare
Water use reduction, 196
Wellness, as healthcare focus, 196
Willowbrook hepatitis study, 110, 303
Workplace, covenantal, 69–70, 298
Workplace justice
as board of directors' responsibil-
ity, 66–68
as healthcare boards' focus, 62
Work relationships, transactional, 70

ABOUT THE EDITORS

Gary L. Filerman, PhD, is recognized as one of the most influential architects of the profession of health services administration. He was the first CEO of the Association of University Programs in Health Administration (AUPHA), founding executive of the organization that preceded the Commission on Accreditation of Healthcare Management Education, founding editor of the *Journal of Health Administration Education*, and a founder of Health Administration Press. He has represented the profession on numerous councils and committees of healthcare delivery institutions, the US government, professional organizations, international agencies, and interdisciplinary education and professional bodies. He has been a consultant or program evaluator to more than 135 governments, colleges, and universities in 39 countries.

Throughout his career, Dr. Filerman has been a forceful advocate for professional health administration education, promoting university and public recognition of the career as a distinct health profession with a defined body of knowledge, professional identity, and mandate to help realize the goal of accessible, high-quality health services. AUPHA's Filerman Prize is the highest recognition of leadership in health services administration education.

Dr. Filerman has also served as interim chairman and professor of health policy and administration at the George Washington University and as chairman and professor of health services administration and of international health at Georgetown University. He was a guest scholar at The Brookings Institution, associate director of the Pew Commission on the Future of the Health Professions, senior advisor at the Academy for Educational Development, consultant to the World Bank, international vice president of Planned Parenthood Federation of America, and advisor to several foundations and international agencies.

Dr. Filerman is the president of the Atlas Health Foundation, an advisor to Joint Commission International, and a member of the Institute of Medicine Forum on Drug Discovery, Development and Translation. He earned his bachelor's degree, master of health administration, master of arts (public administration), and PhD at the University of Minnesota, which honored him with the Regent's Distinguished Contribution Award.

Ann E. Mills is cofounder of IP Advantage, LLC. The company, founded with a grant from the National Institutes of Health, provides easily accessible legal information for students and professionals working in healthcare-related fields. She previously served as an assistant professor at the University of Virginia's Center for Biomedical Ethics and Humanities and codirector of its program in policy and ethics in healthcare systems.

Mills has written or coauthored more than 80 cases, journal articles, and book chapters. She has published in the areas of clinical ethics, healthcare organization ethics, quality improvement, and patent reform. Her work has appeared in journals such as the *New England Journal of Medicine, Nature Biotechnology,* and *Science.* She is coauthor or coeditor of three books, including the seminal *Organization Ethics in Healthcare,* published by Oxford University Press (2000). *Organization Ethics in Healthcare* was one of the first books in the healthcare ethics literature to explore the importance of an ethical climate and culture in healthcare organizations.

Mills has helped numerous ethicists begin or strengthen their organizational ethics programs. In addition she has consulted on patent reform with organizations including the Biotechnology Industry Organization.

Mills received her undergraduate degree from Sarah Lawrence College, her master of economics from London School of Economics, and her master of business administration from James Madison University.

Paul M. Schyve, MD, is senior advisor, healthcare improvement at The Joint Commission, where he was senior vice president from 1989 until 2011. Prior to joining The Joint Commission, Dr. Schyve was the clinical director of the State of Illinois Department of Mental Health and Developmental Disabilities, a system of 22 hospitals and residential facilities.

Dr. Schyve is certified in psychiatry by the American Board of Psychiatry and Neurology and is a distinguished life fellow of the American Psychiatric Association. He is a founding advisor of Consumers Advancing Patient Safety, the chair of the Ethical Force Oversight Body of the Institute of Ethics at the American Medical Association, a former trustee of the United States Pharmacopeial Convention, and a former board director of the National Alliance for Health Information Technology. He has served on numerous advisory panels for the Centers for Medicare & Medicaid Services, the Agency for Healthcare Research and Quality, and the Institute of Medicine of the National Academies. Dr. Schyve has published in the areas of healthcare ethics, quality improvement, and organizational leadership as well as psychiatric treatment and research, patient safety, cultural and linguistic competence, and health literacy.

Dr. Schyve received his undergraduate degree from the University of Rochester, where he was elected to Phi Beta Kappa. He completed his medical education and residency in psychiatry at the University of Rochester and has subsequently held a variety of professional and academic appointments in the areas of mental health and hospital administration, including as clinical associate professor of psychiatry at the University of Chicago and director of the Illinois State Psychiatric Institute, a psychiatric research and teaching hospital.

ABOUT THE CONTRIBUTORS

Katherine L. Acuff, JD, PhD, has more than 20 years' experience in law and health policy, including serving as vice president of policy and education of the National Public Health and Hospital Institute; legal and policy advisor to the Medical Assistance Administration; consultant to the director of the US Department of Health and Human Services' Office of Women's Health; adjunct professor at Emory University's Rollins School of Public Health; consultant to The Carter Center's Mental Health Program; and consultant to the chair of Virginia Supreme Court's Commission on Mental Health Law Reform. She also serves on the boards of the University of Virginia Physicians Group and Mental Health America Charlottesville/Albemarle. Acuff has a law degree from Georgetown University Law Center and a master's of public health and PhD from The Johns Hopkins Bloomberg School of Public Health.

Carolyn Long Engelhard is a health policy analyst and the director of Health Policy Medical Education in the Department of Public Health Sciences at the University of Virginia School of Medicine. Engelhard's academic activities include studying and monitoring changes in health policy at the federal and state governmental levels and teaching in both the Graduate School of Arts and Sciences and the School of Medicine.

Elizabeth G. Epstein, RN, PhD's area of expertise is nursing ethics, particularly preventive ethics and end-of-life issues in neonatal and pediatric intensive care. She currently serves as cochair of the Moral Distress Consult Service, and she is a member of the Ethics Consult Service.

Ann B. Hamric, PhD, RN, FAAN, is the associate dean for academic programs at Virginia Commonwealth University and a professor in the School of Nursing. She received degrees from Vanderbilt University (BSN), the University of California at San Francisco (MS), and the University of Maryland at Baltimore (PhD in nursing with a concentration in ethics). She has served as senior editor of seven books, two on the clinical nurse specialist role, and four on advanced practice nursing. Dr. Hamric has served on five interdisciplinary ethics committees and currently is a member of Virginia Commonwealth

University Health Systems' Ethics Committee. In 2008, she was awarded the Substantive Contribution to Nursing Ethics from the American Society of Bioethics and Humanities Affinity Group for Nursing.

Carrie R. Rich is the cofounder and CEO of The Global Good Fund, a nonprofit organization that identifies and accelerates the development of high potential young leaders to achieve outsized social impact. Rich served as the senior director of managed care business integration at Inova. She was the healthcare specialist at Perkins+Will architecture firm and taught as an adjunct faculty member at Georgetown University, where she developed a healthcare sustainability curriculum that is the first of its kind to teach sustainable operations to healthcare leaders. She is the coauthor of *Sustainability for Healthcare Management: A Leadership Imperative* (Routledge 2012).

Mary V. Rorty has a PhD in philosophy and a master's degree in clinical ethics. She is associated with the Stanford Center for Biomedical Ethics and is coauthor of *Organization Ethics in Health Care* (Oxford University Press 2000).

J. Knox Singleton is CEO of Inova Health System. He previously served as executive vice president for the Fairfax Hospital Association. He is a Phi Beta Kappa graduate of the University of North Carolina, where he earned a bachelor of science degree in business administration in 1970. He received his master's degree in health administration from Duke University in 1973.

Edward M. Spencer, MD, spent the first 20 years of his medical career in the private practice of pediatrics. In 1990 he joined the staff of the University of Virginia's Center for Biomedical Ethics, where he developed a number of programs aimed at bringing the developing field of clinical ethics to healthcare organizations away from the University. Since 2007, he has been semi-retired, but he continues to act as a consultant in clinical ethics to a number of healthcare organizations. He also writes and lectures on the application of clinical ethics to the healthcare system.

Seema S. Wadhwa is the director of sustainability at Urban Ltd. and also serves as the director of sustainability for Inova Health System. Wadhwa is responsible for the creation and adoption of sustainable management practices at Inova. Prior to her role with Inova, Wadhwa spent several years managing engineering design projects. She serves as an adviser about best practices in green building as prescribed by her status as a Leadership in Energy and Environmental Design accredited professional (LEED AP).

John F. Wallenhorst, PhD, is vice president, mission and ethics for Bon Secours Health System, a not-for-profit health system of 20,000 employees serving people in multiple communities in six states. He oversees the organization's ethics program and leadership of mission activities throughout the system, including mission integration, community benefit, ethics, pastoral care, advocacy and government relations, and ecological stewardship and global ministries. He contributes regularly to leadership development in advancing mission, ethics, and values-based leadership competencies. As adjunct assistant professor, Wallenhorst teaches healthcare management ethics at Georgetown University. His areas of professional interest include leadership development, ethics integration, and organizational culture. He serves on the boards of two healthcare organizations.

Mark H. Waymack, PhD, is associate professor of philosophy at Loyola University Chicago. He is also an adjunct associate professor at Northwestern University's Feinberg School of Medicine Program in Medical Humanities and Bioethics. His interests include healthcare organizational ethics, research ethics, ethics and aging, and philosophy of medicine.

Leonard J. Weber, PhD, professor emeritus at the University of Detroit Mercy, is an ethics consultant to healthcare organizations. He received his PhD from McMaster University in Hamilton, Ontario, and was a full-time member of the faculty of the University of Detroit Mercy from 1972 to 2006. His two most recent books are *Business Ethics in Healthcare* (2001) and *Profits Before People? Ethical Standards and the Marketing of Prescription Drugs* (2006), both published by Indiana University Press. He was an associate editor for the third edition of the *Encyclopedia of Bioethics* (MacMillan 2003).

Patricia H. Werhane is the Wicklander Chair of Business Ethics and Managing Director of the Institute for Business and Professional Ethics at DePaul University and professor emerita at the University of Virginia. Werhane has published numerous articles, is the author or editor of more than 20 books, and is former editor-in-chief of *Business Ethics Quarterly*, the journal of the Society for Business Ethics.

Kenneth R. White, PhD, RN, ACNP, FACHE, FAAN, is associate dean for strategic partnerships and innovation at the University of Virginia Medical Center and professor of nursing at the UVA School of Nursing in Charlottesville. White has 40 years of experience in healthcare organizations in clinical, administrative, governance, and consulting capacities. He spent 13 years with Mercy Health Services as senior executive in marketing, operations, and international healthcare consulting. He served as the associate director of the MHA and MSHA programs at Virginia Commonwealth University (VCU) and as the director of the MHA program. He served as VCU's inaugural Charles P. Cardwell, Jr., Professor of Health Administration from 2006 to 2008 and the inaugural Sentara Healthcare Professor from 2012 to 2013. He is a Fellow, former Regent, and member of the Board of Governors of the American College of Healthcare Executives. He is a visiting professor at the LUISS Business School in Rome, Italy, and the Swiss School of Public Health in Lugano, Switzerland.